THE
EMERGENCY DEPARTMENT TECHNICIAN HANDBOOK

THE EMERGENCY DEPARTMENT TECHNICIAN HANDBOOK

Robert Shesser, MD, MPH
Professor and Chair
Department of Emergency Medicine
George Washington University
Washington, District of Columbia
United States

Ali Pourmand, MD, MPH, RDMS
Professor
Department of Emergency Medicine
George Washington University
Washington, District of Columbia
United States

Amy Keim, MS, PA-C
Associate Clinical Professor
Department of Emergency Medicine
George Washington University
Washington, District of Columbia
United States

ELSEVIER

Elsevier
1600 John F. Kennedy Blvd.
Ste 1800
Philadelphia, PA 19103-2899

THE EMERGENCY DEPARTMENT TECHNICIAN HANDBOOK   ISBN: 978-0-323-83002-7

Notice

Content Strategist: Kayla Wolfe
Content Development Specialist: Akanksha Marwah
Publishing Services Manager: Shereen Jameel
Project Manager: Gayathri S
Design Direction: Ryan Cook

Printed in India

Last digit is the print number: 9   8   7   6   5   4   3   2   1

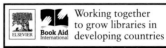

Working together
to grow libraries in
developing countries

www.elsevier.com • www.bookaid.org

Dina Abdelsamad, MPH, PA-C
Physician Assistant
Department of Emergency Medicine
George Washington University
Washington, District of Columbia
United States

Lindsey Abraham, BS, EMT-B
Emergency Department Technician
Emergency Department
George Washington University Hospital
Washington, District of Columbia
United States

Yasmin Al-Atrache, PA-C
Physician Assistant
Department of Emergency Medicine
George Washington University
Washington, District of Columbia
United States

Lareb Altaf, BS, AS
Emergency Department Technician
Emergency Department
George Washington University Hospital
Washington, District of Columbia
United States

Ksenya Badashova, MD, MBA MFA
Department of Emergency Medicine
George Washington University
Washington, District of Columbia
United States

Sonal Batra, MD, MST
Assistant Professor
Department of Emergency Medicine
George Washington University
Washington, District of Columbia
United States

Kamilla Beisenova, BBA
Emergency Department Technician
Emergency Department
George Washington University Hospital
Washington, District of Columbia
United States

Keith Boniface, MD, RDMS, RDCS
Professor
Department of Emergency Medicine
George Washington University
Washington, District of Columbia
United States

Kiara Brooks, Paramedic
Emergency Department Technician
Emergency Department
George Washington University Hospital
Washington, District of Columbia
United States

Brandon Chaffay, MD
Resident Physician
Department of Emergency Medicine
George Washington University Hospital
Washington, District of Columbia
United States

Aileen Chowdhury, BS
Emergency Medicine Technician
Department of Emergency Medicine
George Washington University Hospital
Washington, District of Columbia
United States

Emmanuel Chukwuma, ED-T
Emergency Department Technician
Emergency Department
George Washington University Hospital
Washington, District of Columbia
United States

Sara Cogswell, MSHS, PA-C
Physician Assistant
Department of Emergency Medicine
George Washington University
Washington, District of Columbia
United States

Margeaux Connealy, PA-C
Physician Assistant
Department of Emergency Medicine
George Washington University
Washington, District of Columbia
United States

Cassidy Craig, ED-T
Emergency Department Technician
Emergency Department
George Washington University Hospital
Washington, District of Columbia
United States

Sarah Cronin, RN, MSN, CEN
Clinical Educator
Emergency Department
George Washington University Hospital
Washington, District of Columbia
United States

Steven Davis, MD
Associate Professor
Department of Emergency Medicine
George Washington University
Washington, District of Columbia
United States

Elizabeth Dearing, MD
Assistant Professor
Department of Emergency Medicine
George Washington University
Washington, District of Columbia
United States

Crystal Donelan, MD
Emergency Medicine Physician
Department of Emergency Medicine
George Washington University Hospital
Washington, District of Columbia
United States

Aaran Drake, MD
Assistant Professor
Department of Emergency Medicine
George Washington University
Washington, District of Columbia
United States

Eleanor Frye, PA-C
Physician Assistant
Department of Emergency Medicine
Washington, District of Columbia
United States

Christina Gallerani, MD, MPH
Emergency Medicine Resident
Department of Emergency Medicine
George Washington University
Washington, District of Columbia
United States

Carin Gannon, BS
Lead Emergency Department Technician
Emergency Department
George Washington University Hospital
Washington, District of Columbia
United States

Sara Ashton Garcia, MSN, APRN, NP-C
Nurse Practitioner
Department of Emergency Medicine
George Washington University
Washington, District of Columbia
United States

Jason Gray, EMS, AAS
Emergency Department Technician
Emergency Department
George Washington University Hospital
Washington, District of Columbia
United States

Alexander Gregory Hastava, NREMT-B, NTA
Emergency Department Technician
Emergency Department
George Washington University Hospital
Washington, District of Columbia
United States

Sarah Hocutt, MPAS, PA-C
Physician Assistant
Department of Emergency Medicine
George Washington University
Washington, District of Columbia
United States

Megan Hoffer, DO
Resident Physician
Department of Emergency Medicine
George Washington University
Washington, District of Columbia
United States

Jenny Huang, EMT-B
Emergency Department Technician
Emergency Department
George Washington University Hospital
Washington, District of Columbia
United States

Sarah Ingram, BS
Emergency Department Technician
Emergency Department
George Washington University Hospital
Washington, District of Columbia
United States

Breanne Jacobs, MD, MA
Assistant Clinical Professor
Department of Emergency Medicine
George Washington University
Washington, District of Columbia
United States

Cody Johnson, MD
Fellow of Disaster and Operational Medicine
Department of Emergency Medicine
George Washington University
Washington, District of Columbia
United States

Amy Keim, MS, PA-C
Associate Clinical Professor
Department of Emergency Medicine
George Washington University
Washington, District of Columbia
United States

Margaret Klein, BA
Emergency Department Technician
Department of Emergency Medicine
George Washington University
Washington, District of Columbia
United States

Joseph Kunic, MSHS, PA-C
Assistant Clinical Professor of Emergency
    Medicine
Department of Emergency Medicine
George Washington University
Washington, District of Columbia
United States

Lexington Lemmon, BS
Emergency Department Technician
Emergency Department
George Washington University Hospital
Washington, District of Columbia
United States

Owen Ligas, BS, EMT-B
Emergency Department Technician
Emergency Department
George Washington University Hospital
Washington, District of Columbia
United States

Noah Lubin, BS, EMT
Emergency Department Technician
Emergency Department
George Washington University Hospital
Washington, District of Columbia
United States

Rita Manfredi, MD
Associate Clinical Professor
Department of Emergency Medicine
George Washington University Hospital
Washington, District of Columbia
United States

Maggie McEnery, RN, BSN, EMT-P
Registered Nurse
Emergency Department
George Washington University Hospital
Washington, District of Columbia
United States

Jason S. McKay, MPA, NRP, FP-C, NCEE
Adjunct Instructor
Department of Emergency Medicine
George Washington University
    Medicine and Health Sciences
Washington, District of Columbia
United States

Robert L. McKinney, II, MPAS, PA-C
Clinical Assistant Professor
Department of Emergency Medicine
George Washington University
Washington, District of Columbia
United States

Andrew Charles Meltzer, MD
Professor
Department of Emergency Medicine
George Washington University
Washington, District of Columbia
United States

Elise Milani, MD MFA
Fellow in Disaster Medicine
Department of Emergency Medicine
George Washington University
Washington, District of Columbia
United States

Natalia Monsalve, BS
Emergency Department Technician
George Washington University Hospital
Washington, District of Columbia
United States

Nehal S. Naik, MD
Resident Physician
Department of Emergency Medicine
George Washington University
Washington, District of Columbia
United States

Trent Nayve, NRP, EDT
Emergency Department Technician
Emergency Department
George Washington University Hospital
Washington, District of Columbia
United States

John Organick-Lee, MD
Resident Physician
Department of Emergency Medicine
George Washington University
Washington, District of Columbia
United States

Christopher Payette, BS, MD
Resident Physician
Department of Emergency Medicine
George Washington University
Washington, District of Columbia
United States

Ayal Pierce, MD
Resident Physician
Department of Emergency Medicine
George Washington University
Washington, District of Columbia
United States

Margarita Popova, MD
Resident Physician
Department of Emergency Medicine
George Washington University Hospital
Washington, District of Columbia
United States

Matthew Pyle, BS, MD
Assistant Professor
Department of Emergency Medicine
George Washington University Hospital
Washington, District of Columbia
United States

Claudia Ranniger, MD, PhD
Associate Professor
Department of Emergency Medicine
George Washington University
Washington, District of Columbia
United States

Stephen Robie, MSHS, MPH, PA-C
Physician Assistant
Department of Emergency Medicine
George Washington University Medical
    Faculty Associates
Washington, District of Columbia
United States

Colleen Roche, MD
Residency Program Director
Department of Emergency Medicine
George Washington University
Washington, District of Columbia
United States

Madeleine Rosenstein, EDT, EMT
Emergency Department Technician
Emergency Department
George Washington University Hospital
Washington, District of Columbia
United States

Eleanor Rubin, EDT
Emergency Department Technician
Emergency Department
George Washington University Hospital
Washington, District of Columbia
United States

Zeina Saliba, MD
Assistant Professor and Medical Director for
  Hospital Mental Health Services
Department of Psychiatry and Behavioral
  Sciences
George Washington University
Washington, District of Columbia
United States

Jordan Selzer, MD
Fellow in Disaster Medicine
Department of Emergency Medicine
George Washington University
Washington, District of Columbia
United States

Robert Shesser, MD, MPH
Professor and Chair
Department of Emergency Medicine
George Washington University
Washington, District of Columbia
United States

Leah Steckler, BS, MD
Assistant Professor
Department of Emergency Medicine
George Washington University
Washington, District of Columbia
United States

Ryan Strauss, MPH, MSHS, PA-C
Director of Advanced Practitioners
Department of Emergency Medicine
George Washington Medical Faculty Associates
Washington, District of Columbia
United States

Alexa Tovsen, MSHS, PA-C
Assistant Clinical Professor of Emergency
  Medicine
Department of Emergency Medicine
George Washington University
Washington, District of Columbia
United States

Jesús Treviño, MD, MBA
Assistant Professor
Department of Emergency Medicine
George Washington University School of
  Medicine and Health Sciences
Washington, District of Columbia
United States

Fletcher Vilt, EDT
Emergency Department Technician
Emergency Department
George Washington University Hospital
Washington, District of Columbia
United States

Andzie Warrington, EMT
Emergency Department Technician
Emergency Department
George Washington University Hospital
Washington, District of Columbia
United States

Michael West, DO
Resident Physician
Department of Emergency Medicine
George Washington University
Washington, District of Columbia
United States

Naja Wilson, EMT-B
Emergency Medical Response Group
George Washington University
Washington, District of Columbia
United States

Mary Taylor Winsten, MD
Department of Obstetrics and Gynecology
MedStar Washington Hospital Center
Washington, District of Columbia
United States

Samuel Winsten, MD
Resident Physician
Department of Emergency Medicine
George Washington University
Washington, District of Columbia
United States

Julia Xavier, BSPH
Emergency Department Technician
Emergency Department
George Washington University Hospital
Washington, District of Columbia
United States

David Yamane, MD
Assistant Professor
Department of Emergency Medicine
Department of Anesthesia and Critical Care
   Medicine
George Washington University
Washington, District of Columbia
United States

I would like to dedicate this book to my wife, children, and grandchildren. Sue, Mark, Rebecca, Juli, Madison, and Ella, I love you all.

Robert Shesser

To the loves of my life: Parmis, Amir, and Reza.

Ali Pourmand

In memory of Russell Eggleton, first responder and ER technician, educator, and role model.

Amy Keim

The current US healthcare system includes a large number of hospital emergency departments. These units are supported by all varieties of high-tech diagnostic equipment and are staffed by thousands of wonderful physicians, advanced practice providers, nurses, and a host of other different types of professionals, all of whom are dedicated to providing compassionate care delivered in a timely manner. Despite all that has been invested, many of us know that periodic staffing shortages and other hospital operational issues have significantly undermined our ability to provide excellent, timely care.

We believe that one way to help improve care is to invest in the recruitment, retention, and education of the emergency department technician. This group currently plays a significant role in most EDs and with more advanced training could contribute even more. It is our hope that the *Emergency Department Technician Handbook* can play a major role in the augmentation and further professionalization of the ED technician workforce, leading to an expansion of the technician's scope of practice that will help mitigate the shortages of registered nurses that many organizations experience. ED technicians play an important role in our ED, and more technicians with better training will help us all immensely.

Robert Shesser
Ali Pourmand
Amy Keim

CONTENTS

Video 16.1 – Transverse view with compression. In this view, four anechoic circles can be identified, and with gentle compression three of these circles (paired deep brachial veins and more superficial basilic vein) collapse, while the deep brachial artery is observed to pulsate. Just below the vessels and to the right, a bright "honeycomb" appearance is characteristic of a nerve.

Video 16.2 – Transverse view with Doppler. This view demonstrates the artery from Video 1 with red flow toward the probe (due to slight angulation of probe directed toward the patient's shoulder), and blue veins that collapse with probe pressure.

Video 16.3 – Out-of-plane insertion technique. Narrated video demonstrating insertion of needle, following of needle down to level of vessel, then "train in tunnel" technique to ensure threading of the angiocath.

CHAPTER 1

The Role of the Hospital Emergency Department and the Specialty of Emergency Medicine

Ksenya Badashova ■ Sarah Ingram ■ Robert Shesser

The Organization of the Hospital

A hospital is a complex institution in which patients are treated by members of the hospital's medical staff, that includes, but is not limited to, physicians, advanced practice providers (such as physician assistants [PAs] and nurse practitioners), psychologists, and oral surgeons. Hospitals vary in size and complexity according to the needs and demographics of the communities they serve. There are about 5500 hospitals in the United States today, and this number has been dropping for the past decade due to consolidation of medical services into larger institutions.

Within the United States, there are three major types of hospitals: nonprofit, for-profit, and government-owned. The majority of hospitals in the United States are nonprofit organizations. They are licensed by their state and are deemed to provide essential services to their community. As such, they are effectively owned by the communities in which they are located. They do not pay any federal or state taxes, they can borrow money by issuing tax-exempt bonds, and they reinvest surplus revenues to improve their organization and services. They are led by boards of directors that are self-sustaining and most often comprise a group of business and civic leaders in their communities. For-profit hospitals, which represent roughly 15% of hospitals nationwide, are owned by shareholders who receive some of the profits in the form of dividends. They do pay taxes and borrow money at higher rates than not-for-profit organizations. Despite these major organizational and financial differences, both types of institutions look very similar to the average patient. US government-run hospitals include the Veteran's Affairs, Military, and Indian Health Service systems; this type of hospital is also exempt from paying taxes.

Hospital Type	*Controlling Body*	*Taxes*	*Surplus Income*
Nonprofit	Board of directors	Exempted	Reinvested in the organization
For-Profit	Shareholders	Taxed	Profits shareholders (dividends)
Government-Owned	Government	Exempted	Not applicable

Teaching is an additional aspect that differentiates hospitals. Academic medical centers are institutions committed to training future healthcare providers and facilitating cutting-edge medical research. They are often large, comprehensive medical enterprises that are frequently associated with medical, PA, and nursing schools. Many community hospitals have relationships with educational programs as consistent with their missions and locations.

Medical Staff

The concept of an independent and autonomous hospital medical staff has evolved over time in the United States. Unlike systems in many other countries, until recently, US physicians have infrequently been employed by the hospital. It has been recognized by multiple professional and regulatory organizations, including the American College of Surgeons (ACS) and the Joint Commission, that a medical staff structure independent of the hospital's administration is an important component in guaranteeing quality patient care.

The organized medical staff is responsible for creating criteria for who can practice in the hospital, what their scope of practice is, and supervising a system of due process for responding to situations where concerns about the professionalism or medical quality of medical staff members have been raised. The medical staff is often led by a medical staff president elected by their colleagues. There may also be a hospital medical director who has a dual reporting relationship to both the hospital administration and medical staff. Each of the recognized specialties in the hospital is lead by a department chair who may either be elected by medical staff members in that discipline or appointed by a senior executive according to the hospital's structure.

Many of the departments or service lines in the hospital have a dual structure, with a service-line medical director working together with an administrative partner appointed by hospital administration. The medical staff leaders meet in a monthly medical executive committee (MEC), and the entire medical staff of the hospital generally meets quarterly. In addition, there are various medical staff committees to review matters of medical staff credentialing and quality that are approved by the MEC and ultimately the hospital medical staff as a whole.

Hospital Administration

The hospital's executive management team generally consists of a chief executive officer (CEO), chief medical officer (CMO), chief financial officer (CFO), and a chief information officer (CIO). Thus the area in which they all work is often termed "the C suite." The CEO establishes and oversees the implementation of strategic development initiatives that are aligned with the hospital's mission, vision, and goals. The CMO acts as a liaison between the medical staff, governing bodies, and department chairs to coordinate medical services of various departments. The CFO manages the revenues and expenses. The CIO oversees the information and technology department, ensuring that the hospital's and patients' information is protected and that technology is utilized in accordance with the state regulations. The CEO additionally reports to the hospital's board of directors. Fig. 1.1 describes a typical hospital organizational structure.

Nursing is a critical part of every hospital system. The chief nursing officer (CNO) oversees the management of the nursing division and implementation of hospital strategies related to nursing. In the emergency department (ED), the nursing functions are overseen by the ED nursing director. A charge nurse is appointed on a shift-by-shift basis and maintains managerial responsibility over the nursing functions within the ED on that shift. Registered nurses are responsible for the nursing duties required for direct patient care during a shift. Certain responsibilities of patient care are divided between nurses and technicians within the ED. This division varies significantly among institutions in different jurisdictions.

Another facet of ancillary care that is vital to the smooth functioning of the ED is the hospital staff, who registers the patients and obtains their insurance information. Certain larger hospitals have a nonprovider, professional manager to whom the ED nursing director reports. Other systems have the registrars reporting to the CNO, and in other cases, the registrar reports to the CFO.

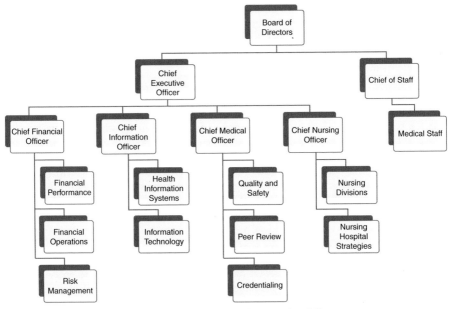

Fig. 1.1   Example of Hospital Organizational Chart.

Regulatory Environment

Hospital care is highly regulated by multiple levels of government and by a series of private organizations to whom hospitals voluntarily submit data. The primary responsibility for hospital licensure rests with the states, but hospitals also partner with county health authorities for certain public health and emergency medical services matters.

The federal government, through the Centers for Medicare and Medicaid Services (CMS) management of the Medicare program, is the largest payer of healthcare in the United States. Medicare participation is virtually universal among US hospitals. Medicare covers most retirees, disabled persons, and patients requiring hemodialysis. Medicare has been gradually replacing strict fee-for-service payments to hospitals with a series of financial incentives to "substitute volume for value." The Medicaid program is a partnership between federal and state governments to provide care for low-income patients. Although much of the financial support and structure is provided by the federal government, Medicaid is administered by the states, and eligibility requirements and covered services vary among the different state programs.

Several important federal regulations affect the hospital. The Health Insurance Portability and Accountability Act (HIPAA) is a privacy act that governs how hospitals (and every related organization) safeguard patient information, particularly electronic information. There are steep fines for HIPAA violations, and every hospital employee has an affirmative duty to protect patient privacy.

The Emergency Medical Treatment and Labor Act was issued by Congress in 1986 after several well-publicized instances of "patient dumping," where unstable patients received inadequate or no care due to financial reasons. This act requires hospitals participating in Medicare to provide a medical screening exam (MSE) to all patients seeking emergency care and to provide the needed treatments to stabilize patients who are found to have an emergent condition or who are in active labor. The MSE cannot be delayed for financial reasons. The MSE must be sufficiently detailed to allow the physician to exclude any emergent condition(s), and would therefore need to include labs and/or imaging in certain patients. Hospitals may transfer patients after stabilization if the hospital does not have the capacity to properly treat the patient. Similarly, hospitals are required to accept emergent transfer patients from hospitals lacking necessary care capabilities regardless of the patient's insurance status.

Hospitals are voluntarily accredited by a group of national organizations. The major organization for general accreditation is the Joint Commission. Joint Commission standards are developed for a wide variety of structure and process measures that are validated through an onsite inspection every few years. The Joint Commission manages several specialty designation programs including the accreditation processes for comprehensive stroke center, heart attack centers, and ventricular assist device center designations. The accreditation standards are set by various organizations. For example, the ACS has developed an extensive trauma center verification process, as well as an extensive quality initiative (the National Surgical Quality Improvement Program) for multiple surgical disciplines. The National Institutes of Health, on the other hand, is responsible for a cancer center designation initiative that involves both hospital and outpatient care.

The Specialty of Emergency Medicine

Emergency medicine is one of the newest medical specialties. It developed as an evolutionary process in which a full-time, professional cadre of career-committed emergency physicians (EPs) replaced a system in which part-time physicians trained in other specialties staffed hospital EDs. The American College of Emergency Physicians is a major specialty society that was established in 1968. The first dedicated emergency medicine residency training program was established in 1970 at the University of Cincinnati. In September 1979, emergency medicine became the 23rd recognized medical specialty, and the first board examination was administered in 1980.

The specialty has grown significantly, as ED volume in the United States has continued to rise steadily over the past 50 years. It is estimated that there are about 145 million ED visits in the United States per year (about 430 visits per 1000 people), demonstrating the need for providers who are trained in the evaluation and treatment of the undifferentiated patient and are experts in resuscitation. There are currently over 250 ED residency programs and a large number of professional societies and journals.

The practice arrangements for EPs are quite varied. Emergency physicians may be employed by the hospital (unusual) or the parent health system in integrated delivery systems that include hospitals, ambulatory facilities, and all the medical providers in one organization. Emergency physicians are frequently employed by regional or national "single-specialty" groups that contract with the hospital to provide physician (and frequently Advanced Practice Provider) coverage for the ED. Regardless of the employment relationships, much of the financial support for EPs comes from their billing the patients for a "professional fee" that is separate from the amounts that the hospital charges the patients (or their insurance companies), which are called "technical fees."

Emergency Medicine Training
PHYSICIAN TRAINING

Physicians are expected to have completed a bachelor's degree with certain premedical prerequisites. Prior to entering medical school, they have often participated in medical research, gained clinical experiences by working as a scribe or technician, and may have performed community service. Emergency medicine (EM) training characteristically begins in medical school. Medical schools throughout the United States have created clinical rotations in the ED with dedicated curricula revolving around the various diagnostic and treatment approaches to common emergency patient presentations, with a special focus on resuscitative measures.

Emergency medicine residencies, accredited by the Accreditation Council for Graduate Medical Education, are designed to teach both cognitive and procedural skills necessary to practice independently. Emergency medicine residency programs are either 3 or 4 years in length. Core rotations are in the ED under the supervision of practicing (attending) EPs. Residents also rotate through intensive care units, coronary care units, certain inpatient services, anesthesiology, and labor and delivery.

Although many physicians begin practice directly after residency, fellowships are a means for EM physicians to establish themselves as subspecialty content experts. Fellowships are available in multiple areas, including ultrasound, administration, international, toxicology, simulation, and pediatric EM.

PHYSICIAN ASSISTANT TRAINING

Physician assistant programs most frequently are organized as a 2-3 year master's program into which candidates enroll after obtaining a bachelor's degree with the necessary prerequisite classes. As with medical school, successful PA applicants often have prior healthcare experience. Curriculum in physician assistant schools is split fairly evenly into preclinical and clinical education. During clinical time, PA students follow a similar rotation pattern as third and fourth year medical students, including at least one EM rotation.

NURSE TRAINING

Becoming a registered nurse (RN) involves either obtaining an associate's degree in nursing (ASN) or a bachelor of science degree in nursing (BSN). Although the length of programs can vary, a BSN typically requires 4 years of university studies, the last 2 of which are focused specifically on nursing. After completing the required coursework, a nurse must pass the National Council Licensure Examination to gain licensure and to begin working within the ED. An ED nurse can additionally obtain a Certified Emergency Nurse certification, the requirements of which are developed and supervised by the Board of Certification for Emergency Nursing, an independent, private, voluntary, professional organization.

PATIENT CARE TECHNICIAN TRAINING

Technicians in EDs are hired by the hospital, which develops its own prerequisites for the job. Many hospitals require their ED technicians to be emergency medical technicians (EMT) in their jurisdiction; they may be certified by the National Registry of Emergency Medical Technicians and state reciprocity programs. Many hospitals prefer ED technicians to have prior clinical experience as an EMT on an ambulance prior to their hire, but there is tremendous heterogeneity among different institutions.

Emergency Department Organization and Flow

Crystal Donelan ■ Christopher Payette ■ Fletcher Vilt

The emergency department (ED) is a complex organization in which care is provided by health-care providers with a variety of different types of training, employment relationships, heirarchy of roles, and job descriptions. The staff includes a group that is dedicated entirely to ED patients and a group that works throughout the hospital and responds to the ED when requested.

Emergency Department Organization

PROVIDERS

The generic term "provider" is applied to practitioners who are members of the hospital medical staff and exercise independent medical judgment. This category includes physicians (either doctors of medicine [MDs] or doctors of osteopathic medicine [DOs]), physician assistants (PAs), and nurse practitioners (NPs). Providers may be employed either by the hospital, a staffing company, or other medical practice organization that has an arrangement with the hospital for staffing providers. Providers are licensed by the state, credentialed by the hospital medical staff (see Chapter 1), and have passed a series of examinations administered by nongovernmental professional societies. Providers generally report to an ED medical director, who is most frequently a physician.

NURSES AND TECHNICIANS

Nurses are employed by the hospital, licensed by the state, and may also have additional certifications (such as certified emergency nurse) from private professional organizations. They report to an ED nursing manager who often (depending on the size and complexity of the hospital) reports to the chief nursing officer or designee. The ED technicians (EDTs) most often report to the ED nurse manager and are directly supervised by nursing staff while working.

PHARMACISTS

Many EDs have in-person pharmacy support for all or part of the day. The pharmacist helps both the providers and nursing staff with the selection and administration of medications.

REGISTRARS

The registration team, is responsible for entering patient demographic information into the hospital's management system and collecting insurance information from the patient. Additionally, they will often have the patient sign a consent to be treated and may document whether a patient has an advance directive.

UNIT CLERKS

The role of the unit clerk is crucial for smooth, efficient ED operations. Their characteristic duties are as follows:

- Answering the main ED department number for general inquiries
- Directing phone and foot traffic to the proper personnel in the ED
- Directing health provider phone calls from outside facilities to the attending MD
- Helping coordinate logistics for patient transfers
- Scanning paper copies of charts, results, or emergency medical services (EMS) run sheets into patients' electronic medical records (EMRs)
- Helping coordinate discharge arrangements for special patient categories

The importance of the role cannot be undervalued and one that the EDT may be tasked with on occasion.

Table 2.1 describes characteristic roles of providers, nurses, and EDTs.

Hospital Personnel Responding to Emergency Department Consultations

SPECIALTY CONSULTANTS

Each hospital develops a relatively unique pattern of specialty physician response to the ED. In larger institutions, there will generally be greater on-site presence of specialists, and there will often be specialty residents (physicians in training) or fellows (subspecialty trainees) who are the first responders to consultations. Smaller community hospitals will have physicians on their medical staff whose availability for bedside ED consultation varies with their other practice demands. Many hospitals have recently hired PAs in a variety of specialty areas who support physician-specialists with postoperative care in hospital patient management, assist in the operating room, and provide in-person ED consults.

Certain specialty consults (most frequently stroke neurology and psychiatry) may be done by off-site physicians via telemedicine. Many initial behavioral health consults will be done by hospital-employed psychiatric social workers who are licensed by the state but are not members of the hospital's medical staff.

TABLE 2.1 ■ **Characteristic Roles of Providers, Nurses, Emergency Department Technicians**

Providers	Nurses	ED Technicians
Medical evaluation	Patient triage	Venipuncture and IV insertion
Ordering labs and x-rays	Nursing assessment	Rooming patients
Assignment of a diagnosis	Medication administration	Obtaining an ECG; initiating cardiac monitoring
Calling consults	Patient education	Wound care
Writing prescriptions and discharge instructions	Managing IV drips	Taking vital signs
Performing bedside procedures		Splinting
Coordinating care with the patient's primary care and specialist physicians		

ECG, Electrocardiogram; *ED*, emergency department; *IV*, intravenous.

CASE MANAGEMENT

As many ED patients have significant, acute social service needs, most EDs have a social worker or case manager assigned to the ED. Some of their duties include coordinating patients' housing and home care needs, arranging transportation, facilitating acquisition of medications or durable medical equipment, and (depending on their backgrounds), helping with psychiatric screening and assessments.

SPECIALTY HOSPITAL SERVICES

Electrocardiogram Technician

In some EDs, electrocardiograms (ECGs) are performed primarily by the EDT, but in others, a central hospital technician will perform some or all of the ECGs on ED patients.

Respiratory Therapy Technician

Helping with ventilator and advanced airway management is the core of this professional category. They may also assist nursing with other functions such as administration of nebulized medications or suctioning intubated patients.

Physical Therapy

Many ED patients with acute or chronic skeletal injuries can benefit from a physical therapy (PT) visit in the ED. A PT evaluation is most helpful in making disposition decisions on patients with movement or balance challenges and in patients with acute vertiginous dizziness.

Emergency Department Administration

The day-to-day administration of an ED is generally a partnership between the medical and nursing leaders. Each leader has primary responsibility for hiring and scheduling members of their group, defining shift length, and creating a back-up system to help ensure adequate staffing at all times. The leadership team develops a synthesis of views on patient arrival patterns and creates schedule templates for providers and nursing that attempts to best fit the available staffing to the patient arrival patterns.

The reporting structure for the physician medical director will vary significantly with the type of hospital. There is always accountability for credentialing and quality issues to the hospital medical staff committees and ultimately to the hospital medical staff executive committee. Administratively, the ED physician leader could report to an administrator or to another physician such as the hospital medical director or vice president of medical affairs.

The ED nursing director most frequently reports to the hospital's director (vice president) of nursing or its designee. Depending on the size and complexity of the organization, the ED nursing director may have administrative oversight over ED registration and may report through the hospital's administrative structure for those functions. Some hospitals will have centralization of functions, such as ED technical charge capture and coding (billing for the hospital) but in others, an ED administrator or ED nurse manager would supervise staff.

The "charge nurse" is a key operational role that is often rotated among a group of experienced nurses. The charge nurse is responsible for managing the operational efficiency of the ED in real time. They help manage the ED patient flow, are usually responsible for calling in additional staff as needed, and coordinate the operations of the ED with those of the rest of the hospital. Table 2.2 describes the types of functions that are required of the ED administrative team.

TABLE 2.2 ■ **Roles of Emergency Department Administration**

Medical	Nursing	Administrative
Hiring physicians and Advanced Practice Provider	Hiring nurses, technicians, clerks	Hiring registrars
	Annual performance reviews Managing patient complaints Nursing scheduling	

TABLE 2.3 ■ **Principles of Registration**

1. The patient should be registered and a new visit should then be populated on the ED tracking board. This way, at the very least, the medical team will now be able to access this patient's electronic visit.
2. The patient should have some form of identifier on their person; typically this is a hospital wristband that will contain patient identifiers, medical record number, and financial number (discussed in later chapters).
3. Finally, patients will need to go through further registration past the creation of a visit. This typically entails gathering financial and contact information for the patient (i.e., health insurance) so the patient or their insurance can be billed for their visit. After the patient is registered, the ED technician can also be involved in the logistics of patient flow in the ED.

ED, Emergency department.

Emergency Department Patient Flow

INITIAL ASSESSMENT AND REGISTRATION

Patients enter the ED in two major categories: ambulatory and ambulance. The two key initial functions that must occur are patient registration and patient assessment. Most EDs have separate entrances and procedures for the assessment and registration of ambulatory and ambulance patients. Generally, sicker patients arrive by ambulance, but procedures must be flexible enough to rapidly assess disease severity in all ambulatory arrivals and prioritize ambulance arrivals to their appropriate place in the queue if there is a wait.

A key function during the first few minutes of a patient's arrival is to register the patient in the hospital's EMR system because all orders, clinical observations, and procedures must be entered into the EMR (other than during computer downtime). The basic registration information is generally the patient's name and date of birth, and these two identifiers are generally adequate to begin a record or determine whether the patient has been in the hospital before. Table 2.3 describes key points for EDT participation in the registration process.

The initial assessment, called triage, is performed by a registered nurse (RN). It requires interviewing the patient, taking a set of vital signs, and assigning the triage category using the Emergency Severity Index (ESI) in the United States. In addition, most EMRs have a series of screens to be completed as a result of the triage nurse's interview.

Patient Intake and Front-End Operations

There is tremendous heterogeneity among different EDs in the precise way the ambulatory arrivals are managed when there are no empty or staffed treatment spaces. If there are available treatment spaces, ambulatory arrivals will generally be quickly placed in an open spot and seen by providers. During times of high demand or when available spaces are filled with boarding patients, EDs use

TABLE 2.4 ■ **Strategies to Improve Emergency Department "Front-End" Processing (*adapted from Wiler et al.*)**

Immediate bedding
Bedside registration
Advanced triage protocols and triage-based care protocols
Physician/practitioner in triage
Dedicated "fast track" service line
Tracking systems and "white boards"
Wireless communication devices
Personal health record technology
Team approach patient care: "Team Triage"
Resource-based triage systems
Waiting room design enhancements
Full/surge capacity protocols
Incentive-based staff compensation
Time to evaluation guarantee
Referral to next-day care

a variety of strategies to improve performance as described in Table 2.4. Many of these front-end strategies will involve some input from providers, nurses, and EDTs. Emergency department technician roles in front-end operations could include registration tasks, venipuncture, intravenous (IV) access, wound care, and patient transport.

Patient Logistics and "Rooming Strategies"

Emergency department technicians are often tasked with escorting patients to their rooms as directed by the triage or charge nurse. Before placing a patient in a room, the EDT should ensure that the room is clean and ready for a new patient. A technician may also assist in the prioritization process, and there are a few key concepts to bear in mind. These include patient acuity, the patient's pain score, and the room type available (e.g., cardiac monitor or negative pressure).

Admission and Discharge

After the provider team has fully evaluated a patient, they will decide whether the patient should be admitted to the hospital or discharged. The EDT may facilitate the discharge home by helping to print out discharge paperwork, removing any IV catheters, taking the patient off the monitor, helping the patient dress, splinting injured extremities, completing any needed wound care and dressing, obtaining provider signatures on prescriptions, placing the patient in a wheelchair if needed, and coordinating where to meet their ride home. In most EDs, the exit interview is performed by an RN, but some EDs may permit this to be done by the EDT, particularly in patients with minor traumatic injuries.

If patient is to be admitted, the EDT can assist the nurse in the transition to another hospital unit by placing the patient on portable monitor, getting a movable source of oxygen, ensuring the belongings accompany the patient, and providing any wound care or splinting needed, as mentioned earlier.

Patient Tracking Board

Although there is some variability among EMRs, a central feature of all systems is the ED tracking board. This portion of the application can be viewed on individual computers and sometimes on a large, centrally located wall monitor. Different categories of ED staff may have different views of the board, and a series of filters allows each person within a category to individualize their view. The tracking board will have a view with the patient's name, chief complaint, geographic location within the ED, and a variety of other information that can be quickly viewed and are depicted by different colors, text, or a variety of icons. Other common information on the tracking board can include ESI level, vital signs, critical lab test results, point-of-care orders, status of provider's documentation, allergies, the patient's primary care physician, status, lab and x-ray orders, disposition, and length of stay.

References

Wiler J, Gentle C, Halfpenny J, et al. Optimizing emergency department front-end operations. Annals of Emergency Medicine. 2010;55:142–160. doi:10.1016/j.

CHAPTER 3

Medical Terminology

Dina Abdelsamad ■ Robert McKinney ■ Jenny Huang

Introduction

Medical terminology is the common language that healthcare providers use to communicate signs, symptoms, exam findings, diagnoses, and medical procedures, as well as anatomic positions, movement and relationships. Its proper and consistent use ensures that shared information, whether it is in a medical textbook, a discussion between providers, or documentation in a patient chart, is concise, specific, and universally understood by anyone in the medical field. Over 60% of all English words have Greek or Latin roots. For science and technology terms, that figure increases to 90%. It may seem a daunting task to learn such an extensive new language, but it is fairly straightforward. This chapter will introduce the most important building blocks of medical terms: the word parts. These word parts (roots, prefixes, and suffixes) are combined to build medical terms. We will also include common medical abbreviations and terms important in describing anatomic planes, positions, and relationships.

Structure of Medical Terms

Medical terms can often be divided into a prefix, word root, and suffix. Not all medical terms are composed of all three aspects, but most will have at least two. The parts of the terms are often connected by combining vowels.

Word Roots

The word root is the fundamental meaning of the term. The word root tends to refer to an area of the body. There can be multiple root words for the same body part or term, such as *ophthalm/o* and *opt/o*, which are both word roots for "eye." Root words can be found anywhere in a medical term, depending on whether a prefix or suffix is present. Additionally, some words have more than one word root in them. Common word roots that are seen in the emergency department (ED) are shown in Table 3.1.

Not all medical terms have a word root. For example, apnea is composed of just a prefix (*a-*, "without") and a suffix (*-pnea*, "breathing").

Prefixes

Prefixes are modifiers that are found at the beginning of a word. They change the meaning of a word. For example, the term "emesis" by itself means vomiting. When the prefix *hyper-*, which means "above," is added to emesis to make the term *hyper*emesis, the new word means excessive vomiting. Common prefixes that are seen in the ED are shown in Table 3.2.

TABLE 3.1 ■ Common Word Roots, Definitions, and Examples

Word Root	Definition	Example
Cardi(o) Cardi(a)	Heart	Cardiologist (heart specialist)
Derm(a) Derm(o) Dermat(o)	Skin	Dermatitis (inflammation of the skin)
Gynec(o)	Female	Gynecology (study of conditions related to women)
Hemat(o)	Blood	Hematuria (blood in urine)
Lymph(o)	Lymph vessel	Lymphadenopathy (disease of the lymph nodes)
Muscul(o) My(o)	Muscle	Musculoskeletal (pertaining to the muscles and skeleton)
Neur(o)	Nerve	Neuropathy (disease of the nerves)
Opt(o) Ophthalm(o)	Eye	Ophthalmology (study of the eye)
Oste(o)	Bone	Osteopenia (low bone mass)
Ot(o)	Ear	Otoscope (tool used to examine the ear)
Path(o)	Disease	Pathology (study of disease)
Thorac(o)	Chest	Intrathoracic (within the chest)
Vascul(o)	Blood vessel	Vasculature (relating to blood vessels)

TABLE 3.2 ■ Common Prefixes, Definitions, and Examples

Prefix	Definition	Example
Brady-	Slow	Bradycardia (slow heart rate) Bradypnea (slow breathing)
Tachy-	Fast	Tachycardia (fast heart rate) Tachypnea (rapid breathing)
Dys-	Difficulty	Dysuria (difficulty and pain with urination) Dyspnea (difficulty breathing)
A-	Without	Anuria (inability to make urine) Apnea (lack of breathing)
Poly-	Many	Polyuria (frequent urination)
Hyper-	Over, Above, Excessive	Hyperemesis (excessive vomiting) Hypertension (high blood pressure) Hyperglycemia (high blood sugar)
Hypo-	Below	Hypotension (low blood pressure) Hypoglycemia (low blood sugar)
Intra-	Within	Intraosseous (within the bone) Intradermal (within the skin) Intramuscular (within the muscle)
Inter-	Between	Intercostal (between the ribs)

Suffixes

Suffixes are found at the end of a word and change the meaning of the medical term. For example, the root word *bronch/o* relates to the bronchial tubes that carry air to the lungs. The suffix *-itis* means infection or inflammation. Adding the suffix *-itis* to *broncho* creates the term bronchitis, which means infection of the bronchial tubes.

Note that in this example the suffix *-itis* begins with a vowel, so the combining vowel in *bronch/o* is dropped. In the word "bronchodilator" *(bronch/o/dilat/or)*, *dilat/o* is a word root that begins with a consonant, so the combining vowel is kept. Additionally, the suffix *-or* begins with a vowel, so the combining vowel is dropped in between those terms, or else the word would be "bronchodilatoor."

Suffixes can be added to a root word to make a complete word. For example, the term "optic" is the root word *opt/o* combined with the suffix *-ic*. *Opt/o* means "eye," and *-ic* means "relating to." When putting the two together to make "optic," the word means "relating to the eye."

The suffixes in the following box all mean "pertaining to." What medical terms can you think of that have these suffixes?

> *-ac, -al, -an, -ar, -ary, -eal, -ical, -ior, -ory, -ose, -ous, -tic*

The suffixes in Table 3.3 are all related to surgical procedures. The examples are medical terms you may encounter in the ED. The suffixes in Table 3.4 are descriptive and refer to conditions or diseases as well as expertise.

Combining Vowels

When combining word parts together, the word root is often modified to make the medical term smoother and more cohesive. Let's use the root word *cardi* as an example. It is found in such medical terms as "cardiology," "cardiomyopathy," and "cardiovascular." As you can see in these terms, *cardi* is connected to the other parts using an *(o)*.

As a rule of thumb, when a root word is connected to another word part that starts with a consonant, a combining vowel, such as *(o)*, *(i)*, or *(a)*, is used. Looking at the preceding examples, "cardiology" is a root word (*cardi*, "heart") and suffix (*-logy*, "study of") combined using an *-o*.

TABLE 3.3 ■ **Common Surgical Suffixes, Definitions, and Examples**

Suffix	Definition	Example
-centesis	Puncture to remove fluid	Abdominal paracentesis (procedure to remove fluid from the abdomen) Pericardiocentesis (procedure to remove fluid from the sac around the heart)
-ectomy	Removal	Nephrectomy (procedure to remove a kidney)
-ostomy	Opening	Thoracostomy (chest tube placement; creates an opening to release air or blood) Colostomy (procedure to create an opening to the colon)
-otomy	Cut into	Thoracotomy (cutting into the chest)

TABLE 3.4 ■ **Common Suffixes, Definitions, and Examples**

Suffix	Definition	Example
-itis	Infection or inflammation	Cellulitis (infection of the skin) Meningitis (inflammation of the meninges in the spine and brain)
-logy	Study of	Neurology (study of the nervous system)
-logist	One who studies	Radiologist (one who studies medical imaging)
-pathy	Disease	Neuropathy (disease of the nerves)
-pnea	Breathing	Hypercapnia (excessive carbon dioxide in the system caused by issues breathing)
-uria	Urine	Hematuria (blood in urine)

"Cardiomyopathy" is a root word + root word + suffix (*cardi*, "heart") + (*my*, "muscle") + (*-pathy*, "disease") meaning disease of the heart muscle. Because *my* and *-pathy* both begin with consonants, combining vowels are used to connect the word parts.

When a root word or suffix begins with a vowel, a combining vowel is not used. For example, the word "cardiovascular" is a root word + root word + suffix: *cardi/o*, *vascul/o*, and *-ar*. The suffix *-ar* begins with a vowel, so no combining vowel is used between *vascul/o* and *-ar*. *Vascul/o*, the second word root, starts with a consonant, so *cardi* and *vascul* are connected using the combining vowel (*o*).

This pattern is consistent with most medical terms. For example, when connecting *rhin* and *-rrhea*, the term would *not* be "rhinrrhea." Because *-rrhea* starts with a consonant, the combining vowel (*o*) is used to make rhinorrhea. When connecting *rhin* and *-itis*, the term would *not* be "rhinoitis." A connecting vowel would not be used because *-itis* begins with a vowel, so the (*o*) would be dropped.

Putting It Together

Practice the concepts you've learned in the following questions:

1. Separate the word parts in this term "Otorhinolaryngologist" with slashes. Then, identify if the word part is a prefix, word root, suffix, or combining vowel. Lastly, define the term.

Ot /	o /	rhin /	o /	laryng /	o /	-logist
Word root	Combining vowel	Word root	Combining vowel	Word root	Combining vowel	suffix

   If it is difficult to define this word, start with the word roots and their meanings. *Ot/o/rhin/o/laryng/o/logist* = ear + nose + throat + one who studies; that is, one who studies the ear, nose, and throat (otherwise known as an ENT). Using context clues (if someone studies the ear and nose, what else might they study?) or anatomic knowledge (*laryng/o* comes from "larynx") can help decipher word components that are unfamiliar.

2. Someone presents to the ED with postop (postoperative) complaints 2 days after their appendix was removed. It was removed because it was inflamed.
   a. What is the medical term for the surgical procedure they underwent 2 days ago?
   b. What is the medical term for the reason why it was removed?
   Answers:
   a. Appendectomy (removal of the appendix)
   b. Appendicitis (inflammation of the appendix)

Medical Abbreviations Commonly Used in the Emergency Department

Abbreviations are commonly used in the ED as a time-saving tactic. Sometimes the abbreviations are universal; however, not all specialties use the same medical abbreviations, and some abbreviations may mean different things in different contexts. For example, LBP can mean "low back pain" or "low blood pressure." It is critical to use abbreviations only in situations where there is no ambiguity. A small sample of common abbreviations used in EDs is shown in Table 3.5.

Although ED technicians do not administer medications, understanding the abbreviations for medication routes can help the flow of the ED (see Table 3.6). How can this information be useful? Many medications are administered in different ways. Hydromorphone (Dilaudid), a pain medication commonly given in the ED, can be administered intravenously (IV), intramuscularly (IM), or subcutaneously (SQ). For some patients, the provider will not order blood work but will order medications for pain management. With IM and SQ hydromorphone, there is no need for

TABLE 3.5 ■ Common Abbreviations and Definitions

Abbreviation	Definition
LUQ	Left upper quadrant of the abdomen
RUQ	Right upper quadrant of the abdomen
LLQ	Left lower quadrant of the abdomen
RLQ	Right lower quadrant of the abdomen
LUE	Left upper extremity (the arm)
RUE	Right upper extremity
LLE	Left lower extremity (the legs)
RLE	Right lower extremity
CHI/TBI	Closed head injury / traumatic brain injury
U-preg	Urine pregnancy test
CXR	Chest x-ray
I&D	Incision and drainage—a procedure to manage abscesses
LP	Lumbar puncture—a procedure to gather CSF (cerebrospinal fluid)
USIV	Ultrasound-guided IV
IVF	IV fluids
PIV	Peripheral IV
ASA	Aspirin
NTG	Nitroglycerin
NPO	Nothing by mouth; no food or liquids by mouth
BIBA	Brought in by ambulance
MI	Myocardial infarction (heart attack)
CP	Chest pain
SOB	Shortness of breath
OD	Overdose
ETOH	Alcohol intoxication
AMS	Altered mental status
Aox3	Alert and oriented to person, place, and time
LOC	Loss of consciousness
MVC	Motor vehicle collision
GSW	Gunshot wound
UTI	Urinary tract infection
LMP	Last menstrual period
URI	Upper respiratory infection
ARDS	Acute respiratory distress syndrome
CHF	Congestive heart failure

TABLE 3.6 ■ Abbreviations for Medication Administration Routes and Definitions

Abbreviation	Definition
IM	Intramuscular, or within the muscle
IN	Intranasal, or within the nose
IO	Intraosseous, or within the bone
IV	Intravenous, or within the vein
PR	Per rectum
SL	Sublingual, or under the tongue
SQ	Subcutaneous, or under the skin

PO Definition: By mouth

an IV for the patient. However, if IV hydromorphone is ordered, an ED technician can place an IV while a nurse prepares the medication.

As an example, if the triage note reports that SL NTG was given to the patient, you know that sublingual nitroglycerin was administered.

Anatomic Relationships

Terms describing body planes and anatomic relationships are used to accurately and consistently describe the location of a structure or point of importance on the human body. We conventionally start with standard anatomic position, in which the patient is standing with their arms by their side and with their palms and toes facing forward (see Fig. 3.1).

Directions are always given from the perspective of the patient. For example, the patient's right hand, though on the observer's left side, is described as the right side of the patient (see Fig. 3.2).

Body Planes

There are 3 anatomic planes (cross sections) commonly used to describe relationships: sagittal, transverse, and frontal (see Fig. 3.2).
- Sagittal – separates the body (or an organ) into right and left sections
- Transverse (horizontal) – separates the body (or an organ) into top and bottom sections
- Frontal (coronal) – separates the body into front and back sections

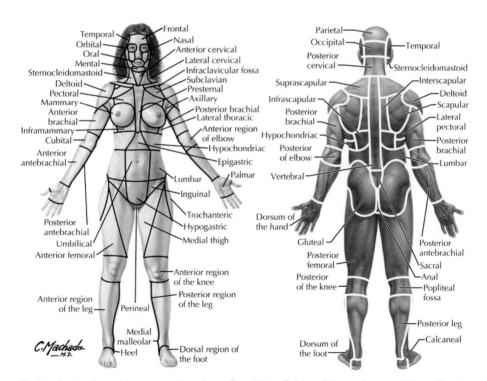

Fig. 3.1 Anatomic position, anatomic regions. (From Netter F. *Atlas of Human Anatomy*. 7th ed. Elsevier; 2018:plates 2 and 3.)

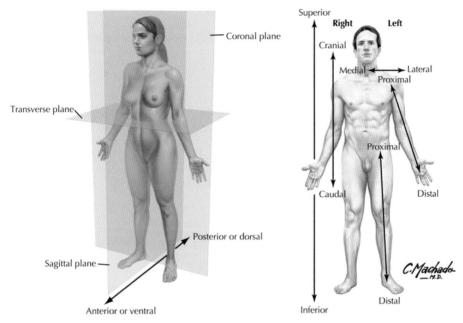

Fig. 3.2   Body planes, key anatomic relationship terms. (From Netter, F. *Atlas of Human Anatomy*. 7th ed. Elsevier; 2018:plate 1.)

Directional Terms

- Anterior (front) versus posterior (back). For example, the chest wall is anterior to the heart.
- Superior (above) versus inferior (below). For example, the knee is superior to the ankle.
- Proximal (closer) versus distal (farther), described in relation to the trunk. For example, the knee is proximal to the ankle.
- Superficial (closer) versus deep (farther), described in relation to the body's surface. For example, the skin is superficial to the muscle.
- Medial (closer to) versus lateral (farther out), described in relation to the midline of the body. For example, the ears are lateral to the nose.
- Ventral (front) versus dorsal (back). For example, the palm is the ventral side of the hand.

Locations are often described in relation to anatomic structures. For example, a laceration may be described as a deep puncture to the left anterior medial forearm, just distal to the elbow. Providing such a specific description also conveys a significant amount of information such as the scope of the potential injury (the ulnar nerve and artery pass through that area) and what type of evaluation is required (a physical exam testing the integrity of the ulnar nerve and artery) and prepares providers for a potential emergent intervention (control of ulnar arterial bleeding).

References for Additional Reading

Cohen BJ, Jones SA. Concepts, suffixes, and prefixes of medical terminology. In *Medical Terminology: An Illustrated Guide*. 9th ed. Burlington, MA: Jones & Bartlett Learning; 2021:4–5.
Netter F. Atlas of Human Anatomy. 7th ed. Elsevier; 2018.

CHAPTER 4

Teamwork and Communication

Noah Lubin ▧ Sara Ashton Garcia

Team Dynamics in the Emergency Department

Team dynamics play a vital role in the emergency department (ED) because teamwork and coordination allow for the highest-quality care possible. Individual skills are important, but without teamwork, the best level of care will never be achieved. As an ED technician (EDT), you play a critical role as a member of an interdisciplinary team. Depending on the scope of your practice and your training, the tasks you perform facilitate the treatment of patients and enable the rest of the team to perform their roles successfully.

Communication and Patient Safety

Communication is the transfer of information from one person to another. In an ED, information must be transmitted quickly and efficiently because lives are on the line. Therefore good communication skills are necessary to be an effective team member. Good communication enhances patient safety and reduces the chance of medical errors. In the ED, good teamwork and communication allow for everyone to work together effectively and use all possible resources, which leads to the best patient outcomes.

The *Joint Commission* is an accrediting body that was established to assess healthcare organizations with the ultimate goal of improving patient care. Their stamp of approval shows that an organization is compliant with national standards for quality of care and patient safety. In their research, they found that communication errors were the cause of 60% of sentinel events (patient safety events that result in death, permanent harm, or significant temporary harm). In these cases, it was the team's failure to communicate well that resulted in serious harm to the patient.

The ED is a dynamic and fast-paced workplace environment where decisions need to be made quickly. Working with such constant activity may lead to errors that cause patient harm. For example, critical information about patients can be missed, or the wrong dose of a medication may be administered. As a result, various systems have been put into place to help reduce medical errors and improve patient outcomes. One such system is *TeamSTEPPS:* Team Strategies and Tools to Enhance Performance and Patient Safety. TeamSTEPPS is an initiative by the Agency for Healthcare Research and Quality, Department of Health and Human Services, and Department of Defense designed to improve patient safety using an evidence-based teamwork system. The system relies on five key principles: team structure, communication, leadership, situation monitoring, and mutual support.

TEAM STRUCTURE

When caring for a patient, multiple teams must work efficiently together to provide the highest-quality care and ensure patient safety. The ED patient care core team is typically made up of physicians, physician assistants, nurse practitioners, nurses, and technicians. The core team is assisted by the coordinating team and other support services. The coordinating team can be thought of as the attending/supervising physicians and the charge nurse. Their role is to oversee and coordinate care for all of the patients in the department. The support services include everyone outside of the core that may be required to assist in the care of the patient. This includes specialists, medical imaging, clerks, and environmental services, among others. All of these roles are supported by the hospital administration, which creates policies and procedures for the hospital staff to follow. As a new EDT, it is helpful to understand the team structure of the ED, as it will help you navigate your new workplace.

COMMUNICATION

The role of communication between staff members is to relay critical information to other members of the care team. Nurses and providers should promptly be made aware of any important changes in the patient's status. For example, if a patient develops a new symptom or develops abnormal vital signs, it is important that whoever notes this information shares it with the entire team. Ensuring that all team members are current on the patient's condition as it changes throughout their ED stay enables providers to make well-informed decisions and respond appropriately to the needs of the patient.

Critical patients often arrive by ambulance. Prior to arrival, emergency medical services (EMS) will radio in to the ED with important information concerning the patient's condition. This includes the patient's complaint (why the ambulance was called) and condition (e.g., "alert and oriented" or "unresponsive"), vital signs, electrocardiogram (ECG) results, and any other critical information (e.g., trauma requiring imaging, surgeons, anesthesia, and an operating room) that will help the ED prepare for the patient. Before the patient's arrival, the ED team will have a *huddle*. During the huddle, the team leader will identify themselves, and each member will introduce themselves and state their roles and specific responsibility. For example, "Noah, EDT, IV [intravenous] access." If members do not already have assigned responsibilities, the team leader will assign them. The team leader is responsible for making sure that all providers know their roles and have the proper skill level to perform them. If a provider is not able to perform the assigned role, they must inform the team leader immediately so a different assignment can be made. During the huddle, the team leader will also provide the team with the information provided by EMS and state the patient management plan.

Effective communication is complete, clear, concise, and quick. Only state the relevant information and avoid superfluous details. Use standard terminology and not acronyms. Be brief. Never delay giving information. Last, make sure the information is received with verbal confirmation from the receiver. Critical situations are often noisy, which is why *call-outs* are used. A call-out is meant to provide critical information to all team members in the room. The team leader will either request certain information, or a team member will provide new information as it is available. Here is an example:

Leader: "Are the pads on the patient"

Technician: "The pads are on the patient."

Leader: "Thank you, pads are on"

Information must always be acknowledged by the receiver. This is called *closed-loop communication*. Closed-loop communication occurs when a sender calls out information to a specific receiver and the receiver confirms back to the sender that the instruction has been received and when the action has been completed. This communication method reduces errors by making others aware of the information or instructions and confirming that the information or instructions are received and acted upon. Here is an example:

Leader: "Kamilla, administer 1 mg of epinephrine."

Nurse: "Administering 1 mg of epinephrine.

Nurse: "1 mg of epinephrine in."

Notice that the leader named the team member to whom the instructions were directed. This helps avoid ambiguity and confusion.

Closed-loop communication also allows for the receiver and other team members to clarify instructions, thereby reducing medical errors. Here is an example:

Leader: "Kamilla, administer 10 mg of epinephrine."

Nurse: "Did you mean 1 mg of epinephrine?"

Leader: "Yes. Thank you. Administer 1 mg of epinephrine."

Nurse: "Administering 1 mg of epinephrine."

Nurse: "1 mg of epinephrine in."

In critical situations, you will often overhear providers discussing the patient's condition. They typically use the *SBAR* method, which stands for situation, background, assessment, and recommendation. It is a technique mainly used by providers to summarize the critical information and develop a plan of action.

Situation: Describe the problem.

"The patient is unresponsive and his wife said he was shaking his whole body and then lost control of his bladder."

Background: Overview of the situation.

"He has a history of diabetes. EMS found his blood sugar to be 30 mg/dL. He received 1 amp of glucose in the field, but he is still altered."

Assessment: Provider's determination of the problem.

"The patient potentially had a seizure secondary to hypoglycemia. However, the cause of his persistent altered mental status is unclear."

Recommendation: Plan of action.

"Closely monitor the patient's blood sugar and vital signs, obtain a full set of labs including a toxicology screen and cultures, and let's get a STAT head CT."

One of the most important staff-to-staff communications comes when care is transferred from one provider to another. At shift change, a *hand-off* is performed and the outgoing technician provides a summary of each patient's case to the incoming technician. It is important to include the following

Chief complaint

Any pertinent medical history

Important findings from their evaluation

Any remaining workup or

Tasks requiring attention

Critical items to be aware of

The sickest patients, those needing the most attention, should be identified. Last, it is helpful to identify any patients who have particular challenges or needs to better prepare the incoming technician.

LEADERSHIP

Team leaders are typically medical providers. In critical situations, their primary goal is to organize an efficient and effective team. During the huddle, the team leader ensures that all roles are assigned to team members capable of fulfilling their specific roles. Once everyone is assigned a role, the team leader will determine the specific plan of action and prioritize certain tasks. As the situation unfolds, it is the job of the team leader to collect information from team members through call-outs, analyze the environment for any issues or changes to the patient's status, and frequently announce the current patient status. By continually receiving information, they can make any necessary changes to the plan of action. Should anyone in the room have any concerns, or if team members have conflicting opinions, it is the team leader's responsibility to resolve the conflict and get all of the team members on the same page.

When the critical situation is over, the team leader will direct a team debriefing. They will summarize the events that occurred and highlight what went well and what could have been better. They will also call for input and feedback from team members. The goal of a debrief is to identify any negative or positive events that occurred. Identifying and discussing the negative events, and how they could have been better or avoided improves team member knowledge and skills. Identifying and discussing the positive events, what went well and why, reinforces good behaviors and skills.

You can also be a leader in your specific role as an EDT. By modeling professionalism and excellence in your role, you set the tone for your department, your team, and your fellow technicians. As a positive role model among your peers, you become an ambassador for your institution and your profession. Be proud of your role in the team, and look for opportunities to excel as a leader.

SITUATION MONITORING

Situation monitoring involves constantly examining your environment, being aware of the actions of your peers and the status of the patient, and providing feedback to assist the team's performance. *STEP* is an acronym to assist you in remembering what needs to be monitored.

Status of the patient: What are the patient's vitals? How does the patient appear? What is the patient's status?

Team members: Are your teammates accomplishing their tasks? Do they need assistance?

Environment: Is something impairing your team's performance? Are there too many people in the room? Are you missing equipment?

Progress toward the goal: Have you stabilized the patient? Are your interventions working?

Examining and synthesizing what is occurring around patient care creates *situational awareness.* It is an active process and cannot be done passively. Everyone in the room must constantly be engaged in situation monitoring because it helps to keep everyone safe, including the patient and team members. When all team members are practicing situation monitoring, are situationally aware, and are communicating all pertinent information, the team has a *shared mental model.* This means that all team members have the same mind frame: they know what is happening and what the plan is. The team leader is vital in ensuring that a shared mental model is formed. They are constantly collecting information (situation monitoring), analyzing it (situational awareness), and sharing it with the team (communication).

MUTUAL SUPPORT AND ADVOCACY

Emergency medicine is practiced as a team. EDTs technicians continually provide *task assistance* to colleagues toward the common goal of optimal patient care. Nurses have many different responsibilities and are often inundated with multiple different tasks for a variety of patients. Therefore, proactively taking responsibility for tasks within your scope eases their workload and builds teamwork. As you work in the ED, your ability to anticipate what patients will need and how to support your nurses will improve.

In critical situations, task assistance happens frequently. As a team, each person helps each other complete tasks, resulting in higher-quality care that is completed faster. For example, while you are getting IV access on one arm, a nurse who has finished their task may start looking for IV access on the other arm. Fostering a collaborative work environment where colleagues are willing to seek and offer assistance is an important component of teamwork that results in high-quality care.

The second component of mutual support is *advocacy.* Technicians are responsible for the health and well-being of patients and must advocate on their behalf. Unfortunately, an ED can be a busy and even chaotic environment and sometimes a patient's needs can go unnoticed. If you see a patient in pain or if you recognize that the patient requires nursing or provider attention, advocate for the patient by notifying a nurse or provider.

In critical situations, advocating for a patient may require speaking up when something is wrong or asking a clarifying question. For example, an unresponsive patient with pulses is brought in by EMS. The patient is put on the cardiac monitor, IV access is established, defibrillator pads are put on, and vital signs are taken. While the other team members are busy completing their tasks, you notice that the patient has lost a pulse. It is your responsibility, using a clear and assertive tone, to let the team leader know that the patient has lost a pulse and that cardiopulmonary resuscitation must be initiated. *This concern must be voiced until you have verbal confirmation that you have been heard by the team leader.*

Advocating for patients can be a daunting task as there is a well-established healthcare role hierarchy. Technicians work under nurses and providers. Although technicians do not have final medical decision-making authority, everyone is equally responsible for a patient's well-being. Therefore, if a situation requires you to speak up, you must do so. Inexperience is no excuse not to voice concerns or ask clarifying questions. When voicing a concern, use "alert language" (e.g., "concerned," "uncomfortable," or "patient safety"). This will notify the team leader and others that there may be a problem that requires immediate attention.

Identifying medical errors does not mean that you or the team will face punishment, rather the opposite. Your insight and your role in the team may expose something important that no one has addressed. As an EDT, you will find yourself in certain situations that will require you to speak up, and your ability to participate in effective communication may end up saving someone's life.

The five key principles of TeamSTEPPS (team structure, communication, leadership, situation monitoring, and mutual support) are proven evidence-based systems that optimize team performance in the healthcare setting. Working on these skills enables high-quality staff-to-staff communication resulting in enhanced patient safety and a reduction in medical errors.

Patient Communication

The first interaction with patients typically occurs when you enter their room to start a workup. A helpful model for an initial patient interaction is the Studer Group's *AIDET model.* AIDET stands for *Acknowledge, Introduce, Duration, Explanation, and Thank you.* Acknowledge by greeting the patients and family members as you enter. Greeting patients with a smile puts them at ease and demonstrates that you are there for their care. Introduce yourself with your first name, title, and your role of technician. Using a first name is more informal and helps to connect with patients on a more personal level. Often, patients are familiar with doctors and nurses, but they do not know what a technician does. An example introduction would be, "Hi, my name is Noah. I am a technician here and I work with everyone taking care of you today."

Next, let the patient know what to expect during the duration of their stay. Identify next steps and the process of an ED visit. Be specific when possible, but when this is not possible, let the patient know that you will (or another member of the team will) provide them with information as it becomes available. One of the most stressful parts of an ED visit is the waiting experienced by the patient. Recognizing that this is a concern for them establishes trust between you and the patient and alleviates frustration for the families.

Then, tell the patient and family what you are going to do and give an explanation as to why they are being done. It is OK to say that you are not sure and that you will have the provider or the nurse provide further details. Always end by asking the patient for consent to perform the procedures ordered, as they have the autonomy to refuse services if they are of sound mental status. An example explanation would be, "The doctors ordered some blood work so I'm going to get an IV started.

They also want an ECG to see how your heart is doing. Is that OK with you?" Most patients will allow you to proceed; however, if the patient refuses any or all of your workup, it is their right to do so. You can then offer to answer any additional questions or provide a further explanation. If the patient continues to refuse, respect their autonomy and inform the nurse and provider.

The next time you enter a room might be to collect blood work, obtain vital signs, or bring someone to medical imaging. Always obtain a patient's consent before doing anything to them. Often, patients ask for test results or if you know why they are sick. Informing patients of test results is typically left to the providers.

Finally, say thank you. Thank them for being patient during difficult procedures, interventions, and wait times. Expressing gratitude and empathy to your patients and their families shows that you are there to support them and can improve their overall experience in the ED.

Language and Barriers

Patients who do not speak or have limited English proficiency (LEP) are particularly at risk for communication errors. All hospitals receiving federal assistance (including Medicare and Medicaid reimbursements) are legally required by the Affordable Care Act to provide all LEP patients with a qualified (typically certified) medical interpreter in person, by phone, or through a digital platform. Any bilingual staff member who translates for a LEP patient must be formally trained to do so and oral translation must be listed in their job description. Bilingual staff and English-speaking family members who accompany non-English speaking patients may assist the patient, especially in emergent situations where a translator is not immediately available; however, they are not to be relied upon for translation once a translator is obtained.

When relying on family members or friends to translate, keep in mind the following barriers to care:

Privacy: The patient may not want to share sensitive or personal information with the family member. They may be forced to give up their right to privacy or provide inaccurate information to protect their privacy.

Medical terms: Medical terms may not be understood or interpreted correctly by the translator, which can lead to significant medical error and patient harm.

Coercion: The patient may feel inappropriately pressured by the translator to accept or decline certain medical interventions based on costs, beliefs, or other factors.

Special Needs

Under the Americans with Disabilities Act, hearing impaired and deaf patients must legally be provided "effective means of communication." These patients must be asked for their preferred method of communication. A majority of deaf people in the United States use American Sign Language (ASL); however, some may prefer to communicate in writing, especially those with newer hearing loss. Other patients may be able to lip-read and respond verbally. Most hospitals have access to ASL interpreters in person or through a digital platform. Effective communication with visually impaired patients can often be done verbally. As long as effective communication can be achieved, then no special interpreter needs to be provided. However, a blind and deaf patient must be provided a tactile interpreter or some other form of translation services, such as a Screen Braille Communicator, to ensure effective communication.

Health Literacy

Health literacy describes the degree to which a patient can understand complex medical information and terminology in a way that they can use that information to make informed decisions and take appropriate actions concerning their health. Poor health literacy can be attributed to multiple factors including low socioeconomic status, insufficient education, LEP, cognitive barriers, and cultural obstacles (e.g., lack of culturally appropriate information). Patients with poor health literacy have substantially worse health outcomes. Because it is not always apparent which patients may struggle with health information, all patients should be spoken to in a straightforward and respectful manner using words and concepts that are easy to understand. Refrain from using overly complicated medical terminology, acronyms, and the like. Explain procedures in lay terms. For example, instead of saying, "I'm going to obtain a troponin," simplify by stating that you are going to draw some blood for a test that can show if there has been any sudden injury to the heart. Create a safe and nonjudgmental space by asking patients if they have any questions and proactively offering to explain anything they may not understand.

Body Language

Although often overlooked, nonverbal cues are an important form of patient communication within the hospital setting. It is important to pay attention to your body language, including facial expressions, gestures, body positioning, tone of voice, and eye contact. When interacting with patients, try to maintain a relaxed stance, or sit across from them so as not to talk down to them. If a patient is talking to you, devote your full and undivided attention and actively listen. Never cross your arms in front of patients, roll your eyes, or take out your cell phone while patients are speaking with you. These actions make you appear uninterested and unreceptive to the patient's concerns. Consider the patient's nonverbal language as well. If the patient is cueing that they are frightened, avoidant, defensive, or in pain, recognizing these signs enables improved communication and care.

Communication Systems and Technology

As technology has revolutionized the world we live in, so too has it changed the way we communicate in the ED. There are three primary ways that healthcare providers communicate with one another throughout the hospital setting. Hospital radiofrequency (RF) phones and tablets allow staff to communicate urgent or important information through calls or texts via a dedicated network. Encrypted smartphone applications that are compliant with the Health Insurance Portability and Accountability Act (HIPAA) may be instituted hospital-wide, enabling staff to use their own phones as a secure means of relaying important patient information through text messages. Computer- and tablet-based electronic medical record (EMR) programs serve as an electronic form of the patient's chart, documenting their care as they receive it. The EMR is the legal record of a patient's healthcare. Most EMRs provide a way to enter comments or notes for communicating useful nonemergent information that is outside of the permanent patient record. For example, if a patient is taken to x-ray, the technician would note to the team that the patient is in x-ray. Hence, when the nurse goes into the patient's room, they know that the patient is in x-ray as opposed to eloping or being in the bathroom for a concerningly long period of time. Often, multiple forms of electronic communication are used within the hospital, and together they play a critical role in improved patient care.

Conclusion

As an EDT, you are an integral part of the team providing direct patient care. Your ability to treat everyone with respect and empathy and maintain your professionalism will establish trust with your team and patients. Your adherence to safety using the TeamSTEPPS approach, closed-loop communication, good patient communication, and knowledge of your scope of practice and hospital policies ensures that you are performing to the highest level of your role. Whether your goal is to be a lifelong EDT or to use this opportunity as a stepping-stone in your career, you are a vital part of the ED team in delivering excellent and competent care.

References for Additional Reading

Agency for Healthcare Research and Quality. About TeamSTEPPS. AHRQ. https://www.ahrq.gov/teamstepps/about-teamstepps/index.html. Published August 8, 2015. Accessed May 29, 2021.

Bethesda, MD: U.S. Dept. of Health and Human Services, Agency for Healthcare Research and Quality; 2006.

Chen AH, Youdelman MK, Brooks J. The legal framework for language access in healthcare settings: Title VI and beyond. *J Gen Intern Med.* 2007;22;22(Suppl 2):362–367.

Clancy CM, Tornberg DN. TeamSTEPPS: assuring optimal teamwork in clinical settings. *Am J Med Qual.* 2007;22(3):214–217.

Farrell M. Use of iPhones by nurses in an acute care setting to improve communication and decision-making processes: qualitative analysis of nurses' perspectives on iPhone use. *JMIR Mhealth and Uhealth.* 2016;4(2):e43.

Register SJ, Blanchard E, Belle A, et al. Using AIDET® education simulations to improve patient experience scores. *Clin Simul Nurs.* 2020;38:14–17.

Rouleau G, Gagnon MP, Côté J. Impacts of information and communication technologies on nursing care: an overview of systematic reviews (protocol). *Syst Rev.* 2015;4:75.

Seibert K, Domhoff D, Huter K, et al. Application of digital technologies in nursing practice: results of a mixed methods study on nurses' experiences, needs and perspectives. *Z Evid Fortbild Qual Gesundhwes.* 2020;158–159:94–106.

Sherman R, Pross E. Growing future nurse leaders to build and sustain healthy work environments at the unit level. *Online J Issues Nurs.* 2010;15(1). Jan 31.

TeamSTEPPS: *Pocket Guide: Strategies & Tools to Enhance Performance and Patient Safety.*

Thomas CM, Bertram E, Johnson D. The SBAR communication technique: teaching nursing students professional communication skills. *Nurse educ.* 2009;34(4):176–180.

US Department of Justice: Civil Rights Division, Disability Rights Section. ADA Business BRIEF: Communicating with people who are deaf or hard of hearing in hospital settings. 2003. Oct:1–4.

CHAPTER 5

Initial Emergency Department Patient Assessment

Nehal S. Naik ■ John Organick-Lee ■ Andzie Warrington

A systematic approach for the evaluation of a newly arrived ED patient will allow the emergency department (ED) technician to properly evaluate and help prioritize the patient. The ED technician (EDT) may be the first person to have contact with the patient, and the information gathered and the initial decisions made are critical to providing rapid, effective care. Remember, if an ED Tech ever feels uncomfortable about a patient, they should escalate the evaluation to an ED physician or nurse.

Doorway Examination

There is a significant amount of information that can be ascertained simply by seeing a patient for the first time from the "doorway," and this "first impression" is valuable in answering the initial question: "Is this patient sick or not sick?"

Among the observations that the tech should consider are:

■ What do you see, hear, and smell?
■ Was the patient ambulatory?
■ How old do they appear relative to their chronologic age?
■ Do they appear to be in any respiratory distress?
■ Is there any obvious trauma?

The answers to these questions should inform the speed with which a patient should be treated. For example, an older-appearing male with a "gray" appearance who is clutching his chest and breathing hard requires a more rapid response than that of a nondistressed, younger female who walked to her bed, speaks in full sentences, and appears "well." The EDT will refine their clinical judgment as they gain more experience. This chapter will provide guidelines and suggestions to assist with the process of building the EDT's assessment judgment.

Primary Survey: ABCDE

The ABCDE framework provides a systematic method of evaluating and assessing patients for life-threatening conditions. This approach is standard in advanced trauma life support (ATLS), but it has been widely adopted to help evaluate any patient.

The ABDCE approach is stepwise algorithm, meaning that the first step must be addressed before going on to the next (Table 5.1). The sequence is as follows:

A: Airway—Is the airway patent? Are any signs of obstruction?
B: Breathing—Does the patient have symmetric chest rise? Is the patient working hard to breathe, or is their respiratory rate either very slow or very fast?
C: Circulation—Are the patient's extremities cool to the touch? Are you able to feel peripheral pulses (pulses in each extremity should be palpated) ? Is their heart rate unusually rapid or slow?

TABLE 5.1 ■ **Primary Survey, Adapted From Advanced Trauma Life Support and** *Basic Emergency Care* **From World Health Organization & International Committee of the Red Cross (ICRC). Basic emergency care: approach to the acutely ill and injured: participant workbook. World Health Organization. 2018. https://apps.who.int/iris/handle/10665/275635.**

Primary Survey	Assessment	Intervention/Management
A: Airway	Can the patient talk normally? If yes, then the airway is open. If the patient cannot talk normally, listen for: • Air movement from the mouth or nose • Abnormal sounds, such as stridor, grunting, snoring, raspy voice (stridor and swelling/hives suggest a severe allergic reaction, indicating anaphylaxis) Look for: • Fluid, such as blood, vomit, saliva • Foreign body • Abnormal swelling • Signs of trauma	If the patient is unconscious, not breathing normally, and there are no signs of trauma: • Open the airway using the head-tilt and chin-lift maneuver • Use the jaw thrust maneuver Place an oropharyngeal or nasopharyngeal airwayIf the patient is not breathing normally and there *are* signs of or concerns for trauma: Maintain cervical spine immobilization Use the jaw thrust maneuver Avoid adjunct airways if there is suspected injury If a foreign body is suspected: • If the patient is conscious and able to make any meaningful sounds, encourage coughing and keep the patient calm • Remove the object if visible, being careful not to push the object deeper • If the patient is unable to cough or move air (i.e., suspected complete occlusion of airway), use age-appropriate chest thrusts/abdominal thrusts/back blows • If patient becomes unconscious while choking, perform CPR If secretions or vomit are present: • Suction, when available • Place patient in lateral decubitus/recovery position (only after patient has been cleared from secondary survey if trauma is suspected) • If the patient has swelling, hives, or stridor, consider anaphylaxis
B: Breathing	Look for: • Chest rise: is rise equal, or is there an absence of movement on one side? • Effort/work of breathing: nasal flaring, tripod position, accessory muscle use Number of respirations per minute Listen for: • Abnormal sounds such as wheezing or crackling • Absence of sounds on one side (absence of sounds on one side, tracheal deviation, and distended neck veins suggest a tension pneumothorax) • Check O_2 saturation	Start bag-valve mask ventilation for the following scenarios: • Unconscious with abnormal breathing • Either tachypnea or bradypnea with reduced level of consciousness • If patient is hypoxic, place patient on nasal cannula, nonrebreather mask, or bag-valve mask • If there is concern for anaphylaxis or tension pneumothorax, notify emergency medicine physician immediately

Continued

TABLE 5.1 ■ **Primary Survey, Adapted From Advanced Trauma Life Support and *Basic Emergency Care* From World Health Organization & International Committee of the Red Cross (ICRC). Basic emergency care: approach to the acutely ill and injured: participant workbook. World Health Organization. 2018. https://apps.who.int/iris/handle/10665/275635.—Cont'd**

Primary Survey	Assessment	Intervention/Management
C: Circulation	Look and feel for signs of poor perfusion: • Cool, moist extremities • Delayed capillary refill >3 seconds • Low blood pressure • Tachypnea and/or tachycardia • Absent pulses Look for and consider areas of blood loss ("Four and the floor"): • Chest • Abdomen • Pelvis • Thigh compartments • External/extremity bleeds • Check blood pressure as well as peripheral pulses for heart rate • Think about placing ECG leads	For cardiopulmonary arrest, begin performing CPR and make sure to place defibrillator pads on patient's chest Consider removing chest hair or drying chest if moist If there are signs of poor perfusion, obtain IV access in order to give fluids and blood For external bleeding, apply direct pressure to site For distal extremity bleeding, consider applying tourniquets proximal to the bleed If there is suspected internal bleeding due to trauma to the pelvis, consider a pelvic binder
D: Disability	Assess level of consciousness with AVPU scale or, in trauma cases, the GCS See Table 5.2 for determining AVPU and Table 5.3 for GCS Check glucose level for all altered or unconscious patients Check pupils for size, whether they are equal, and whether they react to light Check movement and sensation in all four limbs	If glucose levels are low, then alert the physician and nursing, as glucose should be administered as soon as possible If pupils are constricted and patient's breathing is slow, consider opioid overdose and administer naloxone nasal spray If pupils are not equal, consider increased intracranial pressure and raise the head of the bed to 30 degrees Immobilize the cervical spine if there is concern for trauma
E: Exposure	Remove all clothing either with patient cooperation or, if the patient is unable to, using shears/scissors Examine the entire body for injuries, rashes, bites, other lesions, taking care to maintain C-spine or log-roll precautions	Remove all jewelry, as rings, necklaces, or bracelets can constrict limbs or fingers due to swelling; take care to place clothing and patient possessions into separate bag Cover the patient as soon as possible to prevent hypothermia Remove wet clothing immediately and work to dry patients off While not always possible, attempt to respect the patient and protect modesty during exposure

AVPU, alert, voice, pain, unresponsive; *CPR*, cardiopulmonary resuscitation; *ECG*, electrocardiogram; *GCS*, Glasgow Coma Scale; *IV*, intravenous.

D: Disability—What is the patient's level of consciousness? In most patients, the AVPU (alert, voice, pain, unresponsive) scale is sufficient (Table 5.2). In trauma patients, the Glasgow Coma Scale (Table 5.3) is used.

E: Exposure—What other injuries or deformities might be present on exam? Are there any burns, bullet wounds, signs of bleeding, or other obvious signs of trauma? It is important to completely expose the patient to identify all injuries.

TABLE 5.2 ■ **AVPU Scale**

This is a simple bedside tool to describe the patient's level of alertness.

A = Alert	Patient is fully alert and does not need to be repeatedly stimulated to maintain alertness.
V = Verbal	Patient will not remain alert, but regains alertness in response to verbal stimuli.
P = Pain	Patient will not remain alert, but regains alertness after painful stimuli.
U = Unconscious	Patient will not arouse to either voice or pain.

TABLE 5.3 ■ **Glasgow Coma Scale**

The best score is 15, and the worst score is 3, reported either as the total number or by category (e.g., E4, V5, M6).

Revised Scale	Score
Eye opening (E)	
Spontaneous	4
To sound	3
To pressure	2
None	1
Nontestable	NT
Verbal response (V)	
Oriented	5
Confused	4
Words	3
Sounds	2
None	1
Nontestable	NT
Best motor response (M)	
Obeys commands	6
Localizing	5
Normal flexion	4
Abnormal flexion	3
Extension	2
None	1
Nontestable	NT

Remember that each step of this sequence must be addressed and managed before going on to the next step. In trauma patients, you can quickly assess A, B, C, and D by asking them their name and what happened. If they respond appropriately and speak clearly, there is no major airway compromise, breathing is sufficient as they can generate enough air movement for speech, and their level of consciousness is not significantly decreased because when they related what happened they demonstrate their alertness and orientation. Table 5.1 reviews the ABCDE schema.

If at any point the EDT suspects that the patient is critically ill, they must alert the emergency providers.

Vital Signs

Parallel in importance to the primary survey are the patient's vital signs. They should be checked upon initial evaluation and frequently repeated throughout the patient's ED stay. They are key to assessing a patient's stability and disease progression.

The normal range of vital signs in the pediatric patient varies by age, as outlined in Table 5.4. If the vital signs are outside these ranges, consider the potential for instability.

In adults, the thresholds for minimum blood pressures are:

Systolic blood pressure should be above 90 mm Hg

Diastolic blood pressure should be above 60 mm Hg

For adults, sustained blood pressures above 180/110 mm Hg are above the ceiling threshold for elevated blood pressure, should be repeated frequently, and if the elevation is sustained, need to be addressed by the providers.

The range of temperatures considered abnormal does not vary with age. A temperature below 35°C (95°F) is considered abnormally low (hypothermia) and that above 37.9°C (100.2°F) is considered a fever. Remember in both infants and the elderly, both hypothermia and a fever can be signs of serious infection.

Pulse oximetry, or "pulsox," is often called the "fifth vital sign." It measures the oxygen saturation of hemoglobin in a patient's blood. By placing the pulse oximeter on the finger, earlobe, or forehead, the EDT can rapidly and noninvasively confirm whether there is an adequate amount of oxygen carried on the hemoglobin within the red blood cell to supply the cells' energy needs throughout the body. Although the "pulsox" may be less accurate in patients with darker pigmentation, it has proven to be very useful in the ED.

As the amount of oxygen available in the lungs drops as a result of lung or heart disease (e.g., asthma, chronic obstructive pulmonary disease), there will often be a gradual drop in hemoglobin's oxygen saturation. As seen in Fig. 5.1, when the oxygen saturation drops below 90%, any further impairment of lung performance will lead to a rapid and potentially catastrophic drop in hemoglobin saturation that will lead to severe oxygen starvation for cells throughout the body. That is why it is so important to provide as much supplemental oxygen as necessary to keep hemoglobin saturation above 90%.

Many displays of "pulse ox" also give a pulse rate; failure to have an adequate pulse rate waveform could suggest that the "pulse ox" reading may be inaccurate. Fig. 5.2 is a normal pulse waveform as measured on a pulse oximeter.

Irregular sequences of waveforms may be due to either a cardiac arrhythmia or poor quality of the waveform. Some monitors may have stars on the side of the waveform indicating the quality of the pulse oximetry reading. Ensure you have a good quality waveform when documenting the current pulse oximetry.

Oxygen Delivery

If a patient has a low oxygen saturation, the EDT should consider providing the patient with supplemental oxygen. The EDT should always notify the nurse or ED physician if they are placing

---

TABLE 5.4 ■ **Normal Vital Signs by Age**

Age	Heart Rate	Respiratory Rate
Premature	120–170	40–70
0–3 mo	100–160	30–60
3–6 mo	100–150	30–45
6–12 mo	90–130	25–40
1–3 yr	80–125	20–30
3–6 yr	70–115	20–25
6 yr–Adult	60–100	14–22

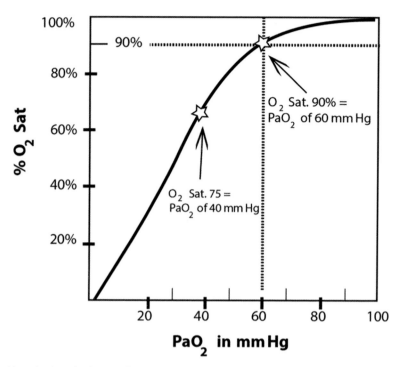

Fig. 5.1   Normal pulse oximeter waveform.

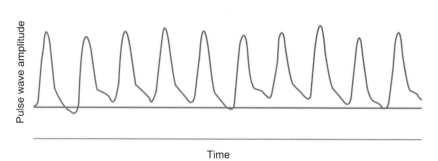

Fig. 5.2   The oxyhemoglobin dissociation curve.

the patient on additional oxygen, but should not delay providing oxygen if the patient seems ill and is hypoxic. Three standard delivery methods and associated oxygen flow rates are described in Table 5.5.

Monitor

Placing the patient on the cardiac monitor quickly allows continuous and onging evaluation of the patient's heart rate and rhythm. Fig. 5.3 describes the lead placement locations for continuous cardiac monitoring.

Intravenous Access

Intravenous access (IV) allows administration of medication and fluids. However, not all patients require an IV. If a patient is unstable, the EDT should place a large bore IV catheter as quickly as possible and inform the providers after successful completion. If a patient is stable, IV access can be established once the need is determined by the ED physician. Choosing the best possible IV size and placement location is based on age and treatment being rendered (Table 5.6). Often if a patient has blood tests ordered, the technician will insert an IV cannula and draw the blood sample through the cannula, then cap the end of the cannula and secure the IV catheter. This way,

TABLE 5.5 ■ Noninvasive Oxygen Delivery

	Nasal Cannula	Face Mask	Nonrebreather
Flow rate	1–6L	6–10L	11–15L
FiO$_2$ provided	21%–40%	40%–60%	60%–80%
Notes			Reservoir must be filled with air for the nonrebreather to be functional

FiO$_2$, Fraction of inspired oxygen.

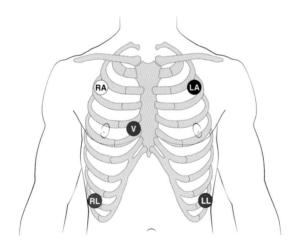

Fig. 5.3   Correct lead placement for 5-lead cardiac monitor.

TABLE 5.6 ■ Appropriate Intravenous Gauge by Age

Age	Intravenous Gauge
Infant (0–1 yr)	22–24
Toddler (1–2 yr)	20–24
Small child (12–18 kg weight)	18–22
Adult + child (>18 kg weight)	18–20

the patient will not have to be stuck a second time if IV fluids or medications are subsequently ordered. Protocols will vary among different EDs.

If a patient is unstable and needs IV access, the largest-bore IV possible should be placed in the antecubital space.

Additional points on IVs include the following:

- Intravenous access in a pediatric patient is much more difficult than in most adults. Generally, EDTs should only place an IV in a pediatric patient if they have received a specific order and specialized training to do so.
- Patients with end-stage renal disease (ESRD) who have an arteriovenous (AV) fistula in place should have an IV placed in the *opposite* arm from their functioning AV fistula.
- Never draw labs from a vein that is proximal to an IV that is infusing fluids.

SAMPLE History

After the ABCDE assessment and IV, O_2, and monitor placement, the EDT may be asked to take a brief history from the emergency patient using the SAMPLE system.

The SAMPLE approach is a standardized method of gathering key components of history of the patient's presenting illness. The EDT can obtain the information from the patient, family members, friends, bystanders, or emergency medical services (EMS) crews.

SAMPLE stands for the following:

S: Signs and symptoms
- A sign is something a family member might notice (e.g., the patient had blue lips).
- A symptom is something the patient describes that they felt.

A: Allergies
- It is often helpful to have multiple members of the healthcare team asking the same question because patients often forget the first time they are asked the question.

M: Medications
- A detailed list of the patient's medications and doses, including recent dose changes, can affect treatment and helps to identify the patient's chronic medical conditions.

P: Past medical history
- A patient's chronic medical problems can help you understand their current illness and affect the patient's management in the ED.

L: Last oral intake
- Record when the last oral intake was, and if it was liquid or solid. If the patient receives sedation or is intubated during their emergency care, a full stomach can increase the risk of vomiting or aspiration.

E: Events surrounding the current illness/injury

Critical Situations

In every evaluation of an ED patient, the biggest question is whether the patient is "sick" or "well." Some specific scenarios are extremely time sensitive and require a multidisciplinary ED team including the EDT, the nurse, and the physician to obtain information and make treatment decisions quickly. In addition to your ABCDE evaluation and SAMPLE history, patients with certain emergencies require additional steps.

Initial Evaluation of Suspected Cardiac Emergencies

Any patient presenting with chest pain, shortness of breath, upper (epigastric) abdominal pain, upper back pain, nausea, vomiting, or neck pain should be considered as potentially experiencing a cardiac emergency. These include, but are not limited to, acute coronary syndrome/myocardial infarction, pericardial tamponade, aortic dissection, pulmonary embolism, pneumothorax. Each of these patients should receive an ECG *immediately*.

The ECG should be promptly reviewed by a physician or their designee. Please ensure that you are aware of your institutional guidelines for the management of patients chest pain and potential cardiac emergencies.

Minutes matter in cardiac emergencies. Recognizing any potential symptoms that may indicate a cardiac emergency can save valuable time in responding to them.

Initial Evaluation of Suspected Neurologic Emergencies

Any patient presenting with facial asymmetry, focal weakness of their arm or leg, speech changes, gaze deviation, or neglect of a certain part of their body may be experiencing an acute stroke.

For rapid evaluation of a stroke, please refer to Chapter 11 and to your hospital's guidelines for initial stroke evaluation. There are multiple stroke evaluation tools that allow ancillary personnel to activate stroke protocols. It is useful to learn the tool used in your hospital.

These evaluation tools often consider a few key exam findings:

- Limb weakness
- Facial muscle weakness
- Speech difficulties
- Neglect of certain part of the patient's body
- Decreased level of consciousness

The other most important question to ask is, when was the "last known normal," or the time that the symptoms began. This can be uncertain if the patient awakened with the findings or if the patient has impaired communication ability and no observer is available. Determining the last known normal is important because certain treatments that dissolve or remove a clot cannot be given if too much time has elapsed after symptom onset.

Rapidly escalate the care of this patient to a physician to assess whether the patient requires rapid intervention. Brain cells that are not being perfused die at an alarming rate. Remember: "Time is brain."

Initial Evaluation of Trauma Patients

While most major trauma patients will come via EMS (ambulance), some may come directly to an ED brought by bystanders, family, or friends. Their initial evaluation is important. ABCDE evaluation is the core of trauma evaluation.

Key Point: Make sure the "C" of circulation includes all the distal pulses of all extremities.

The CDC's Field Triage Decision Scheme as a part of the Guidelines for Field Triage of Injured Patients can be adapted to the initial evaluation of ED trauma patients:

1. Vital signs: Measure vital signs and level of consciousness.
   - If significantly abnormal, notify physician or call a trauma activation per your hospital's guidelines immediately.
2. Injuries: Assess anatomy of injury.
   - Consider trauma activation if a penetrating injury to chest or abdomen, two or more long-bone fractures, crushing or degloving of extremities, amputations proximal to wrist or ankle, open depressed skull fractures, pelvic fractures, or paralysis.
3. Mechanism:
   - Consider trauma activation if patient fell more than 20 ft (for children, >10 ft), high-velocity motor vehicle collision, pedestrian or bicyclist struck by a car, or a motorcycle collision where the motorcycle was traveling in excess of 20 mph.

4. Special populations:
- Consider a lower threshold for trauma activation if the patient is older than 65 years or younger than 10 years, the patient has a bleeding disorder or is anticoagulated, the patient has circumferential burns of an extremity, the patient is dialysis-dependent or has ESRD, or the patient is more than 20 weeks pregnant.

Initial Evaluation of Obstetric Emergencies

Advanced pregnancy in an ED patient presents a challange because patients with certain presentations should go directly to the obstetric department and others should be evaluated/resuscitated in the ED with a rapid obstetric consultation. Exact protocols vary among different institutions.

A few key points about the evaluation of pregnant patients:

The EDT should ensure that the patient's privacy is considered as a pelvic exam is almost always required. The evaluation should occur in a closed or curtained room with a chaperone.

- Start with a brief visual exam without manual inspection: see if the fetal head or other body parts (arm, leg, pelvis) are visible at the vulvar surface. If so, the patient is actively delivering the fetus. Notify physician and nurses immediately.
- How many prior pregnancies has the patient had? Have they had a prior C-section?
  - If the patient has had prior pregnancies and is in labor, the delivery may occur more rapidly. A multiparous patient may require more immediate evaluation by an ED physician before an obstetrician.
  - There is an increased risk of complication for a patient with a prior C-section.
- Is the patient having contractions? How many minutes apart are they? When did they start? The frequency and timing of contractions can help assess at what stage of labor the patient is in.
- Has the patient's " water broken"? The developing fetus is suspended in amniotic fluid during embryonic development. Often at the onset of labor, the sac ruptures and thre is an release of amniotic fluid from the uterus and out the vagina.
- Is there any vaginal bleeding? Significant vaginal bleeding could suggest an obstetric emergency including placental abruption. Notify a physician to help evaluate prior to transport to an obstetric unit.

If the EDT ever feels uncomfortable about a patient, always escalate for evaluation by an ED physician immediately.

References for Additional Reading

ECG Lead positioning • LITFL Medical Blog • ECG Library Basics. Life in the Fast Lane • LITFL • Medical Blog. Published January 31, 2019. Accessed January 12, 2021. https://litfl.com/ecg-lead-positioning/

Guidelines for Field Triage of Injured Patients. Centers for Disease Control and Prevention. Accessed December 20, 2020. https://www.cdc.gov/mmwr/preview/mmwrhtml/rr6101a1.htm

Hastrup S, Damgaard D, Johnsen SP, Andersen G. Prehospital acute stroke severity scale to predict large artery occlusion: design and comparison with other scales. *Stroke*. 2016;47(7):1772–1776. https://doi.org/10.1161/STROKEAHA.115.012482.

Kim J-T, Chung P-W, Starkman S, et al. Field validation of the Los Angeles motor scale as a tool for paramedic assessment of stroke severity. *Stroke*. 2017;48(2):298–306. https://doi.org/10.1161/STROKEAHA.116.015247.

Lima FO, Silva GS, Furie KL, et al. Field assessment stroke triage for emergency destination: a simple and accurate prehospital scale to detect large vessel occlusion strokes. *Stroke*. 2016;47(8):1997–2002. https://doi.org/10.1161/STROKEAHA.116.013301.

McMullan JT, Katz B, Broderick J, Schmit P, Sucharew H, Adeoye O. Prospective prehospital evaluation of the Cincinnati Stroke Triage Assessment Tool. *Prehospital Emergency Care*. 2017;21(4):481–488. https://doi.org/10.1080/10903127.2016.1274349.

Pérez de la Ossa N, Carrera D, Gorchs M, et al. Design and validation of a prehospital stroke scale to predict large arterial occlusion: the Rapid Arterial Occlusion Evaluation scale. *Stroke*. 2014;45(1):87–91. https://doi.org/10.1161/STROKEAHA.113.003071.

Reynolds T. *Basic Emergency Care: Approach to the Acutely Ill and Injured*. World Health Organization; 2018.

Sasser SM, Hunt RC, Faul M, et al. Guidelines for field triage of injured patients: recommendations of the National Expert Panel on Field Triage, 2011. *MMWR Recomm Rep*. 2012;61(RR-1):1–20.

Teleb MS, Ver Hage A, Carter J, Jayaraman MV, McTaggart RA. Stroke vision, aphasia, neglect (VAN) assessment—a novel emergent large vessel occlusion screening tool: pilot study and comparison with current clinical severity indices. *J Neurointerv Surg*. 2017;9(2):122–126. https://doi.org/10.1136/neurintsurg-2015-012131.

Whitten A. *What's The Difference Between Oxygen Saturation And Pao2?* The Airway Jedi. Published December 10, 2015. Accessed January 6, 2021. https://airwayjedi.com/2015/12/09/difference-oxygen-saturation-Pao2/

CHAPTER 6

Triage

Ksenya Badashova ■ Robert Shesser

In the modern emergency department (ED), "triage" is an inclusive term for a series of front-end processes that begin the patient assessment process. Triage helps prioritize which patients are treated when EDs experience treatment space limitations. The Emergency Nurses Association (ENA) notes, "Triage ensures that the most severe acuity patients with the highest need have the correct resources applied as quickly as possible."

The English term "triage" derives from the French verb *trier*, meaning "to sort." The concept was developed and refined in the early 19th century by Napoleon's military to risk-stratify French wounded soldiers on the battlefields. It was recognized that there were three major categories of wounded soldiers: (1) those who were too seriously ill to survive, (2) those with minor wounds that did not threaten life or limb, and (3) those between these two extremes who had injuries that were amenable to treatment given the technology at the time. It was decided that the last group should be taken first, as they could benefit the most from the treatment. This mode of triage is still used in the prehospital setting to prioritize medical responses during disasters and mass casualty events.

Triage Overview

Currently, the term "triage" refers to these steps in the ED patient intake process:

1. *First point of contact for ambulatory patients:* When a patient arrives unannounced, there should be an organized, efficient process by which a patient begins the care process. Although hospitals differ in the details, most place an experienced nurse close to the ED's ambulatory entrance to interact with arriving patients. The nurse performing this process might also be referred to as the "greet" or "pivot" nurse.

2. *First point of contact for ambulance arrivals:* Many EDs have a separate system using a different nurse for receiving the emergency medical services (EMS) report and initiating care for patients arriving by ambulance. This is a much more efficient encounter because the prehospital providers' report is a succinct assessment of the patient's problem that does not involve interviewing the patient. The nurse will often "eyeball" the patient while receiving the EMS report and make a quick judgment that will concur with (or differ from) that of the prehospital provider.

3. *Application of a standardized triage scale to the patient:* This process quantifies the nurse's assessment into a standardized, reliable scale that can be used to
   a. Determine the order in which patients are seen
   b. Allow comparisons to be made over time about longer-term trends in the acuity of a hospital's patient mix

   Most contemporary EDs have a "pull until full" philosophy, meaning if there is an open bed, arriving patients are directly bedded without wait; assignment of the triage score is not needed for prioritization because an open bed is available. However, due to regulatory imperatives and the benefit of understanding long-term trends of arrival acuity, every patient arriving will receive this score.

4. *Initiation of a nursing database:* Over time, and in a manner specific to every institution, documentation requirements of the triage nurse have expanded exponentially. In addition

to documenting a succinct chief complaint and any patient allergies, triage screens may also require that the nurse documents the patient's medications, any history of travel to areas with severe or unusual infectious diseases, whether the patient is a victim of domestic violence, the presence of any recent infectious disease (e.g., tuberculosis) exposures, and any additional questions that may identify other regional health-related issues.

The benefit of a more extensive nursing database development process at triage is the potential for earlier identification of certain medical issues that might involve a higher level of isolation or an earlier mental health consultation. The risk is that this inexorable expansion of required triage fields leads to a longer and more complicated intake process, resulting in either the necessity to devote more workforce to the initial evaluation or to have the triage process become an "entry blocker," leading to increased queuing behind triage.

5. *Segmentation:* This is the process by which certain patient problem categories are managed in a manner specific to that type of problem. The best example is that of a "fast track," where patients with apparent (to the triage nurse) minor problems who can remain vertical (i.e., do not need a stretcher) are sent to a specific area of the ED, often with a higher patient-to-nurse ratio and smaller cubicles with chairs rather than stretchers. The stricter the segmentation process in a given hospital, the greater the requirement for an accurate nursing triage assessment.

Triage Scales

EMERGENCY SEVERITY INDEX

The development of triage severity scales has paralleled the development of emergency medicine. Many hospital EDs started quantifying patient severity by using their own systems that often had three levels (e.g., emergency, urgent, and nonurgent). In the 1990s it was recognized that a better triage scale was needed in the United States, and the 5-level Emergency Severity Index (ESI) was developed by two emergency physicians, Richard Wuerz and David Eitel. The scale was refined by the ENA and the Agency for Healthcare Research and Quality (AHRQ) and is now owned by the ENA.

The scale places patients in the two highest severity categories (1 and 2, with 1 being the most severe) according to the patients' vital signs, mentation, and chief complaint. Patients are divided among the three lower severity categories (3, 4, 5) by the number of resources that the nurse expects the patient will need (see Fig. 6.1). The distribution of patients in each category is outlined in Table 6.1. Unlike many of the other triage scales (see the following sections), the ESI provides more leeway for the triage nurse to use their clinical judgment in assigning the score. It is also the only major triage system that uses resource utilization in assigning the score.

Many studies have shown that the ESI is reliable (i.e., two different nurses would assign a given patient to the same triage category) and can accurately predict the likelihood of ED mortality with high sensitivity. A major weakness is that the ESI 3 group is so large that it does not accurately allow the prioritization of illness severity within this group. Thus some patients with lower-acuity illness might be treated ahead of those with more severe illness who arrived later. The ESI is particularly inaccurate in identifying critical illness in elderly patients, assigning 23% of elderly patients with critical illness to ESI 3 rather than ESI 2. Nevertheless, the ESI has become the most widely used system for triage in the United States.

OTHER TRIAGE SYSTEMS

There are four other major hospital triage systems used worldwide. They are all 5-level systems and, unlike ESI, their major focus is to try to fit patients into categories of how quickly the patient needs to see a physician. A brief description follows for each of these system.

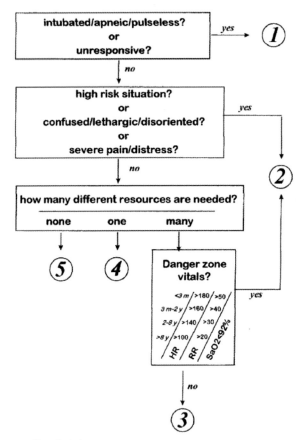

Fig. 6.1 The Emergency Severity Index.

TABLE 6.1 ■ Distribution of Emergency Severity Index Levels in The Average US Hospital

ESI 1	1%
ESI 2	10%
ESI 3	50%
ESI 4	35%
ESI 5	5%

Manchester Triage System

The Manchester Triage System (MTS) is used most frequently throughout Europe. The MTS employs 52 complaint-based flowcharts with 5 possible levels within each one. Its stated objective is to rapidly assess a patient and assign a priority based on clinical need.

Australasian Triage Scale

The Australasian Triage Scale (ATS) is used throughout Australia and has become the basis for numerous international triage systems. The ATS algorithm stratifies patients into 5 categories based on chief complaint, physical appearance, and relevant physiologic findings. The physiologic findings are derived from 79 clinical descriptors, and it is up to the triage nurse to identify the appropriate clinical descriptors. Its stated objectives are to ensure patients are treated in order of clinical urgency and to allocate patients to the most appropriate treatment area.

Canadian Triage and Acuity Scale

The Canadian Triage and Acuity Scale (CTAS) relies on a catalog of standardized chief complaints that determines the time in which the patient should be seen by a provider. The CTAS acuity level corresponds to a set of chief complaints or symptoms that are further subdivided by acuity. Nurses then have the ability to adjust the acuity level according to their clinical judgment. Its stated objective is to provide patients with timely care.

South African Triage Scale

The South African Triage Scale (SATS) is very similar to the other non-ESI scales. The stated objective of the SATS is to prioritize medical urgency in contexts where there is a mismatch between demand and capacity.

Regulatory Environment

The Joint Commission (formerly the Joint Commission on Accreditation of Healthcare Organizations [JCAHO]) is focused on continuously improving patient safety and quality of care. The Joint Commission provides a series of guidelines and mandates that healthcare organizations incorporate into their practice to provide safe and high-quality care. The organization focuses on flow of patients through the ED and does not have a specific set of triage requirements outside of requiring triage competency reassessments for nurses and providers working in triage. Despite this, the Joint Commission has inadvertently shaped triage through general recommendations and mandates.

For example, when the Joint Commission placed emphasis on prompt assessment of pain, many hospitals embedded a pain assessment question into their triage protocols, thus adding to the time to do a triage assessment. After the Joint Commission mandated "screening for suicidal ideation (SI) using a validated tool starting at age 12 and above," EDs across the nation incorporated various SI screening tools into the triage process to maintain best practices. These are just two of many examples of how the Joint Commission has affected triage assessments in EDs.

State and local health departments often request information about the hospital's "triage" process when inspecting hospitals, but as with the Joint Commission, there are frequently no formal requirements mandating that triage be performed in a specific manner.

Emergency Department Technician Roles in Triage

The scope of an ED technician's (EDT's) work varies widely from one ED to another. Emergency department technicians may be trained in patient triage and in some institutions play a vital part in the process, including directing patient flow, obtaining vital signs, and reviewing system protocols with oversight from triage or charge nurses.

References for Additional Reading

Emergency Severity Index (ESI): A Triage Tool for Emergency Department. (2012, September). Agency for Healthcare Research and Quality. https://www.ahrq.gov/patient-safety/settings/emergency-dept/esi.html
Nakao H, Ukai I, Kotani J. A review of the history of the origin of triage from a disaster medicine perspective. *Acute Med Surg*. 2017;4(4):379–384. https://doi.org/10.1002/ams2.293.

Yancey CC, O'Rourke MC. *Emergency Department Triage. [Updated 2021 Jul 30]. StatPearls [Internet].* Treasure Island (FL): StatPearls Publishing; 2021 Jan. Available from: https://www.ncbi.nlm.nih.gov/books/NBK557583/.

Zachariasse JM, Seiger N, Rood PP, et al. Validity of the Manchester Triage System in emergency care: a prospective observational study. *PloS One.* 2017;12(2):e0170811. https://doi.org/10.1371/journal.pone.0170811.

CHAPTER 7

Point-of-Care Testing

Sonal Batra ▪ Margeaux Connealy ▪ Julia Xavier

Introduction

Point-of-care (POC) testing is a term used to describe diagnostic testing that is performed in the patient's unit rather than in the hospital's central lab or outside reference lab. POC testing may be done on blood, urine, swabs from mucosal surfaces, or saliva. In the emergency department (ED), POC testing is typically performed by both ED technicians (EDTs) and nurses. In some jurisdictions, emergency medical services providers use POC tests in prehospital settings. Most hospitals have developed a rigorous quality process for their POC testing programs.

Comparisons With Laboratory Tests

There are pros and cons to POC tests. Point-of-care tests have fewer steps and thus a shorter time between test order and results compared with central lab-performed tests, and patient comfort may be improved by using a smaller sample for testing. The samples required to run POC blood testing are typically no more than 2 to 3 drops of blood. Many POC testing devices also bundle several types of lab tests together so users can obtain multiple results with one sample.

However, decreased accuracy is a potential drawback of POC testing compared with traditional laboratory tests, particularly if the analyte measured is significantly abnormal. For example, when measuring blood glucose levels, a POC test might report a sample as "high," whereas the central lab would report a specific value. Accuracy and reliability vary depending on the type of test. Advantages and disadvantages of POC testing are highlighted in Table 7.1.

It is uncertain whether POC testing decreases medical errors. The simpler process for POC tests may also reduce potential error, such as lost samples and delays in retrieving results. However, in some cases results from POC testing must be manually entered into the facility's database, which may increase the risk of inaccurate results.

Point-of-Care Testing Operation

Although there are various techniques and devices used to perform POC testing on patients, most blood tests are performed on a handheld blood analyzer, such as the Abbott i-STAT device. This device uses cartridges preloaded with the desired tests. The cartridges must be stored at room temperature and they have a specific expiration date. After obtaining a blood sample from a patient, a trained user can follow the prompts on the device to perform the test(s). Fig. 7.1 shows how to operate a typical POC machine.

USING A HANDHELD BLOOD ANALYZER

1. Sanitize hands and don gloves/appropriate personal protective equipment (PPE).
2. Draw the patient's blood into a syringe and attach a blunt-tip needle.
3. Turn on the device (see Fig. 7.1B).

TABLE 7.1 ■ **Advantages and Disadvantages of Point-of-Care Testing**

Advantages	Disadvantages
Quicker results	Increased training for clinical staff
Fewer steps in specimen processing	Increased cost per test
Smaller fluid sample required	Decreased accuracy/reliability of test results
	Limited types of tests available
Decreased patient length of stay	Space requirements for storage and testing

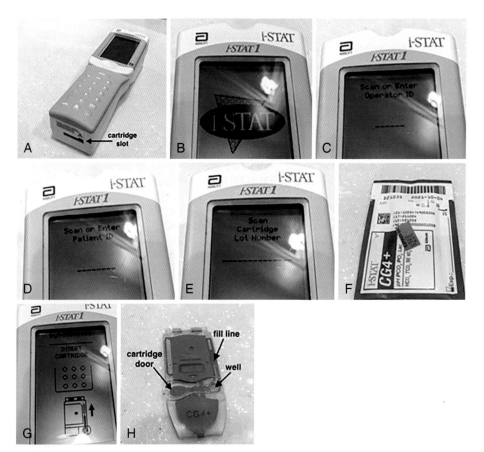

Fig. 7.1 How to use a handheld blood analyzer. (A) An i-STAT machine, a common brand of handheld blood analyzer. The *arrow* indicates the slot where the cartridge will be inserted. (B) Starting up the machine. (C) Scan or enter the operator ID, commonly assigned by a hospital or healthcare facility. (D) Scan or enter the patient ID, commonly found on a patient's hospital armband. (E) Scan or enter the cartridge lot number. (F) Package of an i-STAT CG4+ cartridge, one type of chemistry panel. The cartridge lot number is included on the package. A sticker placed by the laboratory indicates the cartridge expiration date. (G) After entering the appropriate information, the machine is ready for the insertion of a properly filled cartridge. (H) An i-STAT CG4+ cartridge. The *arrows* indicate the well for blood insertion, the fill line indicating when to stop filling the well, and the cartridge door, which the user closes over the well once the cartridge is properly filled. The filled cartridge is inserted in the orientation shown into the cartridge slot, shown in (A). The machine will lock the cartridge in place until the test is completed.

4. Scan and/or manually enter user, patient, and cartridge information for the relevant test, and then place the device on a level surface (see Fig. 7.1C–F).
5. Open the desired cartridge.
6. Waste a few drops of blood from the syringe to ensure the cartridge sample will not contain air bubbles.
7. Fill the cartridge well slowly with blood using the syringe until the blood level reaches the fill line indicated on the cartridge (see Fig. 7.1H).
8. Shut the cartridge door gently and insert it into the slot of the analyzer (see Fig. 7.1G–H). The device will then proceed with running the test; the device screen may indicate "cartridge locked" with the time to results. Leave the device undisturbed on a level surface until the test is complete.
9. After the results display, dispose of the used cartridge and waste materials appropriately.
10. Use the buttons as directed on the device to indicate the type of blood sample used (arterial vs. venous), and enter "comment codes" if any critical values indicate that the results should be reported directly to the provider team.
11. Place the blood analyzer in its appropriate docking station to transmit results and/or document the result manually in the patient's chart. Results can also be printed if needed.
12. Remove and dispose of gloves.
13. Sanitize hands.

TYPES OF POINT-OF-CARE TESTS

Cardiac

See Table 7.2 for a summary of indications for cardiac POC testing.

Troponin I. Troponin I is an enzyme found almost exclusively in heart muscle. In the setting of certain conditions such as a heart attack, levels of troponin I become elevated and can remain so for several days. Typical indications for troponin testing in the emergency setting include chest pain or discomfort, heart palpitations, shortness of breath, fatigue, nausea or vomiting, sweating, dizziness or lightheadedness, and pain radiating to the arm, back, or abdomen.

B-type Natriuretic Peptide. B-type natriuretic peptide is a hormone produced by the heart in response to increased stretch of the heart wall. It is a good marker for both right- and left-sided heart failure.

Respiratory

Arterial and Venous Blood Gases. Arterial blood gas (ABG) and venous blood gas (VBG) tests are used to measure the blood pH and the pressures of oxygen (Pao_2) and carbon dioxide ($Paco_2$)

TABLE 7.2 ■ **Cardiac Point-of-Care Tests**

Test	Indications	Mode of Collection
Troponin	*Acute Coronary Syndrome (Heart Attack) Symptoms:*	Serum
	Chest pain	
	Shortness of breath	
Pro-BNP	*Heart Failure Symptoms:*	Serum
	Shortness of breath	
	Extremity swelling	

dissolved in the blood. These tests are performed on patients with a variety of critical illnesses, such as severe sepsis, diabetic ketoacidosis, acute respiratory failure, acute respiratory distress syndrome, cardiac arrest, or shock.

In most cases, a VBG suffices to answer the clinical question and is easier and safer to obtain. See Table 7.3 for a summary of indications for ABG and VBG testing.

Urinary

See Table 7.4 for a summary of indications for urinary POC testing.

Urine Dipstick. Urinalysis is often the first step in assessing conditions affecting the kidney, bladder, and related organs. This test is typically indicated for a wide range of patient complaints, including urinary frequency, urgency, and abdominal and back pain.

The urine dipstick has a range of tests of varying importance. The tests on the standard dipstick include:

- pH: Although serum pH is tightly controlled, there is a wide range of normal urine pH, and this test is rarely important in the ED.
- Specific gravity: This is an imprecise measure of the patient's level of hydration and fluid balance.
- Glucose: Normally, no sugar is found in the urine. However, when blood sugar rises significantly above normal, the kidney can no longer resorb all the sugar it filters, and sugar spills into the urine.
- Bilirubin: This is a measure of liver function and bile flow integrity. Normally, no bilirubin should be found in the urine.
- Urobilinogen: This is perhaps the least important measure on the dipstick.
- Blood: This test measures hemoglobin, which, although it is found inside of red blood cells (RBCs), it will be present in the urine if any RBCs are in the urinary specimen.

TABLE 7.3 ■ **Respiratory Point-of-Care Tests**

Test	Indications	Mode of Collection
ABG/VBG	*Critical Illnesses:*	Serum:
	Sepsis	Venous or arterial
	Diabetic ketoacidosis	
	Acute respiratory/heart failure	
	Cardiac arrest	

ABG, Arterial blood gas; *VBG*, venous blood gas.

TABLE 7.4 ■ **Urinary Point-of-Care Tests**

Test	Indications	Mode of Collection
Urine dip	*Urinary Tract Infection Symptoms:*	Urine
	Urinary burning	
	Frequency/urgency of urination	
	Blood in urine	
	Diabetes patients	
	Trauma patients	

- Leukocyte esterase: This is an enzyme found on the outside of white blood cells, which, if present in the urine, is abnormal and may indicate a urinary tract infection (UTI).
- Nitrites: These are the result of bacterial metabolism of natural compounds found in the urine. When combined with a positive leukocyte esterase, they are a strong indicator of a UTI.

The exact urine collection technique may vary with the clinical situation and patient's gender. For example, if the specimen will be sent to lab for a urine culture, the patient should clean their external genitalia with a sterile wipe prior to urinating. They should begin urinating into a toilet or bedpan, then stop and redirect the stream into a sterile cup, thus creating a "midstream" sample. This technique will reduce the likelihood of bacterial contamination of the urine sample. An uncontaminated specimen is equally important for dipstick analysis. In clinical situations where gonorrhea or chlamydia is suspected (i.e., sexually transmitted diseases), the initial urinary stream is collected, and the patient should *not* clean their genitals prior to collection.

Performing a POC urinalysis involves the following steps:

1. Sanitize hands, and don gloves and appropriate PPE.
2. Keep the dipstick closed in the appropriate container, and avoid exposure to light until ready to perform the test.
3. Insert the dipstick into the patient's urine sample and quickly remove. Alternatively, use a pipette to place one drop of the patient's urine on each reagent square.
4. Tap excess urine off of the dipstick to ensure the reagent squares do not bleed together and cross-contaminate.
5. The squares can be interpreted within 120 seconds (depending on the brand of dipstick test) by comparing the colors to a reference sheet.
6. Record results on dipstick log and/or patient chart according to department protocols.
7. Dispose of used dipstick, pipette, and gloves.
8. Sanitize hands.

Urine Pregnancy. Urine POC pregnancy testing is required for the assessment of women of childbearing age with abdominal pain and virtually all pelvic complaints. Testing is also done on women of childbearing age before exposing them to ionizing radiation. Point-of-care pregnancy tests measure the presence of the β subunit of human chorionic gonadotropin (hCG), an enzyme secreted almost exclusively by the placenta. In most clinical situations, a random urine test that turns positive about the time of a woman's missed period, is adequate for clinical purposes in the ED. Fingerstick (blood) qualitative POC tests are also available.

Performing a POC urine pregnancy test involves the following steps:

1. Sanitize hands and don gloves/appropriate PPE.
2. Open a POC pregnancy test.
3. Use a pipette to place about 4 drops of the patient's urine in the well on the testing device.
4. After 3 minutes, the result window will either show a + or − symbol, indicating the presence or absence, respectively, of hCG. Ensure that the control window is appropriately marked, indicating that the test is functioning properly. If the control window is empty, discard the test and begin again with a new test.
5. Record results, expiration date, and lot number on the results log and/or patient chart according to department protocols.
6. Dispose of used test, pipette, and gloves.
7. Sanitize hands.

Endocrine

Glucose. Point-of-care glucose testing using a glucose monitoring device (glucometer) is a rapid method of assessing a patient's sugar levels in the home, prehospital, and hospital settings. This test is performed on capillary blood obtained through a finger prick. It is most useful in clinical settings where the blood sugar is suspected of being either very high or very low and following the course of ED diabetes treatment.

Performing a POC glucose test involves the following steps:

1. Sanitize hands and don gloves/appropriate PPE.
2. Turn on the handheld glucometer.
3. Scan and/or manually enter user, patient, and test strip information, similarly to a handheld blood analyzer.
4. Insert the test strip without contaminating the end meant for the patient's blood sample.
5. Massage one of the patient's fingers to increase blood flow.
6. Clean off the finger using an alcohol pad and allow it to dry completely.
7. Use a lancet to prick the side of the finger pad.
8. Wipe away the first drop of blood.
9. Apply gentle pressure, if needed, to obtain enough blood to saturate the end of the test strip. The machine will indicate when the user has collected enough blood. A result will be delivered within 30 seconds.
10. Clean and dress the patient's finger with an adhesive bandage.
11. Remove and dispose of the test strip, lancet, and alcohol pad appropriately.
12. Dispose of gloves.
13. Dock the glucometer in its appropriate docking station to transmit results and/or document the result manually in the patient's chart.
14. Sanitize hands.

Metabolic

See Table 7.5 for a summary of indications for metabolic POC testing.

Creatinine. Creatinine is a waste product of muscle breakdown that is filtered by the kidneys and excreted in urine. Serum creatinine rises when the kidneys are malfunctioning, so this is a rapid way to assess kidney function. Unless the patient is known to have preexisting renal failure, a POC creatinine will be obtained to verify adequate kidney function prior to the patient receiving

TABLE 7.5 ■ Chemistry Point-of-Care Tests

Test	Indications	Mode of Collection
Creatinine	ESRD patients Scans with IV contrast dye	Serum
Chemistry	Altered mental status patients ESRD patients Suspect blood loss/anemia Trauma patients	Serum
Lactate	Respiratory/heart failure Sepsis/septic shock Ischemia (heart, bowel, limb)	Serum – arterial or venous (also on ABG/VBG)
Breathalyzer	Suspect alcohol intoxication in conscious patients	Breath
Urine pregnancy	*Females of childbearing age with:* Abdominal pain Urinary symptoms Vaginal bleeding Nausea or vomiting Missed menses Imaging with radiation	Urine

ABG, Arterial blood gas; *ESRD*, end-stage renal disease; *IV*, intravenous; *VBG*, venous blood gas.

contrast dye for computed tomography or magnetic resonance imaging. Many contrast agents can worsen kidney function in patients with preexisting renal disease so it is very important to verify that the patient has normal renal function before administering IV contrast.

Chemistry. A chemistry panel is a group of tests that can provide the clinician with information about the patient's metabolic status. Although the included tests vary slightly among different platforms, most include the following:
- Sodium: This is the major extracellular cation (positive charge). Sodium abnormalities can reflect the patient's hydration status and kidney function.
- Potassium: This is the major intracellular cation and is present in a much lower concentration than sodium in extracellular fluids such as blood. It must be regulated within a very tight range, as either low or high values of potassium indicate a risk for potentially life-threatening cardiac arrythmias.
- Chloride and bicarbonate: These are anions (negative charge) whose presence fulfills the requirement that the body is electrically neutral, thus there will be an equal number of positively and negatively charged particles dissolved in the serum. Bicarbonate can vary up (alkalosis) or down (acidosis) with the body's acid-base status.
- Hematocrit: This is a measure of the concentration of RBCs in the blood. A low hematocrit indicates anemia and can be an indication of blood loss, decreased red blood cell production in the bone marrow, or increased red blood cell destruction.
- Blood urea nitrogen (BUN): This is similar to creatinine as a measure of the kidney's ability to excrete protein breakdown products. Elevated BUN can indicate renal disease or dehydration.

Lactate. Lactate, or lactic acid, is released in the bloodstream when tissues in the body do not have adequate blood flow or oxygenation. Indications for lactate testing include critical illnesses and severe infections where respiratory or cardiac function may be compromised. A lactate measurement within 3 hours of patient arrival is required to meet sepsis quality guidelines.

Breathalyzer. Breath-alcohol concentration (BAC) is often used in both nonhospital and hospital settings as a rapid, noninvasive, and easily repeatable technique that approximates the individual's blood-alcohol concentration. Screening patients for alcohol use can be important in the emergency setting, particularly if a patient is unable to communicate with staff due to intoxication. Breathalyzers do rely on a patient's cooperation and ability to exhale forcefully.

Obtaining a proper breath sample involves the following steps:
1. Sanitize hands and don gloves/appropriate PPE.
2. Attach a single-use mouthpiece to the machine and turn it on.
3. Have the patient form a seal around the mouthpiece with their lips. The device will indicate when it is time to blow.
4. Have the patient keep the seal and blow for about 5 to 7 seconds, or until the machine indicates that the sample is sufficient.
5. Dispose of the single-use mouthpiece and gloves.
6. Record the result displayed by the machine in the appropriate log and/or the patient's chart.
7. Sanitize hands.

Infectious Disease

COVID-19. Testing for the novel coronavirus (SARS-CoV-2) has rapidly evolved since the start of the COVID-19 pandemic. In the emergency setting, many patients require testing for a variety of clinical or administrative reasons. There are two major types of POC tests for SARS-CoV-2:
1. Polymerase chain reaction (PCR) tests: These tests measure small amounts of viral RNA in a patient's saliva or nasal passages. They are very accurate, although they can remain positive

for weeks after an acute infection when the patient is no longer infectious. This test is performed in the lab in most hospitals, but some manufacturers have developed PCR tests that can be used in nonhospital, ambulatory settings.

2. Antigen testing: Generally, these tests look for specific proteins associated with the virus. They are less accurate than the PCR but much simpler to perform in ambulatory settings.

Different tests can require different collection methods. For many tests, a nasopharyngeal swab is required, but some tests can be run on saliva or buccal or anterior nasal swabs. The swab has a small tip made of synthetic fibers and a flexible plastic shaft (see Fig. 7.2).

Obtaining a deep nasopharyngeal sample involves the following steps:

1. Sanitize hands and don gloves/appropriate PPE.
2. Explain the procedure to the patient.
3. Remove the transport tube and swab from the packaging.
4. Have the patient tilt the head back; slowly insert the swab into the nostril toward the top of the ear, or at an angle parallel to the palate, to reach the nasopharynx.
5. Rotate the swab gently around this spot for about 5 seconds.
6. Retract the swab slowly at the same angle.
7. Repeat the same process on the other side using the same swab.
8. Place the swab into the transport tube and close the cap tightly.
9. Dispose of waste materials and gloves appropriately.
10. Sanitize hands.

Streptococcus. Testing for strep A (a common cause of pharyngitis) can be performed using a rapid strep test. A sample is collected from the posterior pharynx using a swab tipped with cotton, rayon, or similar material (see Fig. 7.3). A rapid strep test can return a result within 15 minutes.

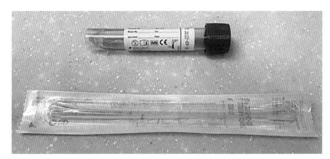

Fig. 7.2 Polymerase chain reaction nasopharyngeal swab and transport tube with liquid medium. After swabbing a patient's nasopharynx, insert the swab into the liquid medium and break off the end of the swab.

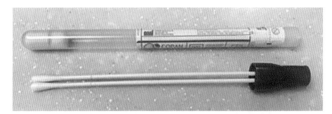

Fig. 7.3 Red-top culture swab and transport tube with sponge. After swabbing a patient's throat, twist off and remove the top of the transport tube and insert the swabs fully into the tube so the tips rests against the sponge.

Although false positive rapid strep tests are rare, the test may have 10% false negatives, so sometimes it is performed together with a throat culture.

Obtaining a proper posterior pharyngeal sample involves the following steps:
1. Sanitize hands and don gloves/appropriate PPE.
2. Explain the procedure to the patient.
3. Remove the transport tube and swab from the packaging.
4. Have the patient open their mouth wide. Depress the patient's tongue using a tongue depressor.
5. Insert the swab to the back of the pharynx and brush the swab against the tonsils and other inflamed regions of the posterior pharynx. Avoid the teeth and tongue.
6. Remove the swab and then the tongue depressor from the mouth.
7. Insert the swab into the transport tube so the swab rests against the sponge at the bottom; close the cap tightly.
8. Dispose of waste materials and gloves appropriately.
9. Sanitize hands.

Influenza. There are several types of POC influenza testing methods. Like rapid strep tests, rapid molecular assays for POC flu testing rarely produce false positives but have some false negative results. The flu swab can be performed using a nasal or nasopharyngeal sample. See the COVID-19 section for instructions on obtaining a proper nasopharyngeal sample.

Obtaining a proper nasal sample involves the following steps:
1. Sanitize hands and don gloves/appropriate PPE.
2. Explain the procedure to the patient.
3. Remove the transport tube and swab from the packaging.
4. Insert the swab into the nostril 1 to 1.5 cm.
5. Rotate the swab gently against the nasal walls several times.
6. Retract the swab slowly.
7. Repeat the same process on the other side using the same swab.
8. Place the swab into the transport tube and close the cap tightly.
9. Dispose of waste materials and gloves appropriately.
10. Sanitize hands.

Respiratory Syncytial Virus. Point-of-care testing is typically performed on nasopharyngeal samples.

HIV. HIV testing has evolved significantly over the last several decades. Point-of-care testing using an enzyme-linked immunosorbent assay technique on blood or a buccal smear to measure antibodies to HIV are commonly used as an initial screen. Confirmatory testing for HIV requires a venous blood sample for laboratory analysis.

References for Additional Reading

Overview of Influenza Testing Methods. *Centers for Disease Control and Prevention.* 2020 Aug; Accessed from https://www.cdc.gov/flu/professionals/diagnosis/overview-testing-methods.htm?web=1&wdLOR=cCDF9F05D-3012-BD44-B9C8-D2CD97AE04CA.

Plebani M. Does POCT reduce the risk of error in laboratory testing? *Clin Chim Acta.* 2009 Jun;404(1):59–64. https://doi.org/10.1016/j.cca.2009.03.014. Epub 2009 Mar 17. PMID: 19298804.

Thompson, G.E., Husney, A., Gabica, M.J. Throat Culture. *The University of Michigan Health Library.* 2020 Sept; Accessed from https://www.uofmhealth.org/health-library/hw204006#:~:text=Rapid%20strep%20test%20results%20are%20ready%20in%2010%20to%2015,infections%20caused%20by%20strep%20bacteria

CHAPTER 8

The Electrocardiogram and Cardiac Monitoring

Breanne Jacobs ■ Stephen Robie ■ Natalia Monsalve

The Electrocardiogram

The electrocardiogram (ECG; also EKG) is an essential component in the evaluation of a patient presenting with cardiac symptoms. It should be obtained simultaneously with, or immediately following, the evaluation of a patient's vital signs. Rapidly obtaining and reviewing the ECG is a vital, time-sensitive step in evaluating all potential cardiac complaints. Professional association guidelines recommend that all patients with suspected coronary heart disease, such as patients complaining of shortness of breath, chest pain, syncope, or palpitations, receive an ECG with physician review within 10 minutes of ED arrival.

The heart is a four-chambered muscle that works as a pump at the center of the body's circulatory system (Fig. 8.1). The heart receives deoxygenated blood from the body's tissues (colored blue) and pumps this blood into the lungs where it is oxygenated, receives this blood back from the lungs (colored red), and then pumps the newly oxygenated blood to the body's vital organs.

The heart muscle contracts and relaxes in an organized manner based upon its own, intrinsic, natural, electrical pacemaker system that sends depolarizing charges to the heart muscle, which mechanically contracts after the heart's membrane is depolarized. Analysis of the ECG allows a clinician to assess the rhythmic patterns and current flows of the electrical system and cardiac musculature. Detailed analysis permits a comparison of the patient's current ECG to the known normal or to the patient's prior ECG, allowing inferences to be made about disease processes affecting the heart. An ECG includes the heart's rate (the number of contractions per minute) and rhythm (area of the heart where depolarizing impulses arise). By analyzing the ECG, physicians are often able to identify regions of the heart that may be receiving inadequate blood flow (such as during a heart attack).

Cardiac Pacemaker and Conducting System

The heart's rhythm is determined by specialized tissues located within the heart that regularly emit an electrical pulse called pacemaker tissues. The main pacemaker of the heart called the sinoatrial (SA) node is located within the right atrium and is largely controlled by the body's nervous system, which can speed it up or slow it down as needed. The cardiac impulse is then conducted throughout the atria until all the atrial cells are depolarized. The impulse then arrives at the atrioventricular (AV) node, where it is delayed for a short period and then released into the His-Purkinje system of the ventricles, which rapidly conducts the impulse throughout the ventricular musculature (Fig. 8.2).

Components of an ECG

The ECG represents current flow between different parts of the heart during the cardiac cycle. To be an effective pump, the heart must contract in an organized manner. The heart's electrical

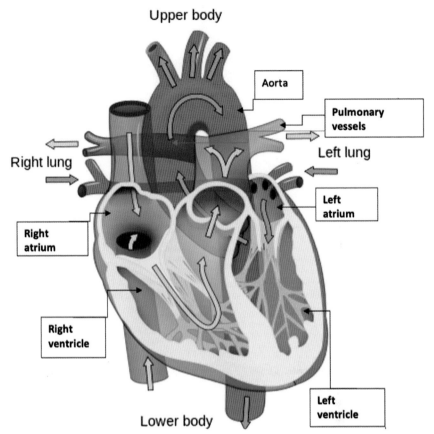

Fig. 8.1 Four-chambered view of heart showing flow of deoxygenated blood *(blue)* and oxygenated blood *(red)* to tissues.

system normally depolarizes cells in a manner to optimize the heart's pumping function. As cells are depolarized, current flows between the depolarized cells and those cells that have yet to be depolarized. The ECG measures this flow on the surface of the chest. The multiple leads that are obtained for the ECG provide the clinician with information about the current flows in different areas of the heart. After all the cells in a given region have depolarized, there is a period when there is no current flow measured, and the ECG returns to its baseline. The heart cells then undergo a wave repolarization in the same order as during depolarization, leading to measurable current flow again until all the cells are repolarized, and the ECG strip returns to baseline of no current flow. Flow of electricity on the cardiac surface *toward* a positive pole on an extremity or chest wall produces an upward deflection in the ECG, whereas electricity flowing *away* from the positive pole produces a negative deflection. Fig. 8.3 depicts these upward and downward ECG images by lead based upon flow of electricity within the heart.

The Cardiac Cycle

The first step of the cardiac cycle is atrial depolarization. This is represented on the ECG by a deflection called the P wave. This deflection can be upward or downward depending on which lead

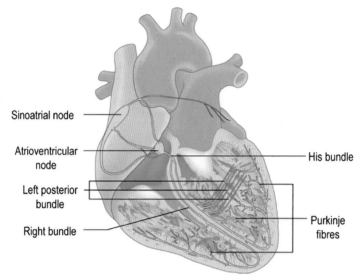

Fig. 8.2 Anatomic aspects of cardiac electrical activity. (Bunce NH, Ray R, Patel H. Chapter 30, Fig. 30.1: Cardiology. In: Feather A, Randall A, Waterhouse M, eds. Kumar and Clark's Clinical Medicine, 10th edn. Elsevier; 2021: 1019-1132.)

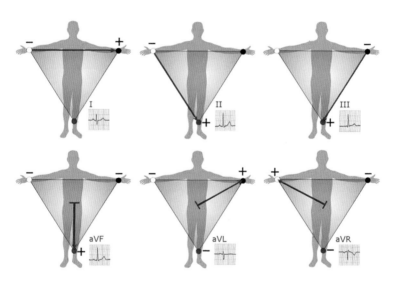

Fig. 8.3 Direction of electric flow within the heart detected by individual leads with graphic electrocardiogram image.

you examine. After all the atrial cells are depolarized, current flow stops, and the ECG returns to its baseline during the period that the impulse is then being delayed in the AV node. This period, the PR interval, is when the atria contract, filling and priming the "ventricular pump" before its contraction. The next set of deflections is called the QRS complex, which represents ventricular depolarization. As there are more cardiac muscle cells in the ventricles than the atria, the QRS complex is often of greater magnitude than the P wave due to the greater current flow that occurs during ventricular depolarization. When all ventricular cells are depolarized, current flow again ceases, and the ECG again returns to its isoelectric baseline during a period known as the ST segment. Ventricular contraction occurs during the ST segment. The final ECG deflection, the T wave, represents ventricular repolarization, after which current flow ceases and the ECG returns to its baseline. The representation of these elements on a normal ECG can be found in Fig. 8.4.

The ECG is produced on specially designed graph paper. When viewed directly, it is an assortment of small squares that are 1 mm wide and 1 mm high. These small squares are further categorized on the paper into larger blocks composed of five small squares in height and width. At a standard paper printing speed of 25 mm/sec, the width of each large block is 0.2 seconds long and each small square is 0.04 seconds long. The vertical aspect of the graph paper reflects voltage. A standard ECG machine is calibrated so that each small square represents 0.1 mV. It is important to be aware of the standard settings on the ECG machine and not to deviate from them, as interpretation can be affected by these changes. Settings can be found printed on the side of a 12-lead ECG or at the bottom of a printed rhythm strip.

Obtaining a 12-Lead ECG

A key task for the emergency department technician (EDT) is to obtain ECGs. This is achieved by placement of external electrodes, referred to as leads, on the patient's skin surface. Some leads are placed on an extremity (limb leads), and some placed adjacent to the chest wall itself (precordial leads). All leads measure current flow in the heart from different positions, resulting in variations among the different leads according to whether the current flow is moving toward the lead (positive deflection) or away (negative deflection). Different leads therefore allow the clinician to study changes in electrical activities for cells located in a specific area of the heart.

To apply the leads, stickers with conductive gel are applied to the skin, and wires transmit the detected electrical impulses to a monitor or ECG machine that can produce 12 simultaneous

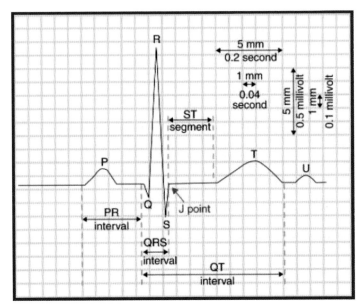

Fig. 8.4 Components of one lead in a normal electrocardiogram.

images measuring the current flows in the different leads. The six limb leads are generated by current flows measured on the extremities, and the six precordial leads are flows that compare the flows measured on the anterior chest wall to those measured on the limbs.

Fig. 8.5 shows the traditional location for appropriate placed limb leads. Usually the leads are applied to the wrists and ankles of the patient, but may also be applied to the anterior shoulder and hips/waist if necessary (this can reduce movement of the wires which can lead to "artifact" or "noise"). The lead wires will often have identification directing the technician to their appropriate placement: right arm, left arm, right leg, left leg.

The wires are also conventionally color coded, with the right arm being white, right leg green, left arm black, and left leg red. Proper placement can often be recalled with the mnemonic "snow over tree, smoke over fire."

The three limb leads and a fourth ground provide six different views of the heart's current flows that are designated I, II, III, AVR, AVL, and AVF. The six precordial leads are designated V1 to V6 (Fig. 8.6). The precordial leads are placed in the following locations: V1 (fourth intercostal space to the right of the sternum), V2 (fourth intercostal space to the left of the sternum), V3 (directly between V2 and V4), V4 (midclavicular line of the fifth intercostal space), V5 (anterior axillary line of the fifth intercostal space in a horizontal line with V4), and V6 (in the midaxillary line of the fifth intercostal space in a horizontal line with V4/V5).

It is important to use anatomic rib spacing to ensure placement in the same location for all patients, as soft-tissue landmarks such as the nipple line can vary according to patient gender and body habitus. When recording, it is important that the patient limit movement and that there are no adjacent electrical instruments in contact with the patient, as these can generate electrical interference that can negatively affect interpretation.

Once properly placed on the skin around the chest wall, the ECG machine will generate a 12-lead ECG graphical printout that shows different vectors of electrical activity throughout the cardiac cycle. Once completed, the 12-lead should be immediately presented to the physician of record for interpretation. Physicians are specially trained to identify an array of cardiac issues, including life-threatening heart rhythms and heart attacks.

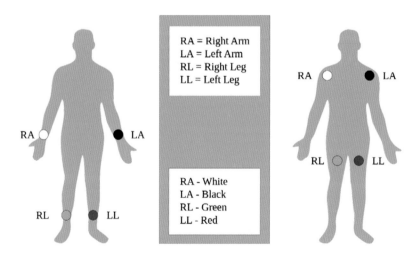

Fig. 8.5 Proper location of limb leads for electrocardiogram.

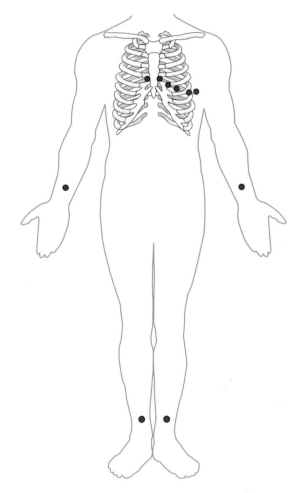

Fig. 8.6   Correct anatomic placement of 10 leads for a complete electrocardiogram.

Cardiac Monitoring

If a 12-lead ECG is a snapshot in time, continuous cardiac monitoring is an assessment of cardiac rhythm in real time. Following the acquisition of a 12-lead ECG, the four limb leads (sometimes accompanied by a single precordial lead) remain on a patient for continuous monitoring. The rhythm from an individual patient is often depicted on both the cardiac monitor in the individual's room and on a monitor in a central station that can allow the clinical team to monitor multiple patients at once (Fig. 8.7).

TIP

Changes in the ST segment may be seen during continuous cardiac monitoring; however, the accuracy of the ST segment for determining changes to the heart's blood flow is significantly limited. If there is concern for this type of change, please notify a physician.

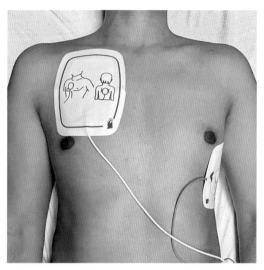

Fig. 8.7   Five-lead cardiac monitor connected to a patient. Note that the *brown* lead is placed where V1 would be on a 12-lead electrocardiogram.

Cardiac Rhythms

Heart rhythm recognition is complex, and interpretation requires some experience. However, EDTs should be familiar with common cardiac rhythms to rapidly identify potentially unstable and life-threatening arrhythmias. Cardiac rhythms can be divided into two basic categories: regular and irregular. Some rhythms in each of these categories can be potentially life-threatening.

REGULAR RHYTHMS

Normal Sinus Rhythm

Normal sinus rhythm (NSR) refers to the cardiac rhythm that is presented by a normal, healthy heart. It has a rate between 60 to 100 beats per minute and typically shows beats at equal intervals from one another. Referring back to Fig. 8.4, there is a P wave, a QRS complex, and a T wave making up each beat, consistent with a sinus rhythm. Fig. 8.8 is an example of a normal 12-lead ECG printout.

Sinus Bradycardia

Sinus bradycardia refers to a sinus rhythm that is slower than NSR. It has a rate that is slower than 60 beats per minute, but beats occur at regular intervals. Although bradycardia can be normal for some individuals, especially the young and physically fit, it can also be indicative of other serious health problems and should not be overlooked. Fig. 8.9 is an example of a 12-lead ECG showing sinus bradycardia.

Sinus Tachycardia

Sinus tachycardia refers to a sinus rhythm that is faster than NSR. It has a rate that is faster than 100 beats per minute, but typically in adults does not exceed 150 beats per minute. Sinus tachycardia can be normal for some individuals as well, but can be caused by other dangerous health conditions. Fig. 8.10 shows an example of a 12-lead ECG with sinus tachycardia.

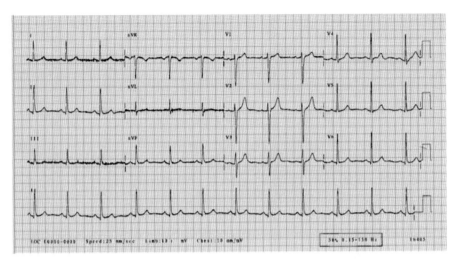

Fig. 8.8   Normal 12-lead electrocardiogram.

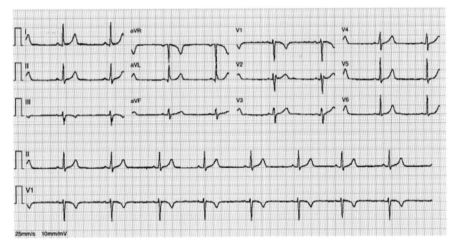

Fig. 8.9   A 12-lead electrocardiogram showing sinus bradycardia.

Supraventricular Tachycardia

Supraventricular tachycardia (SVT) is an abnormal cardiac rhythm that exceeds 150 beats per minute. Most frequently caused by reentry circuits in the AV node that stimulate the ventricles directly, the resulting rhythm is regular, extremely fast (usually around 150 beats/min), and lacks clear-cut P waves (Fig. 8.11).

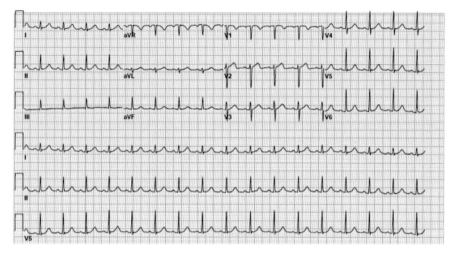

Fig. 8.10   A 12-lead electrocardiogram showing sinus tachycardia.

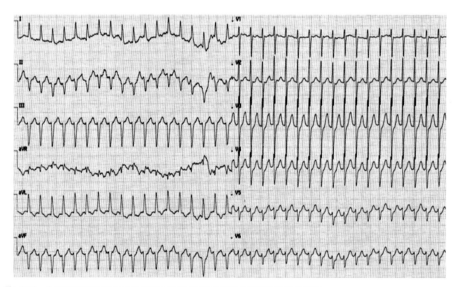

Fig. 8.11   A 12-lead electrocardiogram showing supraventricular tachycardia.

IRREGULAR RHYTHMS

Atrial Fibrillation

Atrial fibrillation (A-Fib) is an irregular cardiac rhythm that is distinguished by a wavering base-line between QRS complexes. Disorganized electrical activity in the atria causes the walls of the atria to "fibrillate" (quiver without effective contraction). This disordered electrical pattern leads to an inability to distinguish clear P waves and causes varying intervals between QRS complexes (Fig. 8.12). A-Fib can be asymptomatic, but the patient often notes palpitations and may have symptoms consistent with low cardiac output, such as weakness or shortness of breath. A-Fib may also lead to stagnation of blood in the atria, leading to a propensity to form blood clots and an increased risk of stroke in certain patient populations.

LIFE-THREATENING ECG PATTERNS

ST-Elevation Myocardial Infarction

A STEMI (ST-elevation myocardial infarction) is the ECG pattern associated with a severe heart attack that involves the full thickness of the ventricular wall. A STEMI often results from a complete occlusion of a coronary artery branch. The name derives from the ECG finding of abnormal current flow during the normally isoelectric period (where the ECG returns to baseline) that elevates the ST segment. This aberrant current flow reflects cellular injury in part of the cardiac musculature resulting from impaired blood flow injuring cells so they can't depolarize and repolarize synchronously with the remainder of the cardiac muscle cells that are not experiencing blood flow disruption. Treatment of this condition requires a breaking up of the acute clot and opening the artery with a stent. These occur during a cardiac catheterization that is often done emergently.

It is extremely important for physicians to be quickly presented with all ECGs to determine whether a STEMI is present. Studies from the American Heart Association (AHA) have shown better outcomes in patients with STEMI who receive early definitive intervention. Thus AHA guidelines recommend that patients with STEMI should be taken to the catheterization lab (where the clot can be treated) within 60 to 90 minutes of ED arrival. Fig. 8.13 shows an example of a STEMI.

Ventricular Tachycardia

Ventricular tachycardia (V-Tach) is an unstable and potentially life-threatening cardiac rhythm characterized by a regular rate that is usually greater than 120 beats per minute with *wide* QRS complexes. This rhythm occurs when electrical activity is originating entirely from the ventricles

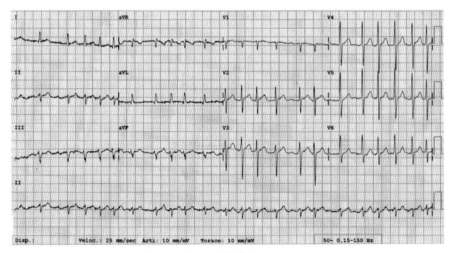

Fig. 8.12 A 12-lead electrocardiogram showing atrial fibrillation.

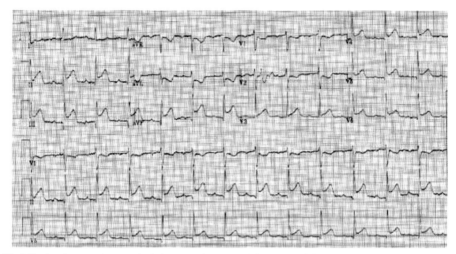

Fig. 8.13   An electrocardiogram displaying anterolateral and inferior acute ST-elevation myocardial infarction.

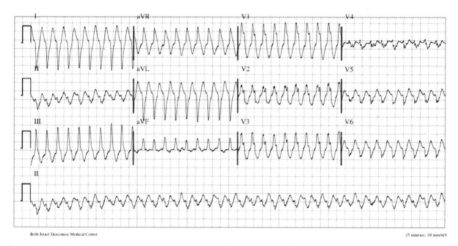

Fig. 8.14   A 12-lead electrocardiogram showing ventricular tachycardia.

and requires immediate attention as it can quickly deteriorate. As seen in Fig. 8.14, there are characteristically no separate P or T waves from the QRS complex. Patients in V-Tach may or may not have a pulse. Regardless, these patients should have defibrillator pads placed on them, as it is a rhythm that may require treatment with an electrical shock to the patient. If the pulse is absent, it is imperative to begin cardiopulmonary resuscitation (CPR) promptly to help the body continue to circulate blood and perfuse vital organs.

Ventricular Fibrillation

Ventricular fibrillation (V-Fib) is a lethal cardiac rhythm characterized by chaotic electrical activity with no discernable pattern. This disorganized rhythm, seen in Fig. 8.15, is the result of

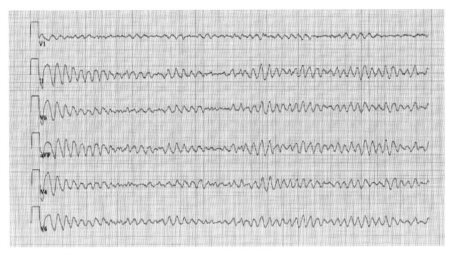

Fig. 8.15 A 12-lead electrocardiogram showing ventricular fibrillation.

disordered conduction in the heart's ventricles resulting in absent cardiac contraction and loss of forward blood flow. Patients in V-Fib require immediate initiation of CPR along with prompt rhythm correction via defibrillation (electrical shock). Defibrillator pads should immediately be placed on these patients to assist in resuscitation.

> **TIP**
>
> If a V-Tach rhythm such as this is perceived on the monitor, but the patient is awake and well appearing, the leads should be assessed because poor skin contact can mimic this rhythm.

Asystole

Asystole occurs in the complete absence of cardiac electrical activity. It is a lethal cardiac rhythm characterized by no visible electrical activity. Asystole presents as a flat line, seen in Fig. 8.16, and occurs when the heart is no longer producing electrical current. Although CPR should be initiated and defibrillator pads should be placed on a patient in asystole, it is not a shockable rhythm.

Summary

The ECG is of equal importance to assessment of basic vital signs in patients presenting to the ED with cardiac disease. A high-quality 12-lead ECG should be obtained and presented to an interpreting physician within the first 10 minutes of anyone presenting with complaints including shortness of breath, chest pain, syncope (fainting), or palpitations. Prompt and accurate 12-lead ECG acquisition is essential for detection and diagnosis of critical conditions and the provision of life-saving interventions. Although interpretation of cardiac rhythms is the domain of a trained physician, EDTs must be familiar with unstable and life-threatening rhythms.

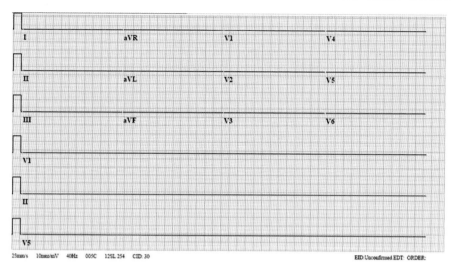

Fig. 8.16 A 12-lead electrocardiogram showing asystole.

References for Additional Reading

Amsterdam EA, Wenger NK, Brindis RG, Casey DE Jr, Ganiats TG, Holmes DR Jr, et al. 2014. AHA-ACC guideline for the management of patients with non-ST-elevation acute coronary syndromes: a report of the American College of Cardiology/American Heart Association Task Force on Practice Guidelines. *J Am Coll Cardiol*. 2014;64:e139–e228.

Johnson F. ECG monitoring leads and special leads. *Indian Pacing Electrophysiol J*. 2016;16(3):92–95.

Park J, Choi KH, Lee JM, et al. Prognostic implications of door-to-balloon time and onset-to-door time on mortality in patients with ST-segment-elevation myocardial infarction treated with primary percutaneous coronary intervention. *J Am Heart Assoc*. 2019;8:e012188.

CHAPTER 9

Cardiologic Emergencies

Breanne Jacobs ▪ Stephen Robie ▪ Owen Ligas

Introduction

The emergency department (ED) technician (EDT) plays a critical role in the initial assessment, triage, workup, and management of patients with cardiac complaints. This chapter provides a framework for understanding and participating in the care of patients with cardiac emergencies.

Cardiac Anatomy

The heart is a four-chambered pump, each chamber separated from the other by two valves. The right atrium and right ventricle, receive deoxygenated blood from the body via the superior and inferior vena cava. This blood is pumped into the lungs from the heart via the pulmonary arteries through the heart's pulmonic valve. The lungs oxygenate the blood and return the blood to the heart via the pulmonary veins. This blood is pumped through the left atrium and left ventricle, which then pump oxygenated blood through the aortic valve into the general circulation via the aorta. (Fig. 9.1).

Understanding of Heart Disease

There are several areas of the heart that can be affected by disease, and although there is usually some overlap, a basic understanding of the specific disease targets will help contextualize the general topic of heart disease.

1. *Coronary artery disease:* The coronary arteries supply the heart muscle cells with oxygen and nutrients. Blockages in the coronary arteries, depending on how rapidly they occur, can reduce the supply of blood to heart muscle cells and in extreme cases lead to cellular death (infarction). The scientific term for heart attack is myocardial infarction (MI). Identification of a patient having a large MI is often straightforward, relying on easily recognized electrical patterns on the electrocardiogram (ECG). However, many patients have much milder symptoms that precede their heart attack by several days, and initially, there may be any of the characteristic findings (Fig. 9.2).
2. *Cardiac muscle disease:* Although a lack of blood flow in the coronary arteries will affect muscular function, many other diseases directly attack and impair the muscle function itself without significant coronary artery blockages. The most frequent result of cardiac muscle disease is congestive heart failure, a condition in which the heart's ability to pump blood is inadequate to meet the body's demands.
3. *Valvular heart disease:* The heart's four chambers are separated from each other and the arteries leading from the heart by four valves, the normal functioning of which is required for adequate blood flow. Conditions that damage a valve can lead to a leaky (insufficient) valve or a tight (stenotic) valve. Both of these situations require greater muscular effort over time to meet the body's demands and can lead to congestive heart failure (Fig. 9.1).

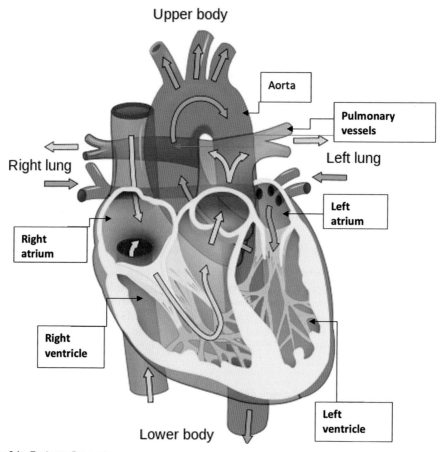

Fig. 9.1 Basic cardiac anatomy.

4. *Pericardial disease:* The pericardium is a tough membrane surrounding the heart separating it from the lungs and assisting the heart's pumping function. When diseased, it can squeeze the heart, decreasing its function (pericardial effusion), and when inflamed, usually by a virus, it can cause chest pain that is hard to distinguish from a heart attack.

Initial Assessment and Triage of the Cardiac Patient

Appropriate prioritization of patients with potential cardiac complaints is important, as many more patients are evaluated for suspicion of heart disease than those who are actually experiencing a cardiac emergency. Patients with cardiac problems can be very unpredictable. A patient with an acute cardiac issue may have relatively minor complaints and normal vital signs initially but can become unstable very quickly; they should be regularly reassessed to quickly identify worsening of their clinical condition.

Initial assessment of all patients should focus on identifying patients who require emergent interventions. Heart disease kills by two major mechanisms:

1. *Arrhythmia:* All forms of heart disease mentioned above can precipitate a sudden disturbance of heart rhythm (either fast or slow), which can suddenly depress or even stop heart function.

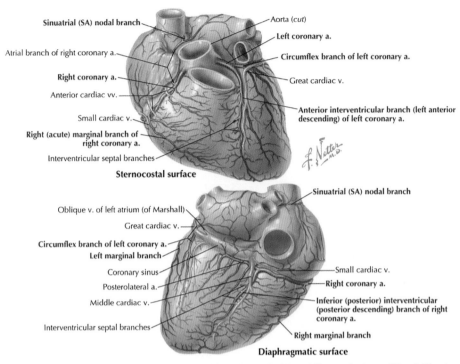

Fig. 9.2 Coronary arteries and cardiac veins. (From Netter F. *Atlas of Human Anatomy*. 7th ed. Elsevier; 2018:plate 222.)

It is therefore vital that anyone with suspected heart disease be placed on a cardiac monitor that will allow the early identification and intervention to identify an arrhythmia quickly.

2. *Loss of cardiac muscle cells:* When the heart loses a significant number of muscle cells (usually from either coronary occlusion or other muscle disease), the heart will no longer be able to pump enough blood to meet the demands. When this happens gradually, a series of compensatory mechanisms ensues that allows some adaptation. If a large amount of muscle dies or ceases to function suddenly (as can happen with a heart attack), the patient can experience a condition called cardiogenic shock. In this situation, the patient often has a low blood pressure, high pulse rate, evidence of poor organ perfusion and appears acutely ill.

Coronary Syndrome

Coronary syndrome is the spectrum of illness that occurs from acute, subacute, or chronic blockages of the coronary arteries. These blockages generally occur at locations where there is a disruption of the wall of the artery by deposition of cells, fats, and cholesterol into a coronary plaque. These plaques can occur in all types of arteries, and the process guiding the plaque development is called atherosclerosis. Major risk factors for atherosclerosis include elevated cholesterol, hypertension, and smoking. Other risk factors include diabetes, kidney disease, male sex, and family history. The arterial walls are in a constant state of motion, responding to differing metabolic needs of the heart muscle. At times, a plaque ruptures, and the body's clotting mechanisms will respond to the plaque rupture by forming a clot at the site of the rupture. There then ensues a dynamic process resulting in either clot expansion (propagation) or dissolution via a natural system that dissolves clots preventing excess clotting (thrombolysis).

When a clot at the site of plaque rupture occurs, the clinical syndrome that ensues will be related to the clot's location in the arterial system, whether the blockage caused by the clot is complete or partial, and how much muscle is supplied by that portion of the artery where flow is impeded. Because both blood supply and the demand of the heart muscle are variable and dynamic, the patient can be expected to have a wide range of symptoms. The three clinical syndromes associated with coronary syndrome are:

- *Angina pectoris*, in which pain results from ischemic heart tissue, where the heart cells have not yet died.
- *ST-elevation myocardial infarction (STEMI)*, where the clot occludes the entire arterial blood supply, severely impairing blood flow and leading to extensive cell death.
- *Non–ST-elevation myocardial infarction (nSTEMI)*, where blood flow at the clot is decreased; there is some cell death but less extensive damage to the heart wall.

Common presenting symptoms of coronary syndrome include the following:

- *Chest pain:* This is a common symptom that can be caused by issues in the heart, lungs, chest wall, pericardium, pleura (membrane surrounding the lungs), ribs, or even problems in the abdomen. The pain from coronary syndrome is generally milder and often has a pressure-like quality. The pain may radiate to the jaw, neck, or down the arm on the ulnar (pinky finger) side. Other symptoms associated with it are shortness of breath and, when severe, nausea, vomiting, and diaphoresis (sweating).
- Other symptoms could include *syncope (fainting), palpitations (sensation of irregular heart beats), pallor,* and a feeling of *"impending sense of doom."* Of note, coronary syndrome in woman may present with atypical chest pain or other less specific symptoms, such as *excessive fatigue.*

Therefore it is important to maintain a high index of a suspicion toward all patients during triage of a potential cardiac emergency.

Heart failure symptoms are variable, but those more frequently expressed by patients include shortness of breath either at rest or on exertion, awakening in the middle of the night with breathlessness, exertional fatigue, and dizziness related to low blood pressure. Heart failure patients often have evidence of fluid retention in the legs (seen on physical exam) or in the lungs (seen on chest x-ray or bedside sonogram).

In patients with all cardiac complaints, the ECG is an early diagnostic test in which a physician analyzes the heart's electrical activity and compares it to normal activity (see Chapter 8).

Measuring leakage of an enzyme only found in heart muscle (troponin) has become an important part of heart disease evaluation. Finding elevated levels of this enzyme in the bloodstream will indicate cardiac cell death (or extreme metabolic strain on heart cells) and will help the physician prioritize the treatment response. This test can either be done as a point-of-care (POC) test or in the hospital lab.

Cardiac Arrest

Cardiac muscle that is diseased or not getting enough blood (ischemic) can become electrically unstable. The heart rhythm can suddenly change from normal to a highly disorganized rhythm called ventricular fibrillation, which leads to a cessation of the heart's organized pumping activity and circulatory collapse (no blood flow to any tissues). Without brain perfusion, respiration will soon stop, and the patient will be in full cardiac arrest (no heart contraction, leading to no pulse or blood pressure and no breathing, or respiratory arrest). These patients are most frequently brought in by emergency medical services; in many systems, they will have their airway controlled and intravenous (IV) access started in the field. For patients who are brought in by basic life support or code in the ED, most EDs have a team approach that includes the EDT, who is often assigned to

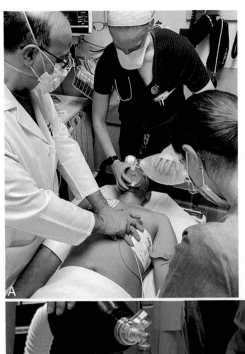

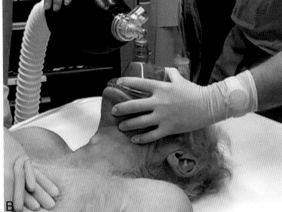

Fig. 9.3 Cardiopulmonary resuscitation. (A) Chest compression and bag valve mask ventilation (B) bag valve mask ventilation.

do chest compressions or obtain an IV line while the physician manages the airway. For those who arrest in the ED, determining their cardiac rhythm and attempting to defibrillate them quickly is of paramount importance (Fig. 9.3).

If your facility has a LUCAS mechanical compression device for administration of CPR, then bring it to the room. There should also be a backboard and stool to facilitate quality CPR compressions. On the wall behind the patient, there should be a working suction machine with a canister and oxygen pump.

Many facilities use POC testing devices for rapid assessment of the patient's blood. For cardiac issues, the most frequent POC test is a measurement of troponin, a muscle-related protein specific for heart muscle that leaks into the bloodstream from damaged heart muscles.

Finally, the cardiac monitor should be fully set up with leads and pulse oximetry monitoring, and the defibrillator, with pads (Fig. 9.4), must be in the room and ready for use.

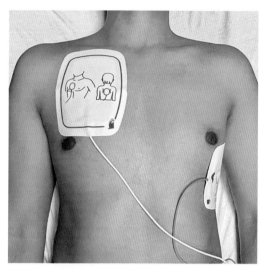

Fig. 9.4   Defibrillator pads placed on a patient.

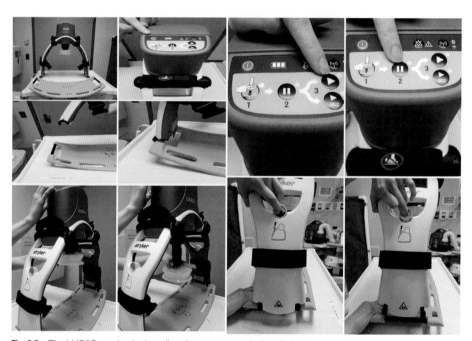

Fig. 9.5   The LUCAS mechanical cardiopulmonary resuscitation device.

LUCAS Device

The LUCAS device is a mechanical compression aid designed to deliver compressions in accordance with CPR guidelines (Fig. 9.5). The goal is to facilitate consistent compression delivery while minimizing interruptions and avoiding human compression fatigue.

Summary

Patients with concern for acute cardiac disease should have a full assessment of vital signs and a 12-lead ECG obtained within their first 10 minutes of ED arrival. Common patient complaints suggestive of coronary syndrome include chest pain (pressure), shortness of breath, sweating, and palpitations. Emergency department technicians may be the first to recognize a patient in distress and are integral in assisting with critical measures, such as alerting the emergency response system, initiating CPR, and facilitating POC testing. They also assist the healthcare team with managing vital equipment, such as the LUCAS device, during a code response.

References for Additional Reading

Basic Life Support (BLS) Provider Manual. 2021 American Heart Association. Available at: https://cpr.heart. org/en/cpr-courses-and-kits/healthcare-professional/basic-life-support-bls-training.

Lichtman J, Leifheit E, Safdar B, et al. Sex differences in the presentation and perception of symptoms among young patients with myocardial infarction: evidence from the VIRGO Study (Variation in recovery: role of gender on outcomes of young AMI patients). *Circulation*. 2018;137:781–790.

CHAPTER 10

Respiratory System Emergencies

Elizabeth Dearing ■ Lindsey Abraham ■ Margarita Popova

Anatomy of the Respiratory System

The primary function of the respiratory system is gas exchange. Oxygen is absorbed by the body from inspired air, and carbon dioxide is removed from the body and released into the environment. Oxygen is used by every cell in the body for the production of energy, and carbon dioxide is a waste product of cellular metabolism that becomes dangerous if accumulated. The body can neither store oxygen nor tolerate elevated levels of carbon dioxide for a long period, so respiratory gas exchange must function continually to support life. The respiratory system's anatomy can be subdivided into three sections: the airway, the lungs, and the muscles of respiration.

THE AIRWAY

The airway is the "A" of the ABC resuscitation mnemonic (Airway, Breathing, and Circulation) and is a passageway through which gases are exchanged. The airway can be further divided into two parts: the upper airway (nasal cavity, the oral cavity, the pharynx, and the larynx) and the lower airway (consisting of the tracheobronchial tree).

Nose, Mouth, and Throat

Air inhalation and exhalation can occur through either the nose or mouth and most frequently through both. Each nostril has three turbinates (shelves of cartilage) that filter, heat, and moisten air. Most conscious adults inspire through the nose.

The mouth is defined as the space between the lips, cheeks, tongue, hard and soft palates, and the throat. The throat, or pharynx, begins behind the nose and ends at the top of the trachea and esophagus (Fig. 10.1). The nasopharynx is the area behind the nose, the oropharynx is the area behind the mouth, and the hypopharynx is the deeper (more caudal) part. At the caudal end of the hypopharynx is the beginning of two important structures: the esophagus (part of the gastrointestinal system) and the larynx (located anteriorly to the esophagus).

Larynx

The larynx, or "voice box," serves two important functions. The first is a conduit for gas exchange, and the second is phonation (speech), which occurs when air passes through movable structures located in the larynx called vocal cords. In order to provide a range of sound, the larynx is relatively narrow at this point, so it can become obstructed in a variety of situations. During inspiration, the epiglottis (a flap of tissue above the larynx) opens like a trap door to allow air to freely pass into the lungs. However, during swallowing, the epiglottis folds back over the laryngeal opening to cover the larynx, preventing food aspiration into the lungs. The epiglottis is an important landmark during endotracheal intubation and can cause severe airway obstruction if it becomes inflamed (epiglottitis).

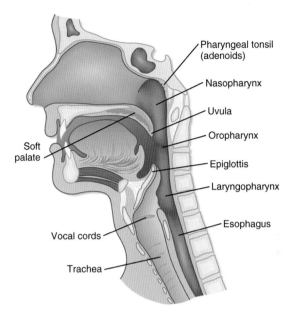

Fig. 10.1 Lateral view of the upper airway demonstrating the sections of the pharynx. (From Koeppen BM, Stanton BA. Introduction to the respiratory system. In: Koeppen BM, Stanton BA, eds. Berne and Levy Physiology, 20th ed. Elsevier; 2018:434–446.)

Lower Airway

Below the larynx is the trachea, a tubular structure supported by cartilage. The trachea splits into the two bronchi, one for each lung, in the upper part of the chest. The bronchi then divide into progressively smaller bronchi (called bronchioles), which terminate at structures called alveoli, where capillaries bring blood very close to the inspired air. There are hundreds of millions of alveoli in the lungs. The alveoli are thin-walled air sacs that look like tiny bunches of grapes. In these structures, oxygen is absorbed from the air, and carbon dioxide is released to be removed from the body by exhalation.

THE PLEURAL CAVITY

The lungs are encased in two thin membranes, called pleura, covering the outer surface of each lung and the inner surface of the chest wall including the muscles and ribs. These membranes are constantly sliding across one another during respiration and help maintain a slightly negative pressure within the chest cavity at rest that helps the lungs stay inflated.

THE MUSCLES OF RESPIRATION

Chest Wall and Ribs

The chest wall is made up of 12 ribs on each side joined at the sternum anteriorly. The intercostal muscles lie between the ribs and pull the ribs together, making exhalation of air easier.

Diaphragm

The diaphragm is the dome-shaped muscle that separates the chest from the abdomen, and it is the main muscle of respiration. During breathing, the diaphragm moves downward until it is flat, creating negative pressure in the chest, which causes air to rush into the lungs. When it relaxes, it tents upward, which causes air to rush out of the lungs during exhalation. The nerve signals to the diaphragm via the phrenic nerve originate in the upper (cervical) spine, which is why upper cervical spinal cord injuries can lead to respiratory failure.

Respiratory Emergencies

Respiratory emergencies can be categorized as traumatic or nontraumatic, as well as by the location of the pathology to the upper or lower airway or the brain. This chapter will focus on nontraumatic causes. Although most patients in respiratory distress arrive by emergency medical services (EMS) and conduct much of the initial evaluation and initial treatment in the field, the following discussion assumes no prehospital care or evaluation.

INITIAL EVALUATION

When evaluating a patient with a potential respiratory emergency, the emergency department (ED) technician (EDT) should evaluate the following:
- The patient's general appearance and the pulse and blood pressure readings
- The natural position that the patient is assuming
- The respiratory rate
- The use of accessory muscles of respiration
- The pulse oximeter reading (or the presence of blueness on the nail beds or the lips, called cyanosis)
- The patient's level of consciousness

The order of evaluation will vary with different clinical circumstances, but the initial actions that should be taken are placing the patient on a cardiac monitor, providing a source of supplemental oxygen, disrobing the patient as appropriate, and positioning the patient on the stretcher in the best possible position (Table 10.1).

RESPIRATORY RATE

The normal respiratory rate is about 12 to 18 times per minute. Most respiratory emergencies present with a rapid rate (>20 breaths/min). We most frequently estimate the rate, and as you gain more experience, you will become proficient at determining who is breathing very quickly (hyperventilation) without taking the time to precisely measure it. Conversely, patients who are breathing very slowly (hypoventilation) are either at an advanced stage of a variety of disease processes or have central nervous system (CNS) depression, often from an opioid overdose and occasionally from

---

TABLE 10.1 ■ **Role of the EDT in the Initial Management of Respiratory Emergencies**

Emergency Evaluation	Initial Tech Management	Additional Adjuncts (if appropriate)
Airway and Breathing	Continuous pulse oximetry Supplemental oxygen (nasal cannula or nonrebreather mask) as directed	Nebulizer Suction OPA/NPA Airway cart/equipment
Circulation	Continuous cardiac monitor IV placement	12-lead ECG
Exposure	Assist patient into gown Provide with blankets if necessary	

ECG, Electrocardiogram; EDT, emergency department technician; IV, intravenous; NPA, nasopharyngeal airway; OPA, oropharyngeal airway.

low blood sugar (hypoglycemia). Patients with severe hypoventilation should be taken to a "code" or resuscitation room, given supplemental oxygen, and have an intravenous (IV) line inserted. Except where CNS depression can be quickly reversed (e.g., naloxone for opioids, IV dextrose for hypoglycemia), these patients will need endotracheal intubation and mechanical ventilation.

PATIENT POSITIONING

Patients with respiratory compromise arriving by EMS will often be sitting up as erect as possible. This will allow for the best diaphragmatic excursion, which will help with pulmonary mechanics and optimize air exchange. Patients with upper airway obstruction may assume the "sniffing position," in which the neck is extended to maximize the airflow through the upper airway.

ACCESSORY MUSCLES

Although the diaphragm is the main muscle of respiration, the muscles between the ribs (intercostal muscles) and some of the neck muscles will be engaged to facilitate respiration during stress from a variety of conditions. Noting whether the patient is engaging these muscles or not may help establish the seriousness of a complaint of shortness of breath.

PULSE OXIMETER

Oxygen saturation is often called the fifth vital sign. A pulse oximeter determines the oxygen saturation of hemoglobin by measuring how certain wavelengths of light are reflected by the capillary beds in the ear or the fingernail. When the amount of oxygen in the lungs drops, there is less oxygen for hemoglobin to capture and distribute to the tissues, and the hemoglobin actually changes color (becoming bluer and reflecting light differently than does fully oxygenated hemoglobin). The pulse oximeter is most often placed on the nail bed and gives a continuous update on the hemoglobin saturation, allowing the clinician to know when the patient is getting worse and also to help regulate the amount of supplemental oxygen provided.

MENTAL STATUS

Increasing confusion in a patient with apparent breathing difficulties is often an ominous sign. It can represent either low blood flow to the brain (hypotension), low oxygen in the blood (hypoxia), elevated amounts of carbon dioxide in the blood (hypercarbia), or some combination of all three. Hypotension and hypoxia will be apparent from bedside measurements, but a lab test is necessary to confirm elevated carbon dioxide levels.

As mentioned, the critical first steps for any patient with respiratory complaints in the ED are placing the patient on both cardiac and continuous pulse oximetry monitors. Supplemental oxygen should also be provided, if needed. A nasal cannula may be applied to patients with mildly increased work of breathing and mild oxygen desaturation. For patients presenting with significantly increased work of breathing or more profound hypoxia, or for any patient who appears to be in distress, a nonrebreather mask may first be applied with maximal oxygen flow (>15 L/min). If there is ever a question of degree of airway assistance needed, place a nonrebreather mask on the patient, as this can always be replaced with a nasal cannula once the patient has been evaluated and stabilized.

AIRWAY ADJUNCTS

Breathing is a two-part process involving both ventilation and respiration. Ventilation is the process of moving air in and out of the lungs, whereas respiration refers to the gas exchange process occurring in the alveoli that oxygenates the blood and supplies oxygen to the cells of the body. If either respiration or ventilation is inadequate, the patient can quickly become hypoxic. Performing additional maneuvers and administering oxygen to the patient can be a lifesaving measure.

The goal of any additional airway maneuvers or application of adjuncts is to maintain airway patency. These techniques are often temporary while awaiting a change in patient's clinical condition or while preparing for a more definitive airway (e.g., intubation).

OPENING THE AIRWAY

Head-tilt, chin-lift: The head-tilt, chin-lift maneuver is used to quickly open the airway of a patient with no suspected cervical spine injuries. The maneuver must be constantly maintained manually or with an adjunct throughout ventilation.

Procedure
1. Place one hand on the patient's forehead and the other under the jaw.
2. Gently apply backward pressure to the patient's forehead while simultaneously lifting the patient's jaw with your other hand. Be careful to only apply pressure to the bony part of the chin. Compressing the soft space under the jaw could create an airway obstruction.
3. Hold the jaw so that the patient's teeth are not touching. It may be necessary to slightly retract the lower lip to keep the airway open.

Jaw-thrust: The jaw-thrust is the preferred method for opening the airway of a patient with a suspected cervical spine injury since it does not require any movement of the cervical spine. Additionally, it may be all that is required to maintain airway patency by moving the tongue forward to decrease airway obstruction.

Procedure
1. Position yourself at the head of the gurney or bed with the patient in the supine position. Place your forearms on either side of the patient's head.
2. Use your index and middle fingers to apply pressure to the angle and back of the jaw (mandible) to push the mandible up. It may be necessary to slightly retract the lower lip with your thumb to maintain an open airway

Nasopharyngeal airway (NPA): The NPA (Fig. 10.2) is an important airway adjunct in patients with altered mental status and an intact gag reflex or in patients with a clenched jaw. The NPA is a flexible tube that is inserted into one of the nares with the distal tip ending in the nasopharynx,

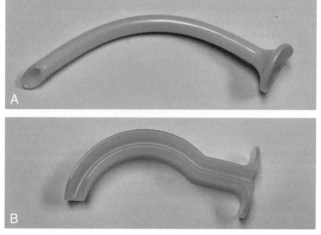

Fig. 10.2   (A) Nasopharyngeal airway (NPA). The beveled end visualized on the left end of the NPA should be inserted into the nares. (B) Oropharyngeal airway (OPA). The curved end of the OPA is inserted into the mouth and behind the tongue.

ensuring rescue breaths have a patent path of travel. It is contraindicated in patients with significant facial trauma, especially nasal trauma.

Oropharyngeal airway (OPA): The OPA (Fig. 10.2) is the preferred airway adjunct for unresponsive patients who do not have a gag reflex. Insertion of the OPA moves the tongue forward to create airway patency while also allowing for suctioning. Insertion of an OPA in patients with an intact gag reflex may result in vomiting and aspiration; therefore it is not indicated in these patients. The OPA is also contraindicated in patients with significant facial injuries.

SUPPLEMENTAL OXYGEN

There are generally oxygen regulators on the walls of most treatment rooms that allow the EDT to regulate the amount of oxygen administered to the patient measured in units of liters per minute (Fig. 10.3). There are various interchangeable administration devices that are connected to the regulator.

Supplemental Device	Oxygen Regulator Setting	Max Inhaled Oxygen Percentage
Nasal cannula	1–6 L/min	24%–44%
Nonrebreather mask	15 L/min	90%
Bag-valve mask	15 L/min	100%

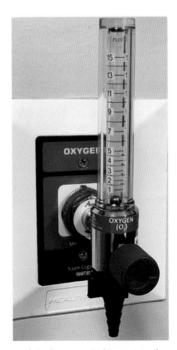

Fig. 10.3 **Oxygen regulator.** The regulator is connected to oxygen through the wall mount with the tubing for supplemental oxygen devices connected through the triangular attachment at the bottom of regulator. A small internal ball will move up or down the numerical gauge (numbered 1 through 15) by turning the dial and is based on oxygen delivery in L/min.

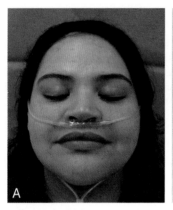
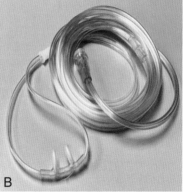

Fig. 10.4   Nasal cannula. (A) Appropriate placement of nasal cannula on patient. (B)Nasal cannula with tubing. Prongs are to be inserted in nares with a slight downward curve. (From King BJ, Megison A, Scogin Z, Christensen BJ. Capnography detection using nasal cannula is superior to modified nasal hood in an open airway system: a randomized controlled trial. J Oral Maxillofac Surg. 2019;77(8):1576–1581.)

NASAL CANNULA

The nasal cannula is used to provide supplemental oxygen to a patient who is breathing adequately. It is the first device used on mildly to moderately ill patients. The nasal cannula consists of long tubing and a flexible plastic piece with two prongs that sit just inside the nares. Inhaled room air is mixed with supplemental oxygen so the nasal cannula provides oxygen concentrations that are between 24% and 44% oxygen (room air is 21% oxygen).

Procedure (Fig. 10.4)
1. Set the oxygen tank regulator between 1 and 6 L/min.
2. Attach the tubing to the regulator and ensure air is being delivered through the prongs.
3. Insert the prongs gently into the patient's nares. The prongs should curve slightly downward when placed correctly.
4. Loop the tubing over the patient's ears and bring both sides together under the patient's jaw.
5. Gently secure the sliding adjuster until it rests just under the patient's chin.

NONREBREATHER MASK

A nonrebreather mask is used to provide higher-concentration oxygen than the nasal prongs. This device consists of a face mask and an oxygen reservoir bag. The face mask has a port on each side that is covered in rubber stoppers. These ports open during exhalation to evacuate the expired air and close during inhalation to prevent room air (21% oxygen) from mixing with the wall oxygen (100% oxygen). Small amounts of room air do leak past the sides of the mask on inspiration, so the nonrebreather mask delivers approximately 90% oxygen.

Procedure (Fig. 10.5)
1. Set the oxygen regulator to deliver 15 L/min or higher.
2. Secure the attached tubing to the regulator and wait for the reservoir bag to completely fill with oxygen. It may be necessary to compress the rubber gasket covering the one-way valve between the bag and mask to completely fill the reservoir.
3. Place the mask over the patient's face and secure the elastic band behind their head. Press down on the metal clip at the top of the mask to form the mask to the patient's nose.
4. Coach the patient to breathe normally and continuously monitor the reservoir to ensure it does not deflate.

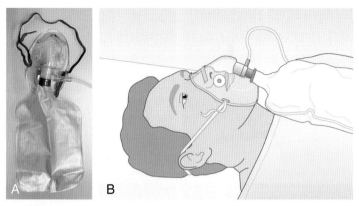

Fig. 10.5 (A) Uninflated nonrebreather mask and (B) oxygen administered using a nonrebreather mask with a reservoir bag. (From Paterson R, Dover AR. The deteriorating patient. In: Innes JA, Dover AR, Fairhurst K, eds. Macleod's Clinical Examination. 14th ed. Elsevier; 2018:339–346.)

BAG-VALVE MASK

The bag-valve mask (BVM) device is used to manually provide breaths to a patient. In the non-intubated patient, the operator tightly seals the face mask over the patient's nose and mouth and assists or provides breaths by squeezing the bag. In the intubated patient, an adapter that articulates with the endotracheal tube is substituted for the face mask. The BVM delivers almost 100% oxygen when attached to an oxygen tank.

Procedure (Fig. 10.6):

1. Position yourself at the head of the patient so that you can clearly visualize the airway.
2. Open the patient's airway using the head-tilt, chin-lift maneuver.
3. Place the narrow portion of the mask over the patient's nose and the widest part just above the chin. Secure the mask to the patient's face by placing your thumb on the mask over the bridge of the patient's nose and index finger over the chin. Apply sufficient pressure to maintain a good seal. Simultaneously use your remaining fingers to pull up on the patient's jaw to maintain the head-tilt, chin-lift position. Check for leaking air during each breath and readjust your hand positioning as needed.
4. Deliver rescue breaths that are sufficient to produce visible chest rise and fall. Breaths should be delivered at a rate of 10 to 12 per minute for adults and 12 to 20 per minute for children.

TROUBLESHOOTING

If you notice the rescue breaths are no longer producing adequate chest rise and fall, you should first check that you are holding an adequate seal. Check for air leaking under the mask and readjust your hand as necessary. Next, confirm that you are maintaining the head-tilt, chin-lift position, and readjust the patient as needed. If neither of these steps corrects the problem, consider an airway obstruction. It may be necessary to suction the patient's airway between breaths to remove secretions or other foreign bodies. Finally, consider inserting an NPA or OPA as appropriate to maintain a patent airway. If none of these measures is effective, intubation may be required.

Special Populations

Pediatric patients: When performing a head-tilt, chin-lift maneuver on a child, it is possible to overextend the neck and create an obstruction due to anatomic differences. It may be helpful to

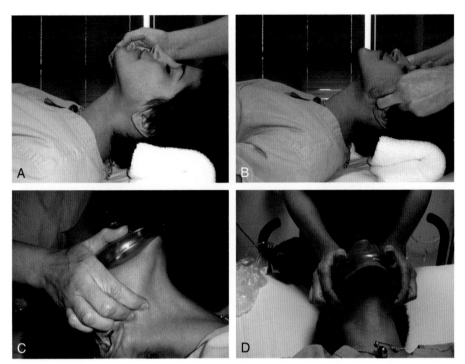

Fig. 10.6 (A) Chin-lift maneuver into sniffing position. (B) Jaw-thrust. (C) Good mask position with one hand. (D) Good mask position with two hands. (From Al-Otaibi Z, Chawla LS.Treatment of medical emergencies. In: Mauro MA, Murphy KP, Thomson KR, Venbrux AC, Morgan RA, eds. Image-Guided Interventions. 3rd ed. Elsevier; 2021:24–28.e1.)

offset the disproportionate size of the pediatric patient's head by placing a small towel under their shoulders. This will elevate the chest and help place the head in a neutral position.

Unresponsive patients: An OPA or NPA may be required to maintain a patent airway.

Suspected spinal injuries: The airway should be opened using the jaw-thrust maneuver to preserve cervical spine integrity. Do not use the head-lift, chin-tilt technique, as this may cause torque on the cervical spine and cause additional injury.

SUCTION

In seriously ill patients, a variety of substances such as blood, vomitus, or mucus can accumulate in the airway. Clearing the airway of these obstructions will improve ventilation and prevent aspiration. Wall-mounted suction devices can be found in most ED patient care rooms (Fig. 10.7). These devices have a container, that receives the aspirate connected to a flexible tube. The actual suction device inserted into the patient is connected to this catheter. The Yankauer catheter is a rigid plastic device that is most frequently used in the ED. Intubated patients need to be suctioned with a smaller, soft plastic suction tube.

THE NEBULIZER

The nebulizer (Fig. 10.8) is used to aerosolize liquid medications to be inhaled for delivery directly to the lungs. Although any liquid medication could be nebulized, this technique is most useful for

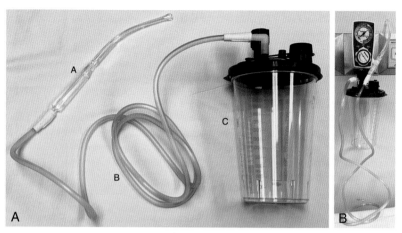

Fig. 10.7   Suction setup. *(Left in)* (A) Suction catheter. (B) Suction tubing. (C) Suction canister. *(Right)* Suction canister attached to wall mount with suction regulator.

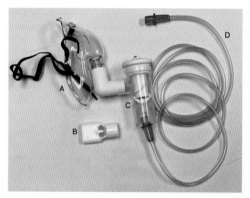

Fig. 10.8   Nebulizer equipment. (A) Facemask with white connector. (B) Mouthpiece (alternative to face mask). (C) Nebulizer. (D) Tubing to connect device to oxygen regulator.

medications for respiratory conditions because inhalation delivers the medication directly to the target tissue. The liquid medication is aerosolized via the nebulizer into a mouthpiece or face mask so that the patient inhales medication with each breath. The nebulizer is most frequently powered by the wall oxygen, or sometimes an oxygen tank.

The two most common medications administered via nebulizer are designed to treat constriction of the bronchial airways, which occurs in diseases such as asthma or chronic obstructive pulmonary disease (COPD). Albuterol, the most frequently used, stimulates receptors (called β2 receptors) on the outside of muscles that surround the bronchi, causing them to relax. Albuterol is often mixed with ipratropium, which works in a different manner by antagonizing a transmitter substance called acetylcholine, which causes bronchoconstriction. Another benefit of nebulizer treatment is that the pressurized oxygen powering the nebulizer will raise the patient's oxygen levels.

Important Respiratory Diseases
UPPER AIRWAY CONDITIONS
Anaphylaxis

Anaphylaxis is a severe, systemic allergic-type reaction leading to release of histamine from certain blood cells that can rapidly lead to upper airway edema and airway compromise. Patients may arrive either ambulatory or by EMS and have a characteristic appearance of facial swelling, respiratory distress, and often a diffuse, reddish skin rash. These patients often have a low blood pressure and rapid pulse. This condition is most frequently caused by an allergy to certain foods or medication, including x-ray contrast dyes.

Epinephrine (adrenaline) given intravenously or intramuscularly is the main treatment for anaphylaxis. Patients need an IV started immediately, and saline should be administered if the patient is hypotensive. Additional treatments often include supplemental oxygen, antihistamines, and nebulized albuterol.

Angioedema

Angioedema appears very similar to anaphylaxis, but there are fewer systemic symptoms and more airway swelling, particularly centered on the lips. Depending on which part of the airway is swollen, severe respiratory distress and airway obstruction can occur. Angioedema in the ED is most frequently associated with a class of drugs called angiotensin-converting enzyme (ACE) inhibitors, which are used to treat hypertension and heart disease. Patients have often taken these medications for some time before the onset of angioedema. Treatment is often quite similar to that of anaphylaxis.

Epiglottitis

Acute epiglottitis is an increasingly rare condition that is usually caused by a bacterial infection of the epiglottis and surrounding tissues. Although traditionally thought of as a disease of children, epiglottitis has now become a disease of adults thanks to the *Haemophilus influenzae* vaccine that is administered during childhood. Patients often have a fever, look sick, and complain of a severe sore throat but have little redness, swelling, or pus on examining the upper throat. As the infection and inflammation progress, the patient will have more difficulty swallowing and may be found to be either drooling on presentation or in the "tripod" position, with their body leading forward supported by their arms and their head upward and neck forward in the "sniffing" position; this position helps to open the airway in the event of upper airway obstruction (Fig. 10.9). Treatment involves antibiotics and airway control, which is often done in the operating room so that an anesthesiologist can attempt intubation; a surgeon stands by to place a surgical airway if the intubation is unsuccessful.

LOWER AIRWAY OBSTRUCTION
Simple Pneumothorax

A pneumothorax is defined as air in the pleural space between the two pleura, and it can cause a partial or complete collapse of the lung. This should not be immediately life-threatening if the patient's other lung is functioning normally. Air enters the pleural space through a communication between the alveoli and the pleural space (e.g., ruptured pulmonary bleb) or communication between the atmosphere and the pleural space (e.g., penetrating chest trauma). On occasion, a pneumothorax can occur when the physician is performing a procedure such as insertion of a central line (iatrogenic pneumothorax), where the needle punctures the pleural space accidentally.

Patients with small pneumothoraces are often asymptomatic, whereas patients with large pneumothoraces may experience symptoms including shortness of breath and chest pain. All patients with a pneumothorax should be placed on high-flow oxygen (either by nasal cannula

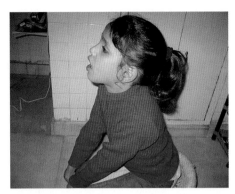

Fig. 10.9　Child in the "tripod" position. (From Subramaniam R. Acute upper airway obstruction in children and adults. Trends Anaesth Crit Care. 2011;1(2):67–73.)

or nonrebreather mask); this has been shown to reduce the size of the pneumothorax through increased rate of resorption of oxygen compared to that of air. Small pneumothoraces may require no additional intervention. Moderate to large pneumothoraces often require insertion of a tube into the pleural space and several days of suction to remove air and help the two pleural membranes adhere together.

Tension Pneumothorax

Tension pneumothorax is a rare but severe condition seen in both traumatic and nontraumatic pneumothoraces, where damage to the lung and pleura causes a one-way valve effect. As the patient inspires, air moves into the pleural space but is blocked from exiting the pleural space during exhalation. Patients with a tension pneumothorax will present with hypotension and respiratory distress with hypoxia and distended neck veins (due to impaired venous return to the heart). Treatment for tension pneumothorax is immediate insertion of a chest tube into the pleural space. Field treatment of a tension pneumothorax is insertion of an 18-gauge catheter into the chest above the second rib in the midaxillary line.

Asthma/COPD

Asthma and COPD are both extremely common respiratory conditions that cause airway inflammation, airway constriction, and, particularly in the case of COPD, destruction of portions of the airway. Asthma is more episodic and the patient's breathing is normal during periods between attacks. COPD is often a result of chronic tobacco smoking and causes more persistent airflow obstruction due to structural changes in the lung. Acute exacerbations of both asthma and COPD will have similar presentations including wheezing, shortness of breath, chest tightness, and coughing, and they are often treated in a similar manner. Oxygen, nebulized albuterol, steroids, and occasionally antibiotics are the mainstays of treatment.

Any patient presenting with respiratory distress should be placed on supplemental oxygen to maintain oxygen saturations above 92%. Nasal cannula can be used for mild hypoxia, whereas a nonrebreather mask with higher flow oxygen should be used for patients with more profound hypoxia (e.g., <85%). Bronchodilators (short-acting β2-agonist and anticholinergic ipratropium bromide) administered through a nebulizer are first-line treatments for both conditions. The medications can be given separately but are commonly given together as DuoNeb. They should be administered in an oxygen-driven nebulizer. Corticosteroids are also considered first-line treatment for acute exacerbations of both asthma and COPD. The patient should be closely monitored for improvement in symptoms or for clinical deterioration requiring additional support.

Respiratory Failure, Noninvasive Positive Pressure Ventilation, and Endotracheal Intubation

Respiratory failure is defined most simply as failure of oxygenation, ventilation, or both. The degree of oxygenation can easily be determined by the pulse oximeter, and a bedside carbon dioxide detector is sometimes used to measure the effectiveness of ventilation.

Patients with respiratory failure of any type are treated with medications and supplemental oxygen, often with subsequent improvement in symptoms. However, in more severe cases, the patient may require further respiratory support as a bridge to allow time for the treatments that alleviate the underlying cause of the respiratory failure to take effect. This can be accomplished through noninvasive means, such as continuous positive airway pressure (CPAP) or bilevel positive airway pressure (BiPAP or BL-PAP), or through invasive means such as supraglottic devices (e.g., laryngeal mask airway or King Airway) or endotracheal intubation.

Noninvasive positive pressure ventilation (NiPPV) most commonly refers to both CPAP and BiPAP, which deliver positive pressure via a sealed mask. CPAP provides a constant positive pressure throughout the respiratory cycle, whereas BiPAP provides higher-pressure support during inspiration and lower pressure during expiration. The benefit of noninvasive ventilation methods is that the patient maintains spontaneous respiration. NiPPV is often used in patients with a normal mental status who are breathing spontaneously and are thought to have an acute but reversible process. Noninvasive ventilation is generally not recommended for patients with altered mental status, as this may lead to increased risk of aspiration of stomach contents. Additionally, noninvasive ventilation will not overcome a decreased respiratory rate or decreased respiratory drive. In these patients, endotracheal intubation and mechanical ventilation is required.

Endotracheal intubation provides maximal respiratory support for patients who require it either for management of critical illness or for airway protection. This procedure does come with risks because the patient's own ability to breathe is stopped by medications for a period of time, and an inability to place the endotracheal tube into the trachea could result in hypoxemia, cardiac arrest, and death. Still, endotracheal intubation is an important procedure for many patients where the benefit outweighs the risk.

To prepare for intubation, the EDT should apply the highest possible oxygen concentration (15 L/min via nonrebreather mask), which should fill the lungs with oxygen. A nasal cannula should be applied in addition to the nonrebreather mask. This preoxygenation helps prevent desaturation during the procedure. The suction should also be set up and turned on to continuous suction. The patient should ideally have two functioning IV lines for administering medications prior to, during, and/or after the procedure. Once the patient is intubated, the respiratory therapist will assist in managing the endotracheal tube and the ventilator. Intubated patients in the ED should be adequately sedated for comfort and should remain on continuous cardiac and pulse oximetry monitors to frequently assess their vital signs for clinical changes because they are no longer able to communicate with the provider.

References for Additional Reading

Adil EA, Adil A, Shah RK. Epiglottitis. *Clin Pediatr Emerg Med*. 2015;16(3):149–153. (accessed December 1, 2020).

Al-Otaibi Z, Chawla LS. *Treatment of Medical Emergencies*. *Image-Guided Interventions*: Elsevier; 2021: 24–28 e1.

Arshad H, Young M, Adurty R, Singh AC. Acute pneumothorax. *Crit Care Nurs Q.* 2016; 39(2):176–189. https://doi.org/10.1097/CNQ.0000000000000110. PMID: 26919678.

Bintcliffe O, Maskell N. Spontaneous pneumothorax. *BMJ.* 2014;348:g2928. https://doi.org/10.1136/bmj. g2928. PMID: 24812003.

Bork K. Angioedema. *Immunol Allergy Clin North Am.* 2014;34(1):23–31. https://doi.org/10.1016/j. iac.2013.09.004. Epub 2013 Oct 20. PMID: 24262687.

Carey MJ. Epiglottitis in adults. *Am J Emerg Med.* 1996;14(4):421–424. https://doi.org/10.1016/S0735-6757(96)90065-0. PMID: 8768171.

King BJ, Megison A, Scogin Z, Christensen BJ. Capnography detection using nasal cannula is superior to modified nasal hood in an open airway system: a randomized controlled trial. *J Oral Maxillofac Surg.* 2019;77(8): 1576–1581.

Lamba TS, Sharara RS, Singh AC, Balaan M. Pathophysiology and classification of respiratory failure. *Crit Care Nurs Q.* 2016;39(2):85–93. https://doi.org/10.1097/CNQ.0000000000000102. PMID: 26919670.

LoVerde D, Files DC, Krishnaswamy G. Angioedema. *Crit Care Med.* 2017;45(4):725–735. https://doi. org/10.1097/CCM.0000000000002281. PMID: 28291095.

LoVerde D, Iweala OI, Eginli A, Krishnaswamy G. Anaphylaxis. *Chest.* 2018;153(2):528–543. https://doi. org/10.1016/j.chest.2017.07.033. Epub 2017 Aug 8. PMID: 28800865; PMCID: PMC6026262.

Mistovich JJ, Karren KJ, Werman HA, Hafen BQ. *Prehospital Emergency Care.* Hoboken, NJ: Pearson Education; 2018.

Paterson R, Dover AR. The deteriorating patient. *Macleod's Clinical Examination:* Elsevier; 2018:339–346. 14th ed.

Seigel TA. Mechanical ventilation and noninvasive ventilatory support. *Rosen's Emergency Medicine: Concepts and Clinical Practice.* Elsevier; 2017:25–33.

Simons FE, Anaphylaxis *J Allergy Clin Immunol.* 2010;125(2 Suppl 2):S161–S181. https://doi.org/10.1016/j. jaci.2009.12.981. Erratum in: J Allergy Clin Immunol. 2010;126(4):885. PMID: 20176258.

Suau SJ, DeBlieux PM. Management of acute exacerbation of asthma and chronic obstructive pulmonary disease in the emergency department. *Emerg Med Clin North Am.* 2016;34(1):15–37. https://doi. org/10.1016/j.emc.2015.08.002. PMID: 26614239.

Subramaniam R. Acute upper airway obstruction in children and adults. *Trends in Anaesthesia and Critical Care.* 2011;1(2):67–73.

CHAPTER 11

Abdominal and Genitourinary Problems

Christina Gallerani ▪ Alexander Gregory Hastava ▪ Andrew Charles Meltzer

Introduction

Symptoms such as abdominal pain; nausea; vomiting; diarrhea; or painful, decreased, or increased urination are some of the most common emergency department (ED) patient complaints. These symptoms can be caused by a variety of gastrointestinal (GI) or genitourinary (GU) conditions of varying severity.

Initial Evaluation

After triage, simple comfort measures should also be offered. Patients who are actively vomiting should be given an emesis bag. Patients with severe pain should be placed on a stretcher. If a patient asks to use the bathroom, the ED technician (EDT) should proactively offer a urine or stool collection cup in anticipation of future physician orders.

The diagnostic testing plan ordered by the ED physician can vary widely. Clinical findings at triage will guide the physician's workup. For example, fever is often a sign of an infectious process and suggests that testing may include blood cultures, urinalysis, and imaging to try to identify the source of the infection. While awaiting the results of the first round of testing, intravenous (IV) medications can be given for pain and nausea, and fluids can be given to rehydrate the patient without yet knowing the specific cause of the symptoms. All individuals of childbearing age with a uterus should receive a pregnancy test unless the patient is already known to be pregnant. Over time, an astute EDT will be able to anticipate the workup for most patients within the first few minutes of initial assessment.

Brief Overview of the Clinical Assessment of the GI or GU System

CLINICAL ASSESSMENT OF THE GI SYSTEM

Physicians will start by taking a history from the patient. There are certain specific questions that are usually asked to help distinguish among the different causes of the complaints. One simple acronym that can be used to outline some of the typical questions is PQRST.

P: Palliating and provocative factors: "What makes the pain better or worse?"
Q: Quality of the pain: "How would you describe the pain?"
R: Radiation: "Does the pain radiate (start in one place and travel to another)?"
S: Severity: "How bad is the pain?"
T: Timing: "How long has this been going on? What were you doing when it started?"

The physician will then do a physical exam. Having the patient get undressed and into a gown is a critical part of obtaining an adequate physical exam, as direct visualization of the skin is necessary and clothing hinders the ability to auscultate or examine the body part in question.

Ill or elderly patients may need help getting changed out of their clothing. The opening of the gown should be facing the back so that the patient's chest and abdomen are not exposed when they are not being examined, and a patient should be helped to tie their gown in the back. They should be offered a sheet or blanket to feel covered and comfortable.

One notable exception to asking a patient to change is if the patient has come to the ED after a sexual assault. In this case, the patient should be asked to remain in their clothing and to try not to use the bathroom until they are seen by a clinician specifically trained in doing a forensic exam so the best evidence can be collected.

BASIC ANATOMY OF THE ABDOMEN

The organs of the GI and GU systems are predominantly located within or behind the abdominal cavity, (retroperitoneal) the anatomy of which is divided into four quadrants (Fig. 11.1). Note that right and left refer to the patient's right and left, not the clinician's. Abdominal pain can be described in terms of its quadrant (e.g., "right lower quadrant pain"). The reason for this is that the location of the pain may correspond to the anatomic location of the diseased organ causing the pain. For example, the appendix is located in the right lower quadrant, where appendicitis pain is often localized. Gallbladder problems present with pain in the right upper quadrant, where the gallbladder is located.

Other common terms that are used to describe the location of pain may include words like *epigastric*, meaning the upper third of the abdomen; *periumbilical*, meaning around the belly button; or *suprapubic*, meaning the pelvic region above the pubic bone. Again, these descriptors often help predict the cause of the patient's pain. For example, epigastric pain may indicate problems like gastritis or ulcers (described later in this chapter), and suprapubic pain may be caused by a urinary tract infection (UTI).

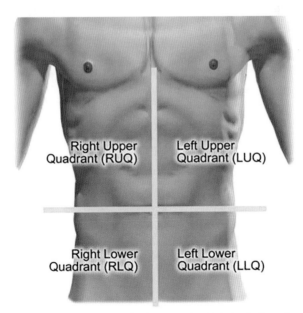

Fig. 11.1 **Labeled zones and boundaries of the four prominent abdominal quadrants.** (From Blausen. com. Medical gallery of Blausen Medical. *WikiJournal of Medicine.* 2014;1(2). doi:10.15347/wjm/2014.010.)

Focused GI Issues in the ED

GI BLEEDING

GI bleeding encompasses complaints of vomiting blood, bleeding from the rectum, or blood seen in the stool, suggesting that there is a source of bleeding from somewhere in the GI tract. GI bleeding can be further categorized as "upper GI bleeding" or "lower GI bleeding." Upper GI bleeding refers to situations where the point that the bleeding originates from is located in the esophagus, stomach, or the beginning of the small intestine known as the duodenaum. Upper GI bleeding most often presents with vomiting of blood (Fig. 11.2). Blood that has been exposed to stomach acid and other digestive enzymes and then vomited up is often described as a "coffee ground emesis," because the vomitus has a dark brown/black and granular appearance, similar to coffee grounds. *Melena* is the name given to black, tarry appearing stools. Similar to coffee ground emesis, the stool appears this way because the blood in the stool has already been partially digested. Melena suggests that the source of bleeding is coming from the upper GI tract because the blood has been acted on by digestive enzymes that are only located in the stomach and intestines.

Common causes of upper GI bleeding include peptic ulcer disease, where the ulcer has eroded into a blood vessel; esophagitis (inflammation in the esophageal lining); gastritis (inflammation of the stomach lining); or tears in the lining of the esophagus. The frequent use of medications like aspirin or ibuprofen can predispose people to developing ulcers and stomach inflammation that can lead to GI bleeding. Forceful vomiting can cause tears in the wall of the esophagus called Mallory-Weiss tears. Chronic ethanol use that leads to liver cirrhosis can also cause enlargement of blood vessels in the esophagus (esophageal varices), which can become a source of potentially life-threatening bleeding. Some upper GI bleeding is more worrisome than others. Patients with bleeding suspected to be from a small tear in the esophagus may be discharged home if they remain stable after a period of ED observation. Most other upper GI bleeding conditions require hospitalization. Smoking and alcohol abuse predispose people to inflammation and irritation in the GI system.

Lower GI bleeding refers to bleeding from the rectum and colon and usually presents with either bright or dark red blood, but not melena. *Hematochezia* refers to bright red blood in the stool.

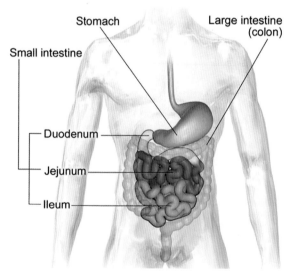

Fig. 11.2   Labeled anatomical reference points of the small intestine. (From Blausen.com. Medical gallery of Blausen Medical. *WikiJournal of Medicine.* 2014;1(2). doi:10.15347/wjm/2014.010.)

The presence of hematochezia means that the blood is coming from the colon or rectum because it has not been partially digested by the time it passes.

Causes of lower GI bleeding range from the relatively benign to the critical. More benign causes of GI bleeding include bleeding from hemorrhoids (dilated veins near the anus), anal fissures (tears in the skin around the anus), and diverticulosis, a condition in which small bulges form in the wall of the colon and can erode into nearby blood vessels. Another consideration in determining the severity of a lower GI bleed is whether the bleeding is ongoing or not. For example, is blood actively leaking from their rectum, or did it occur one time and then stop? Additionally, patient factors like the use of anticoagulant medications and advanced age are important indicators of what actions need to be taken next. If a patient with suspected GI bleeding needs to move their bowels, ask them to use a bedpan, as the physician team may want to visually inspect the stool.

GASTRITIS

Gastritis is an inflammation of the stomach lining. People may experience gastritis acutely or chronically. Patients may present with complaints of nausea, vomiting, feeling full after a small meal (early satiety), bloating or belching, and vague epigastric abdominal discomfort. Common causes of gastritis include bacterial infection from *Helicobacter pylori*; the frequent use of nonsteroidal antiinflammatory drugs (NSAIDs), such as ibuprofen or naproxen; or autoimmune disease. Over time, gastritis can lead to ulcerations in the stomach or duodenum that could cause upper GI bleeding. The treatment of gastritis depends on the underlying cause. For those whose symptoms are caused by *Helicobacter*, antibiotics are needed. Patients using NSAIDs should discontinue their use. Upper endoscopy, a procedure where the physician directly visualizes the stomach and esophagus with a fiberoptic camera, is often performed as an outpatient to help establish the diagnosis.

APPENDICITIS

Appendicitis is inflammation of the appendix. The appendix is a finger-like, blind-ended tube that projects from the first part of the colon *(caecum)*. Most commonly, the appendiceal opening is blocked by small piece of stool *(fecalith)*. Inflammation and infection can then ensue in the appendix, which has become a "closed space." Patients typically present complaining of pain around the umbilicus (early) or in the right lower quadrant (later). Delay in treatment can lead to a perforated appendix, where infectious contents from within the appendix are released into the peritoneal cavity creating a serious infection. Patients with a ruptured appendix may look very ill and uncomfortable. Their abdomen may be exquisitely tender to the touch or even rigid. In general, patients with suspected appendicitis will get bloodwork and some form of imaging. Ultrasound is the preferred means of imaging in children, whereas computed tomography is preferred in adults. Appendicitis is usually managed with antibiotics and surgical removal of the appendix. Appendicitis may also be managed by treating with antibiotics alone, depending on the patient's severity and institutional preferences.

BILIARY EMERGENCIES

The gallbladder is a small, sac-like organ in the right upper quadrant of the abdomen under the liver. The gallbladder stores bile manufactured in the liver and secreted into the small intestine to help with intestinal fat absorption. The gallbladder stores bile until it is needed, which is then released into the small intestine after meals. Stones can form in the gallbladder, leading to a number of problems. The presence of gallstones is called *cholelithiasis*. People can have gallstones and have no symptoms for years. Occasionally, a stone may pass out of the gallbladder and impact within the bile ductal system, blocking the release of bile into the intestines. This can cause the sudden onset of severe pain in the right upper quadrant, or *epigastrium*. Pain from transient passage of a stone is termed *biliary colic*. If the stone remains lodged in the ductal system, there can be ongoing pain and the risk of serious infection. This is termed *choledocholithiasis*. When the gallbladder becomes inflamed and infected, this is called *cholecystitis*. A patient with symptomatic gallstones will need to have the gallbladder removed, the timing of which depends on the patient's clinical situation. People whose gallbladder has been removed have no symptoms or medical needs resulting from the surgery.

URINARY RETENTION

The inability to urinate when the bladder is full is called urinary retention. Patients with urinary retention often present with extreme discomfort in the lower abdomen and may appear to have a very distended abdomen. The most common urinary retention scenario is that of an older man with an enlarged prostate that impedes the passage of urine from the bladder. UTI can be either the cause or result of urinary retention in either men or women. Relief of the urinary retention is achieved by placing a catheter through the urethra to drain the urine from the bladder. A "straight catheterization" is when a catheter is inserted only temporarily to drain the bladder and then removed immediately when the bladder is emptied. An "indwelling" catheter is left in place attached to a drainage bag (Fig. 11.3). Sometimes a patient may be discharged with a catheter in place, with a urine collection bag attached to their leg.

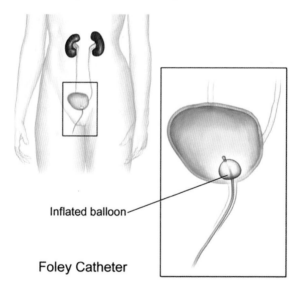

Inflated balloon

Foley Catheter

Fig. 11.3 Location of placement of a Foley catheter in a female patient. (From "File:Foley Catheter.png" by BruceBlaus is licensed with CC BY-SA 4.0. To view a copy of this license, visit https://creativecommons.org/licenses/by-sa/4.0.)

RENAL COLIC

Sudden onset of pain to the left or right flank is often due to a "kidney stone" in the ureter. There are two kidneys, each of which is connected to the bladder by a tube called the ureter (Fig. 11.4). Stones can form in the kidney and lodge in the ureter, blocking urine flow from the kidney causing severe *colic* (pain of varying intensities). Over time this can lead to kidney damage. As most stones pass spontaneously, the goal of treatment is to relieve pain and identify patients who are at risk for complications. If patients have very large stones or a concurrent urinary infection, they may need hospitalization and surgery to have the stone removed.

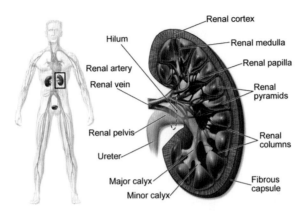

Fig. 11.4 Labeled anatomical reference points of the kidney. (From Blausen.com. Medical gallery of Blausen Medical. *WikiJournal of Medicine*. 2014;1(2). doi:10.15347/wjm/2014.010.)

SEXUALLY TRANSMITTED INFECTIONS

Sexually transmitted infections (STIs) can occur in sexually active patients of any age group. STI-related complaints range from lower abdominal pain, to penile or vaginal discharge, to visible lesions on the genitalia. Patients with complaints involving their genitals should be examined in a private room with a door and should be properly draped. Most patients will need to provide a urine sample as part of the evaluation, and individuals of childbearing age with a uterus will need a pregnancy test. Sensitivity and respect should be practiced regarding the complaint itself. Staff should note that some of these patients may have been victims of sexual assault, even if they have not disclosed this during triage. Lab testing for such infections as gonorrhea, chlamydia, HIV, herpes, and others may be done as part of the evaluation.

Critical Actions for the ED Technician

There are a number of critical ways EDTs assist in the care of patients with GI and GU complaints. Ten important skills and tasks the EDTs should be familiar with are as follows:
1. *Recognize when patients may be very sick:* Clues that may indicate a patient is very sick are abnormal vital signs, especially a low blood pressure, or a patient who is confused or unconscious. As EDTs may be involved in measuring or recording a patient's vitals, they may be the first to identify an ill patient. An EDT should never hesitate to notify a physician or registered nurse if they think a patient needs immediate help.
2. *Place the patient on a monitor:* If a patient is very ill appearing or unstable, a blood pressure cuff, oxygen saturation probe, and cardiac monitor should be applied to the patient and connected to a monitor.
3. *Establish IV access:* IV access is important in nearly every patient with an abdominal complaint. Patients may not physically be capable of eating or drinking or holding down oral medications. They frequently need hydration and IV medications. Additionally, any hemodynamically unstable patient or actively bleeding patient will need two large-bore IVs for

fluids and potentially blood transfusions. If the EDT is unable to establish an IV using surface anatomy, ultrasound guidance may be needed.

4. *Help the patient into a gown:* Patients should be asked to get undressed and into a gown when they are roomed. Gowning is important so that the whole body can be visualized during physical examination. Patients may need help getting undressed and putting on the gown the correct way, with the gown open in the back. The exception is that patients who are presenting after sexual assault and may need forensic examination should be asked to remain in their clothing.

5. *Discourage eating and drinking:* Every patient with an abdominal complaint should be presumed to be nil per os (NPO), meaning they should not be allowed to eat or drink. If a patient whose evaluation is pending asks for food or water, it is safest to advise them to wait until their evaluation is complete. Eating or drinking may delay potential operative care, as an empty stomach is desirable for anesthesia induction. Once an emergency has been ruled out, offering the patient food after physician agreement and ensuring they can keep it down may be an important factor in deciding whether it is safe to discharge the patient. Patients who are unable to hold down fluids are not safe to go home because they risk dehydration.

6. *Know where critical equipment is located in the ED:* EDTs may be asked to bring certain items to a patient's room. The EDT should familiarize themselves ahead of time with where supplies are kept and the names of important pieces of equipment. For example, one specialized piece of equipment that may be required in the event of a critical upper GI bleed caused by esophageal varices is a *Blakemore tube.* The Blakemore tube is a special kind of tube that is inserted into a patient's esophagus and inflated with water in order to compress (tamponade) the bleeding esophageal varices (see Fig. 11.5). Though used rarely, they may be a necessity in a critical situation.

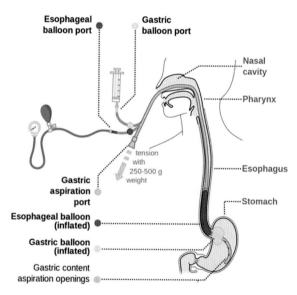

Fig. 11.5 Labeled schematic of the Blakemore tube used in the emergency department to mitigate esophageal bleeding. (From "File:Sengstaken-Blakemore scheme EN.svg" by Olek Remesz (wiki-pl: Orem, commons: Orem) is licensed with CC BY-SA 3.0. To view a copy of this license, visit https://creativecommons.org/licenses/by-sa/3.0.)

7. *Know how to get to other critical areas of the hospital:* In the setting of sudden blood loss, as in a traumatic accident or during a GI bleed, the EDT may need to be the person who physically runs to the blood bank to retrieve the blood needed for an emergency transfusion. Many hospitals in the United States have a tube system to send lab specimens from the rest of the hospital to the laboratory. However, be aware that there are also some special lab specimens that may need to be physically walked down to the laboratory for testing. In some cases, specialized pieces of equipment may not be readily stocked in the ED, and the EDT may be required to obtain it from another unit.

8. *Point-of-care testing:* Point-of-care testing includes rapid blood or urine tests performed at the bedside rather than in the hospital's lab. EDTs will be asked to perform point-of-care tests after obtaining the specimen. Point-of-care tests are described in further detail in Chapter 7.

9. *Transferring and positioning patients:* When an EDT rooms a patient, it is important to ensure that a patient can transfer into bed safely. If a patient is very unwell, they may need to be lifted into the bed or assisted very closely to avoid a fall. A vomiting patient's bed should be positioned with the head of the bed up so the patient does not aspirate while reclining. A patient with a low blood pressure may benefit from lying flat or in the legs-up, head-down position known as the *Trendelenburg position.* Blankets and sheets provide comfort. Give patients with nausea an emesis bag to keep at their bedside. For those who may have difficulty or safety issues getting out of bed, leaving a bedside urinal or a bedside commode is also important.

10. *Ensure privacy, dignity, and safety:* Try to ensure privacy when helping a patient into a gown. Patients who will need a genital or rectal examination should be in a private room with a door whenever possible. When doing sensitive exams, the clinician should ideally also have a third-party chaperone present. Always maintain a nonjudgmental attitude toward whatever complaint the patient comes in with so that they will be reassured they will be treated with respect and dignity.

References for Additional Reading

Macaluso CR, McNamara RM. Evaluation and management of acute abdominal pain in the emergency department. *Int J Gen Med.* 2012;5:789–797.

Silverio L. Abdominal Pain [Internet]. Available from: https://www.saem.org/about-saem/academies-interest-groups-affiliates2/cdem/for-students/online-education/m4-curriculum/group-m4-approach-to/approach-to-abdominal-pain.

O'Brien MC. In: Tintinalli JE, Stapczynski J, Ma O, Yealy DM, Meckler GD, Cline DM. eds. Tintinalli's Emergency Medicine: A Comprehensive Study Guide, 8e. New York, NY: McGraw-Hill.

CHAPTER 12

Endocrinologic Emergencies

Colleen Roche ▓ Brandon Chaffay ▓ Cassidy Craig

The endocrine system is a complex, coordinated, and highly regulated system that helps the body adapt to its constantly changing metabolic needs. One major endocrine-related disease, diabetes mellitus, is frequently seen in the emergency department (ED) and will be reviewed in some detail.

Basic Structure of the Endocrine System

The endocrine system is an interrelated network that enables the body to regulate a series of parameters to maintain a constant internal milieu (homeostasis) (Fig. 12.1). The endocrine system relies on a series of *glands*. Glands are organized collections of cells located throughout the body that can both sense the levels of specific metabolites and secrete proteins, called *hormones*, into the bloodstream. Once released into the bloodstream, hormones circulate throughout the body and act on a variety of target organs. Under normal circumstances, the endocrine glands will either increase or decrease hormone secretion according to their own sensing mechanisms. By doing so, the endocrine system attempts to maintain specific set points for each regulated parameter. Disease occurs when the glands either secrete too much or too little hormone for the body's circumstances at that time.

Signaling

The underlying concept of the endocrine system, autoregulation, is centered on feedback response loops as depicted in Fig. 12.2. Regulation occurs via both positive and negative feedback loops that help maintain homeostasis. For many hormones, an area of the brain called the hypothalamus can sense the level of a given hormone. It can then up- or downregulate its secretion of a "releasing hormone" that acts on the pituitary, which in turn produces another series of hormones that directly regulates the hormone production of many of the endocrine glands scattered throughout the body. Having an elevated serum level of any hormone will generally inhibit its own secretion through a negative feedback loop to avoid an adverse response in peripheral tissues to excessively high hormone levels. Similarly, when levels of that hormone fall, the hypothalamus is triggered to stimulate the pituitary, which in turn secretes a hormone to stimulate the production of the target hormone, creating a positive feedback loop.

Another example of endocrinologic system regulation is when a pair of hormones exists that act in opposite ways. The best example of this is how the body regulates serum glucose levels. When the serum glucose starts to rise, as would happen after a meal, the pancreas will secrete insulin that facilitates the entry of glucose into muscles and fat cells and lowers the blood glucose level. During periods of fasting, blood sugar is maintained by the pancreatic secretion of a different hormone, glucagon, that stimulates release of glucose from storage sites in the liver and other organs.

Some common hormones and their functions are outlined in Table 12.1. The table displays common signs and symptoms of hormone imbalances that can be recognized in the ED. When viewing patients in the ED, some common features listed below require prompt recognition of classic features to allow for expedient management and to ensure these patients are on monitoring early with proper escalation of care.

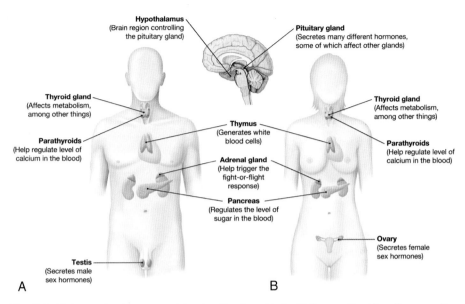

Fig. 12.1 **Major endocrine organs/glands.** (Courtesy Martin Hoffmann, Neu-Ulm, Germany. From Hombach-Klonisch S, Klonisch T, Peeler J. General anatomy. In: Hombach-Klonisch S, Klonisch T, Peeler J, eds. *Sobotta Clinical Atlas of Human Anatomy.* Elsevier; 2019:1–37.)

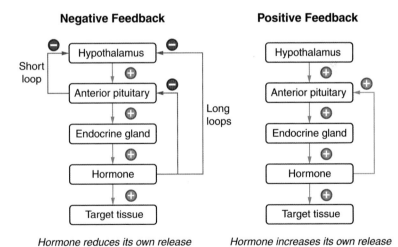

Fig. 12.2 Concept of feedback.

Diabetes

EPIDEMIOLOGY

Diabetes is a chronic illness that is increasing in prevalence both globally and in the United States, and it is the most frequent endocrine system disease seen in the ED. The World Health Organization estimates that the worldwide prevalence of diabetes in adults older than 18 years

TABLE 12.1 ■ Common Hormones Involved in Emergency Department Presentations and the
Consequences of High and Low Levels

Gland	Hormone	Main Functions	Too Much?	Too Little?
Adrenal	Aldosterone Corticosteroids	Regulates salt, water balance, and blood pressure	Hypertension Confusion Hyperglycemia Obesity	Hypotension Confusion Hypoglycemia
Pancreas	Insulin Glucagon	Regulates glucose levels	Hypoglycemia	Hyperglycemia
Parathyroid	Parathyroid hormone	Maintain calcium homeostasis	Kidney stones Abdominal pain Lethargy Confusion	Tingling Muscle aches Seizures Tetany
Pituitary	Multiple	Helps regulate the function of most of the endocrine glands		
Thyroid	Thyroid hormones (T3 and T4)	Regulates cellular metabolism	Tachycardia Tremors Confusion Hypertension Weight loss	Bradycardia Weight gain Lethargy

doubled between 1980 and 2014. In 2018, 10.5% of Americans (34 million) were diabetic, and as many as 88 million may have prediabetes. Diabetes was the seventh leading cause of death in the United States in 2017, with overall direct medical costs in 2018 at $327 billion. The main reasons for these increases are high-calorie, high-fat diets and lack of exercise.

ORGAN INVOLVEMENT AND BASIC PATHOPHYSIOLOGY

Patients with diabetes mellitus (*mellitus* means "sweet" in Latin) have chronically elevated levels of blood glucose that, over time, are toxic to a variety of tissues throughout the body. Major targets of elevated glucose are large and small blood vessels. Blood vessels are dynamic structures that are metabolically active and engaged in both allowing and impeding diffusion of a variety of substances into tissues. Elevated blood glucose levels damage these vessel walls, leading to a cascade of events that decreases the perfusion of and damages the organs that they serve. Organs most affected include the eyes, kidneys, extremities, heart, and the nervous system. Elevated blood glucose can lead to decreased nerve conduction and decreased sensation in the extremities. This alters a patient's perception of all types of pain, subjecting legs and feet to skin and joint damage that can lead to amputation. The major clinical consequences of diabetes are summarized in Table 12.2.

CATEGORIES OF DIABETES

There are two major types of diabetes that have different causes but the same results. For glucose to be used by most cells, it requires the presence of the hormone insulin that is secreted by the pancreas. Insulin stimulates specific receptors on the cell surface to permit the entry of glucose through cell membranes. Without insulin, these cells will not be able to use the glucose for energy, and blood glucose levels will rise. The main types of diabetes are as follows:
  ■ Type 1 diabetes mellitus (T1DM)
    ■ Occurs due to an autoimmune mechanism whereby a patient's own immune system attacks and destroys the pancreatic cells responsible for insulin production

TABLE 12.2 ■ **Major Systems Affected by Diabetes With the Involved Mechanism and Related Clinical Appearance**

Organ	Manifestation
Arteries	Peripheral vascular disease (blockages in large arteries)
Cardiovascular system	Coronary heart disease
	Hypertension
Immune system	Recurrent and chronic infections
Kidneys	Renal failure
	Dialysis
Limbs	Lower extremity ulcers that can lead to amputations
Nerves	Peripheral neuropathy
	Cranial nerve dysfunction
Retina	Vision loss

- Leads to an absolute lack of insulin; requires insulin to treat
- Insulin can be given by intermittent injections or with a pump that administers insulin continuously
- Most often first presents in children and adolescents
- Patients will be insulin dependent and are more prone to having complications such as diabetic ketoacidosis (DKA)
- Type 2 diabetes mellitus (T2DM)
    - Seen most frequently in adults with elevated body mass index (BMI)
    - Due to the patient's elevated weight, there is a need for higher insulin levels to maintain a normal blood sugar
    - Patients initially have elevated levels of blood sugar with elevated levels of insulin
    - Initially, it is most often treated with oral medications
    - Over time, insulin production may decline and the patient may then need to be treated with insulin
- Prediabetes mellitus
    - A blood test called hemoglobin A_{1C} provides physicians with an average of a person's blood sugar for about the prior 90 days. Elevated levels of this type of hemoglobin can indicate that the person is about to become diabetic even if their fasting blood sugars are still within the normal range.

ED-Specific Management

HYPOGLYCEMIA

Hypoglycemia (low blood sugar) can occur in diabetics taking insulin and with those taking certain types of oral antidiabetic medications. Severe hypoglycemia is a clinical diagnosis that is usually seen when the blood glucose level falls below 40 to 50 mg/dL. The symptoms of hypoglycemia can be quite varied, but they occur because the brain relies almost exclusively on glucose for its energy supply (many other tissues can use both fat and sugar for energy). The brain's manifestations of hypoglycemia are called neuroglycopenia. In most cases of hypoglycemia, the patient is confused; in severe cases, the patient may be completely unresponsive and/or perspiring heavily. At times, hypoglycemia can mimic a stroke or cause seizures. Because hypoglycemia can mimic virtually any behavioral or neurologic disturbance, blood sugar is measured on every ED patient with a major behavioral or neurologic disturbance. Fig. 12.3 outlines changes that can be seen in patients with hypoglycemia.

Early adrenergic symptoms	Neuroglycopenic signs
Pallor	Confusion
Diaphoresis	Slurred speech
Shakiness	Irrational or uncontrolled behavior
Hunger	Disorientation
Anxiety	Loss of consciousness
Irritability	Seizures
Headache	Pupillary sluggishness
Dizziness	Decreased response to noxious stimuli

Fig. 12.3 Outlining symptoms possibly exhibited by a hypoglycemic patient.

When patients present with the above symptoms, it is critically important to place them on a monitor and obtain a point-of-care glucose. The subsequent management depends on the mental status of the patient. If the hypoglycemic patient is awake enough to follow directions and swallow, it is appropriate to give the patient a cup of juice. Ingesting approximately 15 g of a rapid-acting carbohydrate for a child or adult or 0.2 g/kg for infants will raise blood glucose levels by approximately 50 to 60 mg/dL in 10 to 15 minutes. There are 15 g of glucose in 4 oz of orange or apple juice, 1 teaspoon of honey, or 2 tablespoons of raisins.

If the patient is unable to safely swallow, they should be given intravenous dextrose. Ideally, administer 0.2 g dextrose/kg body weight. For example, a 70-kg adult would require 14 g, which is approximately half the amount in an ampule of D50 (25 g in a 50-mL syringe). An alternative to intravenous dextrose is the administration of the hormone glucagon, which releases stored sugar from the liver to raise blood sugar. Dosing is based on weight; administer 0.5 mg if the patient weighs less than 25 kg and 1 mg if more than 25 kg. Additionally, glucagon can induce significant nausea. Ondansetron (Zofran) is commonly coadministered for symptomatic relief. Glucagon is not advised for patients with liver disease from ethanol use disorder as these patients often have lower liver stores of glycogen.

After an episode of hypoglycemia, the patient should be monitored for at least 1 hour to ensure that their blood sugar does not drop again. Persistent, recurrent hypoglycemic episodes may require hospitalization.

HYPERGLYCEMIA

The two most serious concerning ED presentations of hyperglycemia are DKA and hyperglycemic hyperosmolar state (HHS). Generally, HHS is seen in older diabetics with T2DM. It evolves gradually, usually as a result of the patient not taking their prescribed medications or having an occult infection. Over time, the blood glucose rises gradually, causing increased urination and ultimately severe dehydration. Diabetic ketoacidosis is often seen in younger patients with T1DM who either stop taking insulin or have an infection. In these patients, the lack of insulin causes a release of fatty acids from the body's fat stores, and the liver responds by metabolizing the fats into ketoacids, which makes the patient's breath smell like acetone. The pH of the blood drops, causing the patient to hyperventilate and often vomit. The EDT should be aware that the decrease in blood pH that occurs with DKA can cause excess potassium to enter the circulation from cells, which in turn can cause cardiac arrhythmias. Every suspected patient with DKA should be placed on a cardiac monitor. These patients will most frequently require fluids (normal saline or lactated Ringer solution), an insulin drip, potassium replacement, and intensive care unit admission.

References for Additional Reading

NaN. Diabetes Mellitus Type 2 in adults, 2022. [Accessed 16 May 2022].

NaN. Dover Anna, Zammitt Nicola The Endocrine System. MacLeod's Clinical Examination. Elsevier; 2018:193–209. 14th ed.

CHAPTER 13

Ear, Nose, and Throat and Ophthalmologic Emergencies

Eleanor Frye ■ Steven Davis ■ Kamilla Beisenova

Otorhinolaryngologic Emergencies

Otorhinolaryngologic emergencies include emergencies of the ear, nose, and throat (ENT), and ophthalmologic emergencies include emergencies of the eye. Injuries and illnesses related to these body parts are commonly seen in the emergency department (ED). ED staff must be proficient at rapidly recognizing these emergencies and initializing appropriate treatment while aiming to preserve function and to avoid complications.

Ear

OVERVIEW OF ANATOMY AND PHYSIOLOGY

The ear consists of the external ear, the middle ear, and the inner ear (Fig. 13.1). The external ear is made up of the auricle and the canal. The canal contains glands that produce cerumen (earwax). At the end of the canal is the tympanic membrane (eardrum), which is the transition between the external and middle ear. The middle ear is full of air and contains the ossicles (three bones: the malleus, incus, and stapes). It also contains the eustachian tube, which connects to the pharynx. The inner ear consists of the cochlea, the semicircular canals, and the distal end of the vestibulocochlear nerve (CN VIII). Behind and below the ear canal is the part of the temporal bone called the mastoid.

The hearing pathway is composed of two phases: the conductive phase and the sensorineural phase. During the conductive phase, sound vibrations from the outside environment are transmitted from the external ear through the canal to the middle ear, where the ossicles transform the vibrations into waves. Next, during the sensorineural hearing phase, the cochlea in the inner ear produces nerve impulses based upon these sound waves, which are then transmitted to the brain via the vestibulocochlear nerve (CN VIII).

The semicircular canals in the inner ear are responsible for helping the body maintain balance and know where it is in space. This information also is transmitted to the brain via the vestibulocochlear nerve (CN VIII).

COMMON EMERGENCY DEPARTMENT PRESENTATIONS

Sudden Sensorineural Hearing Loss

Sudden sensorineural hearing loss (SSNHL) occurs when a patient experiences significant hearing loss ($\geq 30\,$dB over three frequencies) within 72 hours. It can be caused by infection, trauma, or underlying disease, but in 60% to 90% of cases there is no underlying cause identified ("idiopathic SSNHL").

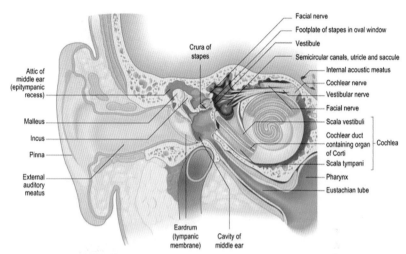

Fig. 13.1 Anatomy of the ear. (From Wareing MJ. Ear, nose and throat. In: Glynn M, Drake WM, eds. *Hutchison's Clinical Methods*. 24th ed. Elsevier; 2018:439-463.)

The first step in the assessment of these patients is to differentiate between unilateral and bilateral hearing loss. Bilateral hearing loss is rarer but has higher morbidity and mortality. A thorough history should be conducted, including asking about associated symptoms, trauma, barotrauma such as flying or scuba diving, and ototoxic medications. The physical examination should visualize the tympanic membrane, including cerumen removal if necessary, as well as a neurologic examination focused on cranial nerves and cerebellar testing. Tuning fork testing is used to help differentiate sensorineural versus conductive hearing loss.

Patients with SSNHL require emergent referral to ENT as well as audiology for formal hearing testing.

Cerumen Impaction

Cerumen is produced by glands in the ear canal and varies in color and consistency. It functions to aid in the turnover of dead skin cells in the canal, keep the canal clean and lubricated, and trap dirt and water. It can also help prevent infection. When cerumen builds up in the canal it can become impacted, which can sometimes be due to the makeup of the cerumen itself or to behavioral factors, such as using cotton swabs to clean the canal (Fig. 13.2A and B).

Patients with cerumen impaction may be asymptomatic or may present with a wide range of symptoms, including itching, ear pain, hearing loss, tinnitus, or dizziness. It also heightens the risk of infection.

If the patient is asymptomatic and the cerumen is not preventing adequate ear examination, it does not require routine removal. However, if the patient is symptomatic or the impaction is impeding assessment of the ear, it should be removed. Removal can be done using any combination of cerumen softening agents (such as liquid docusate or triethanolamine polypeptide), irrigation, or manual removal. Irrigation should not be performed if there is concern for tympanic membrane rupture, previous tympanic membrane surgery, or concern for retained battery in ear (typically from hearing aid). If these techniques are unsuccessful, the patient should be referred

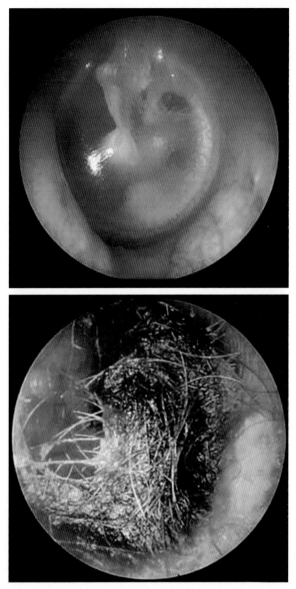

Fig. 13.2   Top: Normal ear canal and tympanic membrane. Bottom: Cerumen impacted ear canal. (A, from Wareing MJ. Ear, nose and throat. In: Glynn M, Drake WM, eds. *Hutchison's Clinical Methods*. 24th ed. Elsevier; 2018:439-463. B, from Swartz MH. The ear and nose. In: Swartz MH. *Textbook of Physical Diagnosis: History and Examination*. 8th ed. Elsevier; 2021:228-248.)

to a specialist. Patients should also be educated regarding proper ear hygiene to prevent recurrence, including avoidance of cotton swabs for cleaning the ears. The ear canals do not require additional cleaning, as they are naturally cleaned via epithelial migration that should suffice.

Ear Canal Irrigation

Equipment (Fig. 13.3)

1. An otoscope to visualize the external auditory canal
2. Water and a cerumen-softening agent (it is important to keep the temperature of the solution close to a patient's natural body temperature in order to avoid unnecessary discomfort such as dizziness)
3. A 30-mL or 60-mL syringe with a 16- or 18-gauge intravenous (IV) catheter attached to the syringe with the needle removed (the catheter should be cut shorter than the length of the canal to prevent inadvertent tympanic membrane injury)
4. Two basins (one to hold the irrigating solution and one to catch what flows out of the ear)
5. Face shield during the procedure for personal safety

Technique

1. Position the patient lying on one side with the target ear pointed up to the ceiling (Fig. 13.4).
2. Fill the ear canal with the cerumen softening agent and let it sit for 15 to 30 minutes before initiating irrigation. Drain the instilled agent into the waste basin.
3. Position the patient on their back with the waste basin under the target ear beside the patient's head (Fig. 13.5). Place an absorbent plastic-lined pad around the patient.
4. Fill up the second basin with warm water. Keep the solution close to human body temperature to avoid discomfort, dizziness, and nausea.
5. Use the syringe to draw up the solution from the basin and attach the IV catheter to the filled syringe.

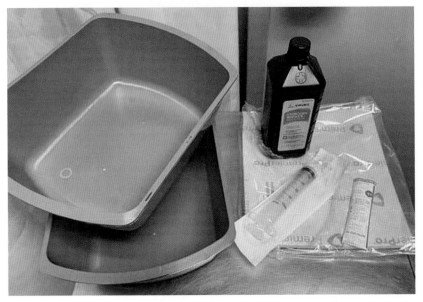

Fig. 13.3 Typical supplies for ear irrigation include water basin, 30-mL syringe, large-bore Angiocath (cut down to 1 in), absorbent pads, and hydrogen peroxide (if alternate solution to break down cerumen is not used).

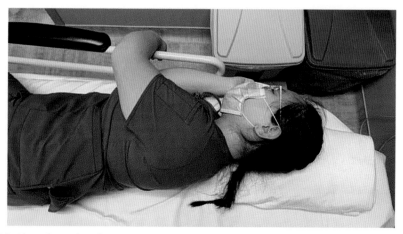

Fig. 13.4 Have the patient lie on the unaffected side with their head supported. Apply the hydrogen peroxide (or alternate solution) into the affected part canal and leave for 10 to 15 minutes or according to product directions.

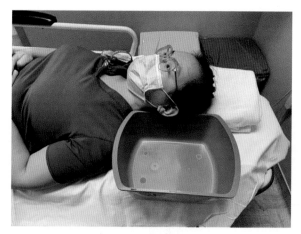

Fig. 13.5 Once you are ready to irrigate, position the patient's ear over an empty basin to collect the irrigant.

6. Position the IV catheter inside the ear canal with the tip aimed at the wall of the ear canal so as not to aim directly for the tympanic membrane, as this can cause perforation (Fig. 13.6).
7. Flush the ear as many times as necessary until no more cerumen comes out.
8. Dry the outer ear with gauze. Repeat the procedure on the second ear if needed.
9. If the ear irrigation was performed successfully, one should be able to visualize the tympanic membrane.

Ear Foreign Body

Foreign bodies in the ear are especially common in children; the most common foreign bodies found in the ear are beads, cotton tips, and insects. Most commonly, patients are asymptomatic

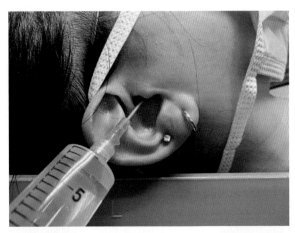

Fig. 13.6   Using a large-bore Angiocath catheter (cut down to 1-in length) and a 30-mL syringe, gently irrigate the canal, taking care not to touch the tympanic membrane with the catheter.

and are brought by the caregiver. Those with symptoms most commonly endorse otalgia, bleeding or drainage from the ear, tinnitus, hearing loss, or a sensation of fullness in the ear.

Foreign bodies should be removed by a medical provider as soon as possible, especially if there is obvious infection or if the object is a disk or button battery. If the foreign body is not tightly wedged in the canal, irrigation with warm water is often effective, but should never be performed if the object is a battery or may expand with water (such as a bean). Suction can also be used if the object is light. For more tightly wedged objects, tools such as an ear curette, wire loop, or hook under direct visualization through an otoscope can be used. Alligator forceps are especially useful for soft objects like cotton. If the foreign body is a live insect, it should be killed before removal by filling the canal with mineral oil or 2% lidocaine. If the patient is uncooperative, removal should be performed under procedural sedation, as sudden movement can cause damage to the middle ear. After removal, patients should be assessed for otitis externa, laceration or bruising of the ear canal, tympanic membrane perforation, and acute otitis media.

Otitis Externa

Acute *otitis externa* is inflammation of the ear canal (Fig. 13.7). It may also affect the tympanic membrane and/or pinna. Patients with acute otitis externa present with rapid onset of otalgia, ear itching, or a sensation of fullness in the ear and on examination have tenderness with movement or palpation of the external ear or swelling or redness of the canal. The most common bacterial causes are *Pseudomonas aeruginosa* or *Staphylococcus aureus*, so it is treated with topical antibiotics that cover those organisms. If the canal is swollen to the point of preventing effective administration of antibiotic ear drops, a Pope Oto-Wick should be placed. The wick will absorb the ear drops and deliver the antibiotic to hard-to-reach places.

Otitis Media

Otitis media is inflammation of the middle ear (Fig. 13.8). It is one of the most common diseases in children. It is often caused by pathogens coming from the nasopharynx into the middle ear through the eustachian tube during an upper respiratory infection (URI). Patients often present with acute ear pain, and associated cold symptoms and fever are also often seen. In preverbal children, pulling on the ear or excessive crying may be the primary presenting symptom, though

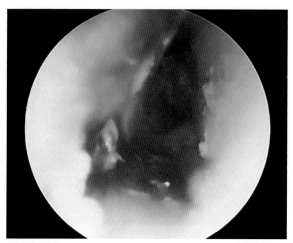

Fig. 13.7   Otitis externa. (From Chi DH, Tobey A. Otolaryngology. In: Zitelli BJ, McIntire SC, Nowalk AJ, Garrison J, eds. Zitelli and Davis' Atlas of Pediatric Physical Diagnosis. 8th ed. Elsevier; 2018:868-915.)

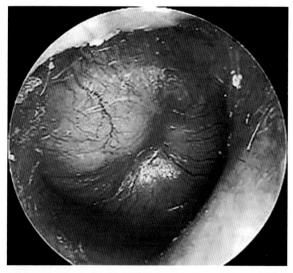

Fig. 13.8   Otitis media. (From Kerschner JE, Preciado D. Otitis media. In: Kleigman RM, Geme JW III, Blum NJ, Shah SS, Tasker RC, Wilson KM, eds. *Nelson Textbook of Pediatrics*. 21st ed. Elsevier; 2020:3418-3431.e1.)

this is nonspecific. The examination reveals a bulging red tympanic membrane. The first-line treatment is pain and fever control with acetaminophen and ibuprofen. Antibiotics are reserved for children younger than 2 years of age with bilateral infection and children with severe, persistent, or recurrent infection because, although routine use reduces the duration of symptoms, the risk of antibiotic resistance and adverse effects outweigh the benefits.

Mastoiditis

Mastoiditis is an infection of the mastoid bone of the skull and is a serious life-threatening complication of otitis media. It can lead to facial paralysis, meningitis, brain abscess, or other serious complications. Patients may present with ear pain with redness, swelling, pain, or fluctuance over the mastoid or behind the ear, or bulging of the external ear. CT imaging of the temporal bone with contrast should be performed. Historically, the mainstay of treatment was surgical mastoidectomy, but newer data supports starting with a conservative approach with IV antibiotics with or without myringotomy.

Nose

OVERVIEW OF ANATOMY AND PHYSIOLOGY

The upper part of the nose is made up of bone (the "bridge"), whereas the lower part is cartilage. On each side of the nose, air travels through the nares to the vestibule and then through the narrow passageway between the nasal septum and the turbinates into the nasopharynx. Turbinates are curved bony structures covered by a mucous membrane that extend into the nasal cavity (Fig. 13.9). The paranasal sinuses are cavities in the bones of the skull near and around the nose that are filled with air and drain into the nasal cavities

The nose has many functions. Through the olfactory system it sends signals to the brain to interpret different smells. It also cleanses, humidifies, and controls the temperature of the air we breathe in before delivering it to our lungs. Mucus produced by the nose works with the small hairs that line the nostrils to capture and filter dust, dirt, and other particles from the air as well.

COMMON EMERGENCY DEPARTMENT PRESENTATIONS

Nasal Foreign Body

Like with the ear, nasal foreign bodies are most often seen in pediatric patients. The most common nasal foreign bodies are those that children find around the house: beans, peanuts, and other foods;

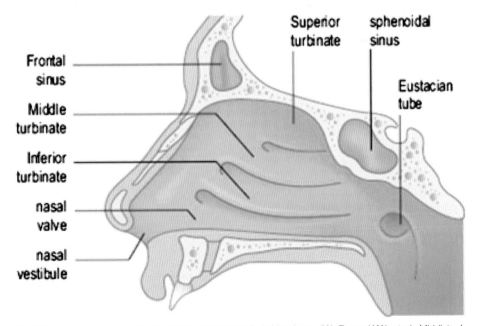

Fig. 13.9 Nasal anatomy. (Modified from Adkinson NF Jr, Yunginger JW, Busse WW, et al. *Middleton's Allergy Principles and Practice*. 6th ed. Mosby; 2003:1412.)

beads; parts of toys; pebbles; paper; and eraser tips. Most patients are brought in by a caregiver after inserting something into their nose. Symptoms may include nasal pain, unilateral purulent nasal discharge, epistaxis, voice change, or malodorous breath, though the vast majority of patients are asymptomatic. The object is usually located just below the inferior turbinate or in front of the middle turbinate and can usually be directly visualized on exam. It is important to take care during removal not to push the object farther back, as this can cause aspiration into the trachea leading to respiratory obstruction.

Depending on the type of object and cooperation of the patient, many different techniques for removal are available, including suction, air pressure, ear curettes, curved hooks, alligator or bayonet forceps, irrigation, glue, or balloon catheter. Pressure techniques ("blowing the nose") are preferred for cases in which there is no edema or infection to reduce the risk of pushing the object farther back during the procedure. For small children who will not blow their own noses, a caregiver may blow air into the child's mouth while occluding the unaffected nostril, forcing the object out of the nose via positive pressure. Another technique for creating pressure is to place oxygen tubing into the opposite nostril at 10 to 15 L/min (called the "Beamsley Blaster technique"). If suction is used, placing a piece of soft plastic tubing over the end of the suction tip can increase success.

Epistaxis

Epistaxis is bleeding from the nose. Causes of epistaxis may include trauma, inflammation, drugs, and structural or hematologic reasons. Bleeding may be from an anterior or posterior source. Anterior bleeding is more common, occurs at Kiesselbach's plexus, and generally presents as visible bleeding from the nose (Fig. 13.10). Posterior bleeding occurs at the sphenopalatine artery and is typically more brisk, difficult to control, and can have less obvious presentations such as nausea, hematemesis, anemia, hemoptysis, or melena. Posterior bleeding is an emergency and can be life threatening. If the patient is hemodynamically unstable, gain vascular access and initiate IV fluid resuscitation immediately.

Epistaxis Management

The first step of epistaxis management is direct pressure with compression of the nostrils for at least 5 minutes and up to 20 minutes and should be initiated immediately (Fig. 13.11).

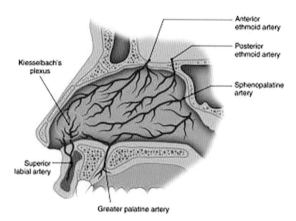

Fig. 13.10 Nasal vasculature. (From Krulewitz NA, Fix ML. Epistaxis. *Emerg Med Clin N Am*. 37(1);2019: 29-39. Courtesy Christy Krames, Austin, Texas.)

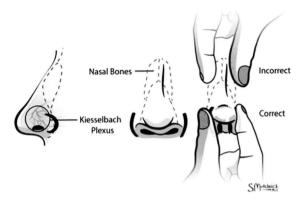

Fig. 13.11 Epistaxis control. (From Svider P, Arianpour K, Mutchnick S. Management of epistaxis in children and adolescents. *Pediat Clin N Am.* 65(3);2018:607-621.)

Ask the patient to pinch the nostrils with a gauze sponge while tilting their head slightly forward to prevent blood from collecting in the posterior pharynx. Gauze or cotton that has been soaked in a topical decongestant (such as oxymetazoline [Afrin], phenylephrine, or 4% cocaine solution) should be inserted into the affected nostril for vasoconstriction. If the bleeding does not respond to these techniques, the source of the bleeding should be identified via direct visualization. If an anterior source is visualized, chemical cautery (silver nitrate) or electrocautery can be applied directly onto the bleeding site for about 30 seconds. Packing the cavity with a hemostatic agent such as Gelfoam or Surgicel may also be effective. If these treatments fail, the anterior nasal cavity should be packed with nonadherent ribbon gauze or a preformed balloon device for up to 5 days. Packing increases risk of septal hematoma or abscess from trauma induced during packing, sinusitis, neurogenic syncope, pressure necrosis, and toxic shock syndrome, so it should be reserved for use after other techniques have failed. Posterior bleeding often requires consultation with ENT and is usually controlled via balloon device or posterior packing. ENT consultation may also be appropriate for refractory or unstable bleeding. The EDT can independently perform nostril compression; as for the remaining procedures, the EDT can only assist in the process.

Throat

OVERVIEW OF ANATOMY AND PHYSIOLOGY

Within the mouth, the gingiva connects to the teeth and the maxilla or mandible. The teeth are numbered 1 to 32, and each has an invisible root within its socket. The tongue sits in the midline with the submandibular glands beneath it. The roof of the mouth is composed of the hard palate (anteriorly) and the soft palate (posteriorly). The pharynx is visible behind the soft palate and tongue, the uvula hangs above it, and the tonsils sit on either side (Fig. 13.12).

COMMON EMERGENCY DEPARTMENT PRESENTATIONS

Pharyngitis

Pharyngitis is sore throat caused by inflammation of the pharynx and the surrounding tissues due to viral, bacterial, or fungal infection. Viral infections are most common and are self-limiting,

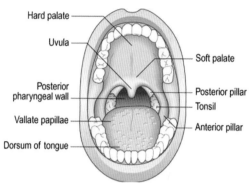

Fig. 13.12   Oral anatomy. (From Hathorn I. The ear, nose and throat. In: Innes JA, Dover AR, Fairhurst K, eds. *Macleod's Clinical Examination*. 14th ed. Elsevier; 2018:171-191.)

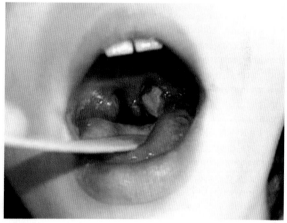

Fig. 13.13   Exudative pharyngitis. (From Kullar P, Yates PD. Infections and foreign bodies in ENT. *Surgery.* 33(12);2015:593-599.)

whereas bacterial infection is commonly caused by *Streptococcus pyogenes* (group A beta-hemolytic streptococci [GABHS]) and requires antibiotic treatment to avoid complications including rheumatic fever and a rare kidney disease called poststreptococcal glomerulonephritis. The cause of infection is often differentiated by history and physical examination findings. Patients with viral infection often present with concurrent URI symptoms and have enlarged tonsils and pharyngeal redness on examination. For those with viral infection, symptomatic treatment is first line, including lozenges, pain-relieving medications, rest, and hydration. In contrast, bacterial infection often does not present with cough or other URI symptoms, and on physical examination patients often have exudates on their tonsils as well as enlarged lymph nodes (Fig. 13.13). A rapid antigen detection test (RADT) is standard for detection of GABHS in the pharynx. The Modified CENTOR Criteria is a scoring system that helps calculate the likelihood of streptococcal pharyngitis and determine the need for strep testing and antibiotic treatment. Generally, testing of patients of 3 years or younger is not recommended as their likelihood of developing a GABHS infection is very low.

Criteria	Points
C—Cough absent	1 point
E—Exudative or swollen tonsils	1 point
N—Swollen and tender anterior cervical lymph nodes	1 point
T—Temperature ≥100.4°F	1 point
O—Often young (age 3–14y)	1 point
R—Rarely old (age ≥45y)	Subtract 1 point

Total Points	Likelihood of GABHS	Action
0–1	(0) 1%–2.5% (1) 5%–10%	No testing indicated
2–3	(2) 11%–17% (3) 28%–35%	Testing indicated
4	51%–53%	Treat without testing

False-negative test results are possible; therefore, if the RADT is negative, a formal throat culture should be sent.

Peritonsillar and Retropharyngeal Abscess

A peritonsillar abscess is the most common deep space infection of the head and neck in adults. It is usually caused by a mixture of different bacteria, starting as a tonsillar cellulitis and subsequently forming an abscess. The abscess forms between the palatine tonsil and the capsule that surrounds it. Prompt recognition and treatment is paramount to avoid complications including airway obstruction, aspiration, and extension of the infection into surrounding muscles, deep tissues of the neck, and neurologic and vascular structures. In addition to sore throat (which is usually unilateral), patients often present with fever, dysphagia, trismus, and a muffled voice. On physical examination the patient's tonsil will be displaced inferiorly and medially, and classically the uvula will be deviated to the opposite side. Imaging with ultrasound or CT is usually indicated to differentiate a peritonsillar abscess from other diagnoses. Treatment of a peritonsillar abscess includes incision and drainage and antibiotic therapy.

Retropharyngeal abscesses are less common than peritonsillar abscesses but potentially more life-threatening as the swelling can promptly lead to sudden airway obstruction. They typically occur in children under 5 years of age but can occur in any patient. Classically, the patient's neck is hyperextended, and they may be in respiratory distress. X-ray imaging of the lateral neck can aid in diagnosis, and a CT scan is the most helpful imaging modality. Emergent airway management and surgical intervention are vital to avoid complications including spread of infection, airway obstruction, and erosion into major vessels.

Pharyngeal Foreign Body

Foreign bodies, such as fish bones, can become lodged in the throat after swallowing. Unlike with ear and nose foreign bodies, which are often asymptomatic, patients presenting with a foreign body in their throat often complain of feeling like they can still feel "something in the throat" when swallowing, which is sometimes painful. The patient may drool or choke or spit up after ingestion of food or liquid as well. They may also complain of difficulty breathing, coughing, or wheezing, which may indicate that the object has been aspirated into the tracheobronchial tree, and a chest x-ray or chest CT scan should be performed. Pharyngeal foreign bodies can lead to partial or complete airway obstruction, and if this is the case, intervention with laryngoscopy for removal is indicated.

Angioedema

Angioedema is swelling of the skin and/or mucous membrane of the respiratory and gastrointestinal tracts (Fig. 13.14). It is sometimes due to an allergic hypersensitivity reaction, and other times it is caused by dilation of blood vessels due to hereditary or drug-induced factors. Allergic angioedema is often accompanied by urticaria or systemic anaphylaxis and typically occurs 1 to 2 hours after exposure to an allergen. Angiotensin-converting enzyme (ACE) inhibitors, a class of anti-hypertensive medications, and nonsteroidal antiinflamatory drugs (NSAIDs) are more common causes of drug related angioedema. If the patient's airway is compromised, emergent cricothyroidotomy may be indicated, as endotracheal intubation is often unable to be performed due to swelling. Epinephrine, diphenhydramine, and IV steroids have also been used for management, but no controlled study has supported their efficacy.

Common ED Technician Procedure: Airway Suctioning

Airway suctioning is performed when a patient is not able to effectively move secretions in the respiratory tract. Suctioning helps prevent airway occlusion and aspiration of secretions into the lungs. It also improves visualization during airway procedures including endotracheal intubation.

Equipment

1. An oxygen source and suction device (Fig. 13.15)
2. A suction container to collect the secretions (Fig. 13.16)
3. A sterile hard suction catheter (Yankauer) (see Fig. 13.16)
4. Tubing to connect the catheter to the container (see Fig. 13.16)

Technique

1. Attach the container to the suction port on the wall.
2. Attach one end of the tubing to the opening in the container on the wall and the other end to the hard catheter. Make sure the rest of the openings in the container are closed.
3. Turn on the wall suction and use the catheter tip to suction the patient's mouth for secretions. Note that posterior suctioning can elicit a gag reflex. The patient can be allowed to hold the suction and suction their own mouth if they are capable.
4. Suctioning should be performed for no longer than 15 seconds for each attempt, and the patient should have some time to recover (10–15 seconds) in between attempts.

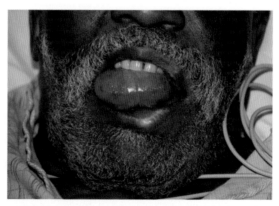

Fig. 13.14 **Angioedema.** (From Gorski EM, Schmidt MJ. Orolingual angioedema with alteplase administration for treatment of acute ischemic stroke. *J Emerg Med*. 45(1);2013:e25-e26.)

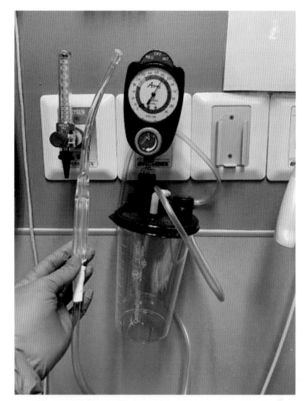

Fig. 13.15 Yankauer suction tip connected to suction canister and wall unit.

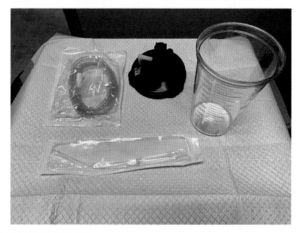

Fig. 13.16 Individual suction supplies.

The Eye

The ED receives patients with eye conditions ranging from minor annoyances to those that threaten vision if not promptly addressed.

ANATOMY AND FUNCTION

The eye is composed of a globe (the "eyeball") (Fig. 13.17); its corresponding arteries, veins, nerves, lymphatics, and muscles; a cushioning fat pad behind the globe; and the bony orbit (the "eye socket") that surrounds these structures and physically isolates them from the remainder of the face (see Fig. 13.17). The globe is a spherical structure responsible for initial processing of light into neural impulses that the brain interprets as visual images. Similar in design to a camera, the front-facing structures first focus incoming light that structures within the globe can process as images in focus. The most anterior component to the globe, the cornea, is a clear membrane. Directly behind the cornea sits the iris, which functions like the aperture of a camera to let in varying amounts of light to adjust for both the brightness of the ambient environment and the distance from the viewed object. Behind the iris rests the lens, which focuses light onto the deeper globe structures. The space between the cornea and the lens is filled with a water-like nutrient bath (aqueous humor) that provides an energy and electrolyte source for the otherwise avascular cornea and lens. Behind the lens sits the vitreous, a translucent gelatinous cavity that comprises roughly 80% of the globe's volume. Behind the vitreous rests the retina, which is composed of light-sensitive cells and neurons that receive and transmit incoming light to the brain. The entire globe, except for the cornea, is coated by the sclera (the "white of the eye"), a strong elastic membrane that maintains the shape of the globe.

Globe structures in front of the vitreous comprise the anterior segment of the globe. Injury or illness to these structures is often associated with eye pain and with some degree of vision

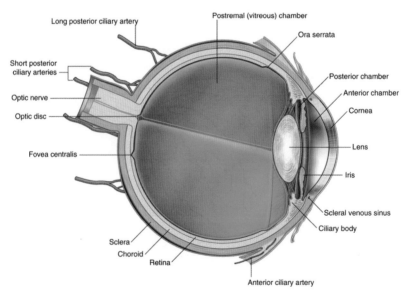

Fig. 13.17 Eye anatomy. (From Drake R, Vogl AW, Mitchell AWM. Head and neck. In: Drake R, Vogl AW, Mitchell AWM, eds. *Gray's Anatomy for Students*. 4th ed. Elsevier;2020:823-1121.e4.)

loss. Injury or illness to the posterior segment of the globe (behind the lens) is often painless and presents with vision loss alone.

Within the bony orbit of the eye, the globe rests on a cushioning posterior fat pad and is suspended and moved by six separate ocular muscles that insert directly into the sclera from the orbital wall. The arteries, veins, nerves, and lymphatics of the eye pass from deep within the skull through a small opening in the back of the orbit and directly into the back of the globe. In front of the globe are two eyelids that may close to protect the globe; these secrete a protective lubricating liquid onto the surface of the cornea.

Injuries or illnesses that affect the eye may involve one or many of the structures above.

THE "EYE ROOM"

Most EDs have a designated room in which patients with eye problems are examined. The room often has a chair that can be raised and lowered as needed and a locked cabinet in which supplies needed for patients with eye complaints are kept. Some of the devices and products with which the EDT should be familiar are as follows:

1. The *slit lamp* is a specialized piece of equipment with which the provider can examine the external portion of the eye, including the cornea and the anterior chamber (Fig. 13.18). The EDT should be aware that the lamp's movable stage should be in the "locked" position between patients and should know how to clean the slit lamp between patients.

2. The *hand-held tonometer* is a device that measures the pressure in the anterior chamber of the eye (Fig. 13.19). Elevated pressures are seen in glaucoma, a disease that affects the production and resorption of aqueous humor, and acute elevations can lead to vision loss (Fig. 13.19). EDTs should be aware of the purpose of this device and how it is cleaned between patients. As the tip touches the cornea, there is often a disposable cover that is placed over the sensor during the examination. There are several brands and designs of tonometers, including those integrated into the mechanism of the slit lamp.

3. *Rust ring remover:* If a piece of metal embeds in the cornea, metal ions can diffuse from the foreign body leaving a metallic stain, called a rust ring, on the otherwise clear corneal surface. The metal is toxic to corneal healing and can impair vision, so it should be removed. Many EDs have a dental burr with a sterile tip that is often referred to as a "rust ring remover" (Fig. 13.20). The EDT should be familiar with where it is stored and how the burr is sterilized.

4. *Fluorescein strip paper:* Fluorescein is a water-soluble, fluorescent dye that is used topically to help diagnose problems of the cornea. Most EDs have small paper strips containing the fluorescein, which are often wetted by the provider and touched to the patient's conjunctiva, distributing the dye over the whole corneal surface (Fig. 13.21). When a blue light from the slit lamp is shined on the cornea, any irregularities or areas of inflammation or trauma fluoresce and can be more easily seen with the slit lamp.

5. *Local anesthetic:* Local anesthetic drops (tetracaine or proparacaine) provide the patient with tremendous relief in painful corneal problems such as corneal abrasions. Many ophthalmologists believe that excessive use of the local anesthetic can impair healing of the abrasion. These drops should never be left in the room and the patient should never be discharged with these local anesthetic drops to go.

INITIAL APPROACH TO THE PATIENT WITH AN EYE PROBLEM

When the EDT is confronted by a patient with an eye issue, they should determine if the patient has a traumatic injury. If eye trauma is part of a multisystem trauma, it is likely that stabilizing the other areas would take precedence over the eye treatment.

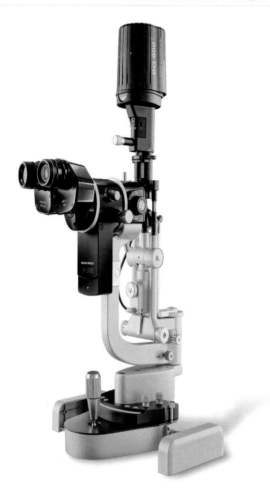

Fig. 13.18   **Slit lamp.** (From: BM 900, Haag-Streit, Mason, OH.)

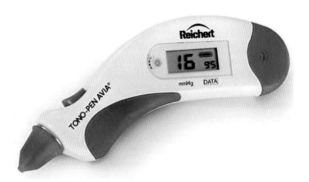

Fig. 13.19   **One type of tonometer.** (Reichert Inc, Tono-Pen AVIA®)

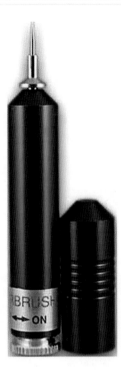

Fig. 13.20   Burr device.

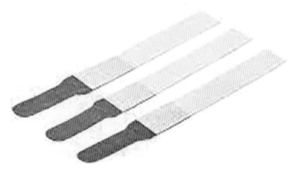

Fig. 13.21   Fluorescein strips.

The major three mechanisms of trauma are blunt, penetrating, and caustic. If the mechanism was either blunt or penetrating, the affected eye should be covered with a metal eye shield that should be taped in place, securing the shield to the bony structures surrounding the orbit (Fig. 13.22). The shield should remain in place until the medical provider sees the patient. If no metal eye shield is available, the EDT can fashion a makeshift shield as shown in Fig. 13.23. The patient should be put in a quiet, dark room with the head of the bed elevated while awaiting the ophthalmologist. The traumatized eye should not be examined or manipulated by the EDT, as there is the potential to worsen the injury if the patient sustained a ruptured globe from the trauma.

In the case of potentially caustic substances contaminating the eye, the EDT may have to initiate potential sight-saving treatment on their own if a physician or nurse is not immediately

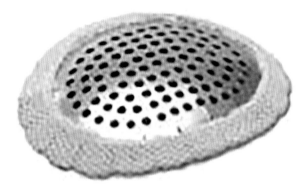

Fig. 13.22   Metal eye shield.

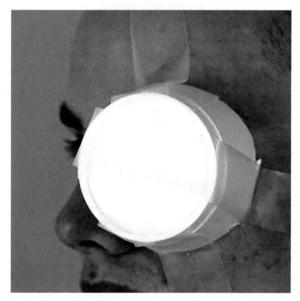

Fig. 13.23   **Makeshift eye shield.** (From: Knoop KJ, Dennis WR. Chapter 62: Ophthalmologic Procedures. In: Roberts JR, Custalow CB, eds. *Roberts and Hedges' Clinical Procedures in Emergency Medicine and Acute Care*, 7th edn. Elsevier;2019:1295-1337.e2.)

available. In this case, copious and continuous irrigation of the eye is the priority. To prevent any delays in management, start with tap water and shift to Lactated Ringers (LR) IV solution as soon as possible. Normal saline (0.9% sodium chloride solution) can be used if LR is not available. The IV fluids can be dripped into the eye through a normal IV administration setup as illustrated (Fig. 13.24).

Another irrigation technique is to use a commercially available product called a Morgan Lens, which is inserted under both eyelids and permits continuous irrigation without the need for a provider to stand by the bedside (Fig. 13.25).

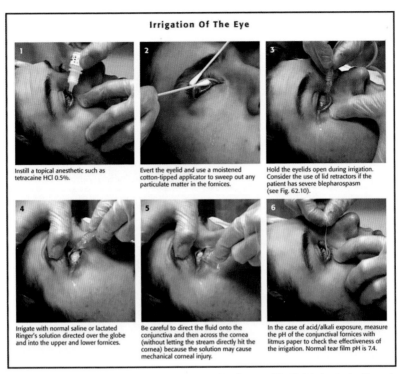

Irrigation Of The Eye

1 Instill a topical anesthetic such as tetracaine HCl 0.5%.	**2** Evert the eyelid and use a moistened cotton-tipped applicator to sweep out any particulate matter in the fornices.	**3** Hold the eyelids open during irrigation. Consider the use of lid retractors if the patient has severe blepharospasm (see Fig. 62.10).
4 Irrigate with normal saline or lactated Ringer's solution directed over the globe and into the upper and lower fornices.	**5** Be careful to direct the fluid onto the conjunctiva and then across the cornea (without letting the stream directly hit the cornea) because the solution may cause mechanical corneal injury.	**6** In the case of acid/alkali exposure, measure the pH of the conjunctival fornices with litmus paper to check the effectiveness of the irrigation. Normal tear film pH is 7.4.

Fig. 13.24   Eye irrigation. (From: Knoop KJ, Dennis WR. Chapter 62: Ophthalmologic Procedures. In: Roberts JR, Custalow CB, eds. *Roberts and Hedges' Clinical Procedures in Emergency Medicine and Acute Care*, 7th edn. Elsevier;2019:1295-1337.e2.)

COMMON EMERGENCY DEPARTMENT PRESENTATIONS

The Red Eye and the Eyelid

Many patients arrive complaining of a red eye, and the EDT should be aware of some of the more common etiologies.

1. *Subconjunctival hemorrhage:* These occur suddenly when a small vessel leaks blood and may be caused by the patient straining or vomiting (Fig. 13.26). The patient's vision is entirely normal, and the anatomy of the eye means that the hemorrhage will be contained over the sclera and will not impair the patient's vision by extending to the cornea. There is no specific treatment needed, and the hemorrhage will resorb over several weeks. As the blood can be rather dense, patients become very anxious about the potential for vision loss and need to be reassured.

2. *Conjunctivitis:* This is caused by inflammation or infection of the conjunctiva, a thin membrane covering both the underside of the eyelids and the surface of the visible sclera (Fig. 13.27). Conjunctivitis may result from allergic reactions, from viral or bacterial infections, or from minor trauma. In all causes of conjunctivitis, the conjunctival capillaries dilate, resulting in the visible reddened appearance of both the visible sclera and the underside of the eyelids. The EDT should be very careful when helping the provider with a patient suspected of having conjunctivitis, as many of its infectious causes are quite contagious.

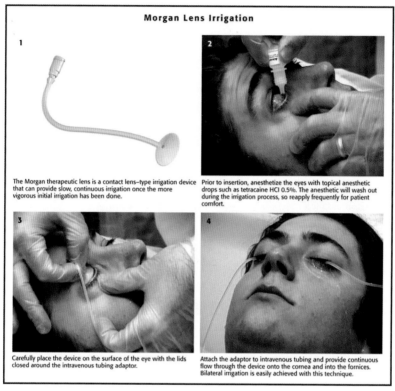

Morgan Lens Irrigation

The Morgan therapeutic lens is a contact lens–type irrigation device that can provide slow, continuous irrigation once the more vigorous initial irrigation has been done.

Prior to insertion, anesthetize the eyes with topical anesthetic drops such as tetracaine HCl 0.5%. The anesthetic will wash out during the irrigation process, so reapply frequently for patient comfort.

Carefully place the device on the surface of the eye with the lids closed around the intravenous tubing adaptor.

Attach the adaptor to intravenous tubing and provide continuous flow through the device onto the cornea and into the fornices. Bilateral irrigation is easily achieved with this technique.

Fig. 13.25 **Morgan lens eye irrigation.** (From: Knoop KJ, Dennis WR. Chapter 62: Ophthalmologic Procedures. In: Roberts JR, Custalow CB, eds. *Roberts and Hedges' Clinical Procedures in Emergency Medicine and Acute Care*, 7th edn. Elsevier;2019:1295-1337.e2.)

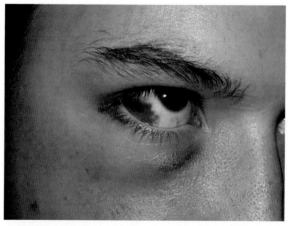

Fig. 13.26 **Subconjunctival hemorrhage.** (From Rutter P. Ophthalmology. In: Rutter P. *Community Pharmacy*. 5th ed. Elsevier; 2021:55-77.)

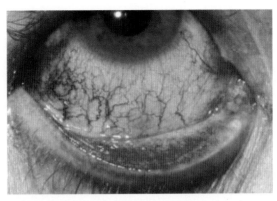

Fig. 13.27   Viral conjunctivitis. (From Mahmood AR, Narang AT. Diagnosis and management of the acute red eye. *Emerg Med Clin N Am.* 2008;26(1):35-55.)

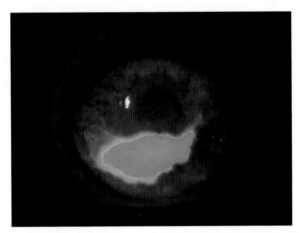

Fig. 13.28   Corneal abrasion with fluorescein uptake on slit lamp examination with blue light. (From Hoffman RS. Corneal abrasion. In: *Ferri's Clinical Advisor 2022.* Elsevier; 2022:446.e2-446.e3.)

Decontamination of the room and equiptment by the ED technician following patient care is essential to preventing spread of infection.

3. *Acute glaucoma:* The patient with a sudden increase in intraoccular pressure may have an intensely painful red eye with vision loss. The patient may describe seeing "halos." The pupil will often be dilated and the cornea is cloudy. This is a true emergency requiring prompt treatment to prevent vision loss. The EDT should be aware of this emergent condition and expedite the patient's care.

4. *Corneal abrasion:* Perhaps the most frequent cause of a painful, red eye seen in ED practice is the corneal abrasion that occurs from direct mechanical trauma to the cornea. At times this can be seen when directly inspecting the cornea, but it is best seen through a slit lamp after applying fluorescein to the cornea and using the blue light to bring on the fluorescence (Fig. 13.28). Most of these abrasions heal on their own. The patients are often treated with

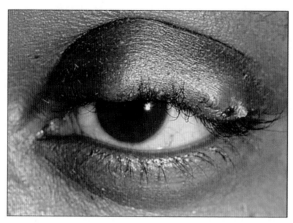

Fig. 13.29   **External hordeolum (lateral lid) and chalazion (medial lid).** (From Neff AG, Chahal HS, Carter KD. Benign eyelid lesions. In: Yanoff M, Duker JS, eds. *Ophthalmology*. 5th ed. Elsevier; 2019:1293-1303.e1.)

topical anesthetic aplication in the ED, antibiotic drops or ointment, and a mild oral pain reliever to go.

5. *Stye:* A stye (or *hordeolum*) is a painful, red, localized swelling of either the upper or lower eyelid and may be seen either on the outside or inside of the lid (Fig. 13.29). This is the result of an infection that was initiated by a blocked hair follicle or eyelid gland. Treatment is usually topical antibiotics and moist warm compresses. Occasionally, the provider will puncture a pustule and drain the infection.

Sudden Loss of Vision

A patient who complains of sudden vision loss is generally considered to be a medical emergency. Painful vision loss can occur with trauma, glaucoma, or any severe condition affecting the cornea. Painless vision loss may occur in a stroke (there will be partial loss of vision in each eye) or an embolus to the artery that supplies the eye (loss of vision in the affected eye only). A tear (detachment) of the retina will usually cause only a partial vision loss and may be associated with sparkling lights. Regardless of the cause, an acute complete or partial loss of vision generally represents a potentially serious situation, and the patient needs prompt evaluation.

TRAUMATIC EMERGENCIES

Hyphema

A hyphema is blood in the anterior chamber (between the cornea and the iris) (Fig. 13.30). Depending on the severity of the trauma, blood may obscure the iris either partially or completely. Treatment is usually conservative but merits specialty evaluation in the ED.

Ruptured Globe

Globe rupture describes a traumatic tear or puncture of the outermost coating of the globe and may involve either the sclera, cornea, or both. Puncture injuries to the sclera or cornea may allow globe contents to leak (in the case of aqueous or vitreous humor) or herniate (in the case of solid internal globe structures) through the traumatic defect. This can lead to a very bizarre-looking pupil (Fig. 13.31).

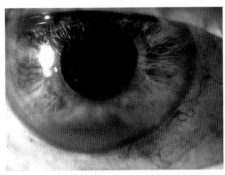

Fig. 13.30 Hyphema. (From Salmon JF. Trauma. In: Salmon JF. Kanski's *Clinical Ophthalmology*. 9th ed. Elsevier; 2020:891-916.)

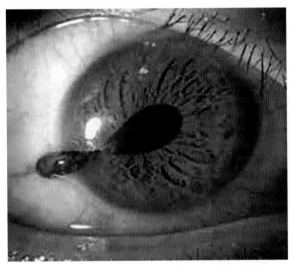

Fig. 13.31 Corneoscleral laceration with iris prolapse and pointed pupil (points in direction of globe injury).

Globe ruptures also increase the potential for globe infection. Whereas very small globe ruptures may fully recover following appropriate treatment, larger globe ruptures are commonly associated with devastating visual loss. Due to the traumatic mechanism of globe ruptures, associated injuries involving the head and body are commonly encountered and may obscure early recognition of eye injuries. Therefore a high index of suspicion for globe rupture is necessary when triaging a patient with facial injuries or trauma, particularly those involving small, high-speed projectiles. Patients with globe rupture may report ocular pain or vision loss, though some patients may have minimal symptoms.

Emergent management of globe rupture requires rapid diagnosis and emergent management by an ophthalmologist.

Retrobulbar Hematoma

Retrobulbar hematoma describes a collection of blood within the bony orbit and behind the globe. Frequently the result of blunt or penetrating trauma, retrobulbar hematomas may also occur in patients with bleeding disorders. Regardless of the inciting event, retrobulbar hematomas may displace the globe forward as the hematoma expands and compress the globe itself, the optic nerve, and the ophthalmic vessels. Without treatment, retrobulbar hematomas can result in permanent vision loss. If this diagnosis is suspected, a bedside procedure (called a *lateral canthotomy*) performed by the emergency provider or ophthalmologist may be needed to relieve the pressure on the eyeball.

Orbital Fracture

Orbital fractures involve the fused facial bones that form the eye socket and house the globe. Other structures such as the extraocular muscles; arteries, veins, nerves, and lymphatics; and the retroorbital fat pad can also be affected by the fracture. Orbital fractures frequently result from high-energy blunt or penetrating trauma, often with associated injury to intraorbital structures (including the globe), the adjacent facial sinuses, and the nose. In some cases, intraorbital structures may herniate through an orbital fracture and into adjacent sinuses, leading to impaired eye movements and double vision.

VISUAL ACUITY

Visual acuity is a measurement of the effectiveness of discriminating two stimuli that are presented in high contrast to the background, giving a basic idea of how well a patient can see. Typically, this test is performed by asking the patient to differentiate letters of different sizes to determine the smallest letters the patient can read on a standardized chart, also known as the *Snellen chart*. Visual acuity charts designed for pediatrics, non-English speakers, or illiterate patients use common shapes or a shape facing different directions instead of letters. Normal vision is described as 20/20 on the chart. The numerator stands for the distance in feet that the patient is from the chart, whereas the denominator stands for the distance from which a patient with normal eyesight can read the letters on the chart. Patients who are unable to read the top line when wearing corrective lenses are termed "legally blind" in the United States.   When recording visual acuity, indentify the eye tested by using OD (oculus dexter) to indicate the right eye, OS (oculus sinister) to indicate the left eye, and OU (oculus uterque) to indicate both eyes. For example, OS 20/40 means that the smallest line of shapes or letters that the patient was able to read with the left eye was the line with the fraction 20/40.

TECHNIQUE

1. Make sure that the room and the Snellen chart are both well illuminated.
2. Stand the patient 20 feet away directly in front of the chart. Depending on the patient's complaint, the patient may keep their glasses on or contacts in (Fig. 13.32).
3. Have the patient cover the unaffected eye and read the letters starting from the top of the chart with the affected eye. Record the fraction listed by the lowest line of letters that the patient was able to read correctly (Fig. 13.33).
4. Have the patient cover the affected eye and, in the same manner, read the letters with unaffected eye. Record the fraction.
5. Have the patient repeat the process with both eyes uncovered and record the fraction. Document all three fraction measurements in the patient's chart.

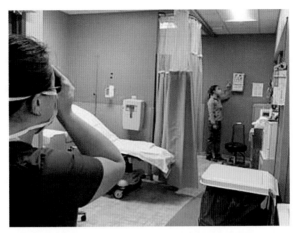

Fig. 13.32   The patient should be positioned 20 feet from the Snellen chart.

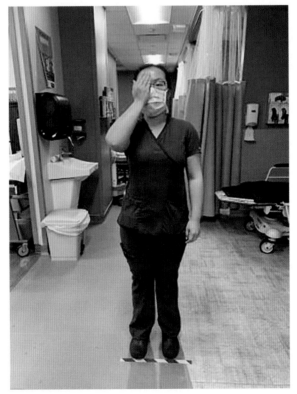

Fig. 13.33   While testing visual acuity, test each eye individually by asking the patient to cover one eye and read the Snellen chart, repeat with the other eye, and then repeat with both eyes uncovered.

References for Additional Reading

Agostoni A, Cicardi M. Drug-induced angioedema without urticaria. *Drug Safety.* 2001;24(8):599–606. https://doi.org/10.2165/00002018-200124080-00004.

Alberti PW. Epithelial migration on the tympanic membrane. *J Laryngol Otol.* 1964;78:808–830. https://doi.org/10.1017/s0022215100062800.

Awad AH, ElTaher M. ENT foreign bodies: an experience. *Int Arch Otorhinolaryngol.* 2018;22(2):146–151. https://doi.org/10.1055/s-0037-1603922.

Azzam D, Ronquillo Y. Snellen chart. StatPearls. Updated June 10, 2020. Accessed June 7, 2022. https://www.ncbi.nlm.nih.gov/books/NBK558961/.

Bas M, Hoffmann TK, Kojda G. Evaluation and management of angioedema of the head and neck. *Curr Opin Otolaryngol Head Neck Surg.* 2006;14(3):170–175. https://doi.org/10.1097/01.moo.0000193202.8 5837.7d.

Beck R, Sorge M, Schneider A, Dietz A. Current approaches to epistaxis treatment in primary and secondary care. *Dtsch Arztebl Int.* 2018;115(1-02):12–22. https://doi.org/10.3238/arztebl.2018.0012.

Bequignon E, Vérillaud B, Robard L, et al. Guidelines of the French Society of Otorhinolaryngology (SFORL). First-line treatment of epistaxis in adults. *Eur Ann Otorhinolaryngol Head Neck Dis.* 2017;134(3):185–189. https://doi.org/10.1016/j.anorl.2016.09.008.

Bickley L, Szilagyi P, Bates B. *Bates' Guide to Physical Examination and History-Taking.* 11th ed. Wolters Kluwer Health/Lippincott Williams & Wilkins; 2013:232–234.

Bickley L, Szilagyi P, Bates B. *Bates' Guide to Physical Examination and History-Taking.* 11th ed. Wolters Kluwer Health/Lippincott Williams & Wilkins; 2013:238–239.

Bickley L, Szilagyi P, Bates B. *Bates' Guide to Physical Examination and History-Taking.* 11th ed. Wolters Kluwer Health/Lippincott Williams & Wilkins; 2013:242–244.

Buttaravoli P, Leffler S. *Minor Emergencies.* Elsevier Saunders; 2012:108–111.

Buttaravoli P, Leffler S. *Minor Emergencies.* Elsevier Saunders; 2012:113–114.

Buttaravoli P, Leffler S. *Minor Emergencies.* Elsevier Saunders; 2012:119–120.

Chandrasekhar SS, Tsai Do BS, Schwartz SR, et al. Clinical practice guideline: sudden hearing loss (update). *Otolaryngol Head Neck Surg.* 2019;161(suppl 1):S1–S45. https://doi.org/10.1177/0194599819859885.

Cheng AW, Mitchell Z, Foote J. Can you hear me? Sudden sensorineural hearing loss in the emergency department. *Can Fam Physician.* 2014;60(10):907–e477.

Cohen EG, Soliman AM. Changing trends in angioedema. *Ann Otol Rhinol Laryngol.* 2001;110(8):701–706. https://doi.org/10.1177/000348940111000801.

Diamond L. Managing epistaxis. *JAAPA.* 2014;27(11):35–39. https://doi.org/10.1097/01.JAA.0000455643.58683.26.

Falcon-Chevere JL, Giraldez L, Rivera-Rivera JO, Suero-Salvador T. Critical ENT skills and procedures in the emergency department. *Emerg Med Clin North Am.* 2013;31(1):29–58. https://doi.org/10.1016/j.emc.2012.09.010.

Fasunla J, Ibekwe T, Adeosun A. Preventable risks in the management of aural foreign bodies in western Nigeria. *Internet J Otorhinolaryngology.* 2006:7. https://doi.org/10.5580/18fe.

Fine A, Nizet V, Mandl K. Large-scale validation of the Centor and McIsaac scores to predict group A streptococcal pharyngitis. *Arch Intern Med.* 2012;172(11):847–852.

Foden N, Mehta N, Joseph T. Sudden onset hearing loss—causes, investigations and management. *Aust Fam Physician.* 2013;42(9):641–644.

Galioto NJ. Peritonsillar abscess. *Am Fam Physician.* 2017;95(8):501–506.

Goldenberg D, Golz A, Joachims HZ. Retropharyngeal abscess: a clinical review. *J Laryngol Otol.* 1997;111(6):546–550. https://doi.org/10.1017/s0022215100137879.

Goldstein E, Gottlieb MA. Foreign bodies in nasal fossae of children. *Oral Surg Oral Med Oral Pathol.* 1973;36(3):446–447. https://doi.org/10.1016/0030-4220(73)90225-9.

Grossman E, Messerli FH, Neutel JM. Angiotensin II receptor blockers: equal or preferred substitutes for ACE inhibitors? *Arch Intern Med.* 2000;160(13):1905–1911. https://doi.org/10.1001/archinte.160.13.1905. Published correction appears in *Arch Intern Med.* 2001;161(2):300.

Guest JF, Greener MJ, Robinson AC, Smith AF. Impacted cerumen: composition, production, epidemiology and management. *QJM.* 2004;97(8):477–488. https://doi.org/10.1093/qjmed/hch082.

Hartmann RW. Recognition of retropharyngeal abscess in children. *Am Fam Physician.* 1992;46(1):193–196.

Heim SW, Maughan KL. Foreign bodies in the ear, nose, and throat. *Am Fam Physician*. 2007;76(8):1185–1189.

Hoffmann JF. An algorithm for the initial management of nasal trauma. *Facial Plast Surg*. 2015;31(3):183–193. https://doi.org/10.1055/s-0035-1555618.

Kalan A, Tariq M. Foreign bodies in the nasal cavities: a comprehensive review of the aetiology, diagnostic pointers, and therapeutic measures. *Postgrad Med J*. 2000;76(898):484–487. https://doi.org/10.1136/pmj.76.898.484.

Kaplan AP, Greaves MW. Angioedema. *J Am Acad Dermatol*. 2005;53(3):373–392. https://doi.org/10.1016/j.jaad.2004.09.032.

Kniestedt C, Stamper RL. Visual acuity and its measurement. *Ophthalmol Clin North Am*. 2003;16(2):155–170. https://doi.org/10.1016/s0896-1549(03)00013-0.

Kucik CJ, Clenney T. Management of epistaxis. *Am Fam Physician*. 2005;71(2):305–311.

Kulthanan K, Jiamton S, Boochangkool K, Jongjarearnprasert K. Angioedema: clinical and etiological aspects. *Clin Dev Immunol*. 2007;2007:26438. https://doi.org/10.1155/2007/26438.

Laulajainen Hongisto A, Jero J, Markkola A, Saat R, Aarnisalo AA. Severe acute otitis media and acute mastoiditis in adults. *J Int Adv Otol*. 2016;12(3):224–230. https://doi.org/10.5152/iao.2016.2620.

Lee SS, Schwartz RH, Bahadori RS. Retropharyngeal abscess: epiglottitis of the new millennium. *J Pediatr*. 2001;138(3):435–437. https://doi.org/10.1067/mpd.2001.111275.

Mondin V, Rinaldo A, Ferlito A. Management of nasal bone fractures. *Am J Otolaryngol*. 2005;26(3):181–185. https://doi.org/10.1016/j.amjoto.2004.11.006.

Ngo A, Ng KC, Sim TP. Otorhinolaryngeal foreign bodies in children presenting to the emergency department. *Singapore Med J*. 2005;46(4):172–178.

Obringer E, Chen JL. Acute mastoiditis caused by *Streptococcus pneumoniae*. *Pediatr Ann*. 2016;45(5):e176–e179. https://doi.org/10.3928/00904481-20160328-01.

Pasrija D, Hall CA. Airway suctioning. StatPearls. Updated June 2, 2020. Accessed June 7, 2022. https://www.ncbi.nlm.nih.gov/books/NBK557386/.

Rosenfeld RM, Schwartz SR, Cannon CR, et al. Clinical practice guideline: acute otitis externa. *Otolaryngol Head Neck Surg*. 2014;150(suppl 1):S1–S24. https://doi.org/10.1177/0194599813517083. Published correction appears in *Otolaryngol Head Neck Surg*. 2014;150(3):504.

Sara SA, Teh BM, Friedland P. Bilateral sudden sensorineural hearing loss: review. *J Laryngol Otol*. 2014;128(suppl 1):S8–S15. https://doi.org/10.1017/S002221511300306X.

Schilder AG, Chonmaitree T, Cripps AW, et al. Otitis media. *Nat Rev Dis Primers*. 2016;2(1):16063. https://doi.org/10.1038/nrdp.2016.63.

Schumann JA, Toscano ML, Pfleghaar N. Ear irrigation. StatPearls. Updated September 25, 2020. Accessed June 7, 2022. https://www.ncbi.nlm.nih.gov/books/NBK459335/.

Schwartz SR, Magit AE, Rosenfeld RM, et al. Clinical practice guideline (update): earwax (cerumen impaction). *Otolaryngol Head Neck Surg*. 2017;156(suppl 1):S1–S29. https://doi.org/10.1177/0194599816671491. Published correction appears in *Otolaryngol Head Neck Surg*. 2017;157(3):539.

Steyer TE. Peritonsillar abscess: diagnosis and treatment. *Am Fam Physician*. 2002;65(1):93–96. Published correction appears in *Am Fam Physician*. 2002;66(1):30.

Tamir S, Shwartz Y, Peleg U, Shaul C, Perez R, Sichel JY. Shifting trends: mastoiditis from a surgical to a medical disease. *Am J Otolaryngol*. 2010;31(6):467–471. https://doi.org/10.1016/j.amjoto.2009.06.003.

CHAPTER 14

Stroke and Neurologic Emergencies

David Yamane ▪ Sarah Hocutt ▪ Aileen Chowdhury

Introduction

The term *stroke* refers to a spectrum of conditions affecting the brain's vasculature that can lead to sudden brain tissue compromise and ultimately brain tissue death. An acute stroke is an emergency in which early intervention can significantly improve outcome. The emergency department (ED) technician (EDT) plays a crucial role in the multidisciplinary response to stroke recognition and treatment.

There are 17 million new stroke cases worldwide annually. Strokes are the fifth-leading cause of death in the United States and the second-leading cause of death worldwide. The stroke mortality rate has been declining over recent years due to treatment advances, but as mortality has dropped, more patients are living with stroke-related disabilities.

A stroke may be:

- Thrombotic: a clot occurs at the site of arterial wall damage (50%).
- Embolic: a clot formed at a distant site travels from that site, impacting an artery supplying the brain (30%).
- Hemorrhagic: an artery bleeds into brain tissue, disrupting the function in the area of the bleed (20%).

Thrombotic and embolic strokes are described as "ischemic" strokes. This means that they occur from lack of blood flow to the area downstream from the blockage. The focus of treatment in these strokes is to restore the blood flow as quickly as possible. By documenting the patterns of dysfunction on the clinical examination, the provider can often infer the location of the blood vessel blockage.

Initial Assessment and Triage

An important role of the EDT is to help the treatment team with the early recognition and response to strokes. Although most stroke patients arrive by ambulance, many will arrive unannounced.

The most common recognizable signs of an acute stroke are described by the acronym FAST (Table 14.1). There are, however, multiple other findings of a stroke not covered by the FAST evaluation, including loss of vision, inability to speak (aphasia), and confusion. A severe headache associated with stroke-like findings suggests a hemorrhagic stroke. Any concerns that a patient is having a stroke should be raised to the nurse or provider, following the hospital's stroke protocol. Though these protocols vary among hospitals, they will facilitate rapid brain imaging and neurologic evaluation.

An example of a stroke protocol is shown in Fig. 14.1.

TABLE 14.1 ■ FAST Symptoms

F	Facial droop: Ask the patient to smile. If one side droops lower than the other, start to think that the patient is having a stroke.
A	Arm drifting: Ask the patient to raise their arms. If one arm drifts lower, again, recognize that this is a potential stoke. Dizziness, loss of balance, and one-sided weakness are commonly associated with stroke.
S	Speech: If speech is slurred or confused, you must rule out stroke vs. altered mental status.
T	Time: Time is brain cells. The longer it takes to get this patient treated, the more brain cells will die, resulting in potential hemiparesis or hemisensory loss.

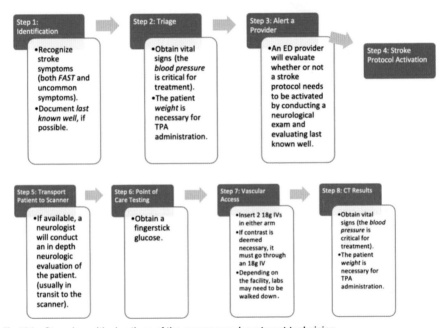

Fig. 14.1   Stepwise critical actions of the emergency department technician.

Ischemic Stroke

Approximately 700,000 US patients experience an acute ischemic stroke annually. The overall mortality of acute ischemic strokes is 15%, but severe strokes have a 75% mortality. Half of patients who experience an ischemic stroke will have a permanent disability, such as weakness or speech difficulties, and will be dependent on others for care.

Ischemic strokes are most often a result of atherosclerosis (plaques of fatty materials on the inside of blood vessel walls). When one of these plaques fissures, an acute clot at that site can form that will compromise flow to downstream tissue. The symptoms and examination findings of a stroke patient vary with the clot's location and the area of the brain it supplies. Brain tissue deprived of blood ceases to function normally, and the physician's physical examination will document the patient's deficits and allow the physician to determine where the clot is located even before seeing damage documented on the brain computed tomography (CT) scan (Fig. 14.2).

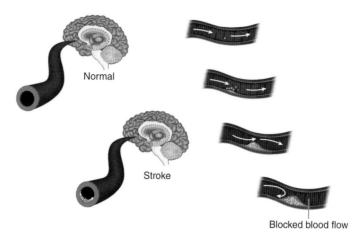

Fig. 14.2 Atherosclerotic plaque causing an ischemic stroke.

Hemorrhagic Stroke

Hemorrhagic strokes are caused by bleeding into the brain or spinal fluid. Although hemorrhagic strokes only comprise about 20% of all strokes, they are more lethal, with a mortality rate of 30% to 55% in the first month.

The major causes of hemorrhagic strokes are from vessel malformations, excessively elevated blood pressures, or tumors. There are two major types of vessel malformations: intracranial aneurysms (ICAs) or arteriovenous malformations (AVMs). An ICA is an outpouching or "ballooning" of the blood vessel, making it prone to rupture. It accounts for 80% of bleeding around the brain; its major risk factors are smoking, high blood pressure, and family history. An AVM is a disorganized collection of arteries and veins that are also prone to bleed (Fig. 14.3). Extremely elevated blood pressures can put excess pressure on the vessels of the brain, causing bleeding into the brain. Tumors in the brain may have weakened blood vessels, making them prone to bleeding as well.

Diagnosis

The diagnosis of an acute stroke is complicated by the fact that many patients with prior strokes present with new symptoms that could either represent an acute new stroke or an exacerbation of their prior stroke symptoms caused by another disease process. Table 14.2 outlines conditions that could mimic an acute stroke. After completing a history and careful neurologic examination, the physician will order a noncontrast brain scan (i.e., CT)

CT can be done rapidly and will identify all hemorrhagic strokes (Fig. 14.4); it may confirm the diagnosis of an acute stroke by demonstrating areas of tissue death within the brain, though an entirely normal CT is often seen early in an ischemic stroke. Magnetic resonance (MR) imaging is a more accurate test for an acute stroke and will likely supplant a CT scan in future years if MR can approach the speed of a CT, which is not yet possible in most settings (Fig. 14.5A–C).

A CT angiogram (CTA) utilizes contrast dye during a CT to highlight the vasculature of the brain. This can affirmatively document the large vessel blockages that cause an ischemic stroke, which may be amenable to therapeutic interventions. In hemorrhagic strokes a CTA can help identify abnormal vasculature that is the cause of the bleed (see Fig. 14.5D).

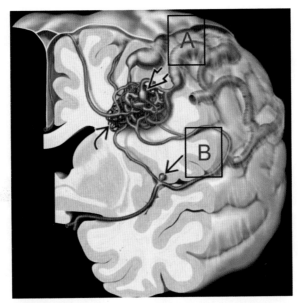

Fig. 14.3 **Vascular malformations causing hemorrhagic strokes.** *(A)* Arteriovenous malformation. *(B)* Intracranial aneurysm. (https://www.clinicalkey.com/#!/search/Digre%20Kathleen%20B./%7B%22type% 22:%22author%22%7D. Imaging in Neurology:117–117.)

TABLE 14.2 ■ **Stroke Mimics**

Hypoglycemia/hyperglycemia
Electrolyte abnormalities (i.e., low sodium)
Brain abscess
Brain tumor
Meningitis/encephalitis
Multiple sclerosis
Seizure with Todd paralysis
Exacerbation of a previous stroke
Ingestions/intoxication
Syncope
Neuromuscular disorders
Generalized weakness due to other conditions (anemia, cardiovascular disease, infection)

LABORATORY TESTING

Laboratory tests should be performed rapidly, but waiting for results should not delay treatment. As mentioned, it is important to rapidly bring the blood samples to the laboratory. Depending on the facility, some may require that blood samples be walked down to the laboratory.

The importance of various laboratory tests is explained below in Table 14.3.

Treatment

Ischemic stroke is the main focus of time-dependent treatment, as the faster that blood flow can be restored, the fewer cells will die ("time is brain"). It is estimated that 2 million brain cells can

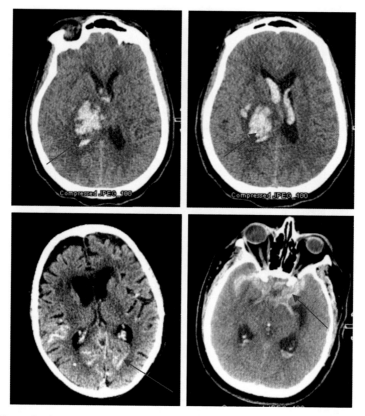

Fig. 14.4 Hemorrhagic strokes shown on noncontrast head computed tomography scans.

die every minute in patients with acute ischemic strokes. The two ways that blood flow can be restored are as follows:

- Administration of an intravenous (IV) drug (tissue plasminogen activator [TPA]) that helps the body break down clots
- Mechanical clot breakdown or removal through interventional neuroradiologic techniques

The management of hemorrhagic stroke is multifaceted, with goals of slowing down the bleeding and preventing complications that can arise.

TISSUE PLASMINOGEN ACTIVATOR

TPA has been the mainstay of ischemic stroke treatment since 1995. It has been shown to improve outcomes if given within 4.5 hours of a stroke's onset. If given too late in a stroke, TPA will be less effective for clot breakdown and will increase the chance that an ischemic stroke will convert to a hemorrhagic stroke, thereby increasing the amount of brain tissue damage. Thus the establishment of the time of the stroke's onset is of paramount importance in the ED for the safe administration of TPA.

Because TPA is administered intravenously, establishing timely IV access is one of the crucial jobs of the EDT.

Other contraindications for TPA treatment of stroke include the following:

- Blood pressures above 185/110 mm Hg that cannot be lowered in the ED with treatment
- Patients with an established bleeding disorder

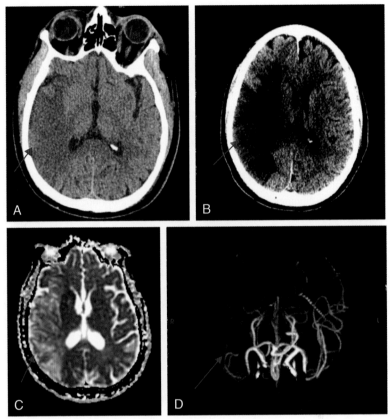

Fig. 14.5 Imaging modalities of an acute ischemic stroke. (A) Noncontrast computed tomography (CT) scan demonstrating early signs of an acute ischemic stroke. (B) Repeat noncontrast CT a couple of days later, demonstrating the evolution of a completed stroke on CT. (C) Magnetic resonance diffusion-weighted imaging, demonstrating an acute ischemic stroke. (D) Three-dimensional reconstruction of a CT angiogram, demonstrating an acute obstruction of the blood vessel causing an acute stroke.

TABLE 14.3 ■ Important Diagnostic Laboratory Testing for Stroke Patients

Point-of-care glucose	Rule out low sugar as a cause for neurologic symptoms.
Point-of-care creatinine	Determine kidney function. Necessary for contrast administration for imaging studies.
CBC	Evaluate platelet levels for TPA administration.
Electrolytes	Evaluate for other causes of neurologic changes (i.e., low sodium). Evaluates renal function with serum creatinine.
PT/INR, PTT	Helps determine anticoagulation use, a contraindication to TPA and must be reversed in hemorrhagic strokes.
Urine analysis	Evaluate for infections that can be causing neurologic symptoms.
Urine toxicology screen	Determine if drugs/alcohol are causing apparent neurologic symptoms.
ECG	Evaluate for arrhythmias such as atrial fibrillation (a potential cause of ischemic strokes).

CBC, Complete blood cell count; *ECG,* electrocardiogram; *INR,* international normalized ratio; *PT,* prothrombin time; *PTT,* partial thromboplastin time; *TPA,* tissue plasminogen activator.

- Patients who have had recent head trauma or certain surgeries
- Patients with existing brain tumors, aneurysms, or other anomalies

The EDT plays a pivotal role in obtaining IV access so that clinicians may provide rapidly acting medications to lower the blood pressure and ensure close monitoring and control of the patient's vital signs. Close monitoring of the post-TPA patient's neurologic status should be done by the nursing staff, and any abrupt changes should be brought to the attention of the treating team immediately.

Although many laboratory tests are important to the patient's care, only a head CT is necessary to start TPA treatment if there are no signs of hemorrhagic stroke. Administration of TPA should generally not be delayed pending laboratory test results.

MECHANICAL THROMBECTOMY

Recent advances in technology have created newer therapeutic options for stroke patients and lengthened the treatment window, the time between "last known well" and treatment. Mechanical thrombectomy is performed by a neurointerventionalist who passes an intraarterial catheter from a puncture site into the arteries in the brain. They then remove the occluding thrombus and can potentially restore blood flow to the brain (Fig. 14.6). Mechanical clot removal can be used in conjunction with TPA but has shown benefits after the 4.5-hour TPA window, making it an option for patients who are ineligible for TPA. Only certain hospitals will have the equipment and personnel to provide this level of sophisticated care, which are identified as "comprehensive stroke centers" by the Joint Commission.

Hemorrhagic Stroke Treatment

BLOOD PRESSURE MANAGEMENT

Many patients with a hemorrhagic stroke may have severely elevated blood pressure on initial assessment, and lowering the blood pressure to a specified goal (typically a systolic blood pressure of <140) will help decrease brain bleeding.

PROCEDURES

Once stabilized, the patient may be taken to the operating room or interventional radiology for a procedure to treat the source of the bleeding. These procedures may include coiling or clipping of an aneurysm or a craniotomy, in which part of the skull is removed to aspirate blood and remove clots (Fig. 14.7).

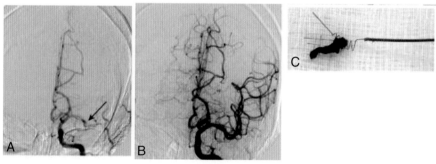

Fig. 14.6 Example of a mechanical thrombectomy with restoration of blood flow. (Grotta J, Albers G, Broderick J, et al., eds. *Stroke: Pathophysiology, Diagnosis, and Management.* 6th ed. Elsevier; 2016.)

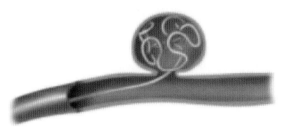

Fig. 14.7 Coiling of an intracerebral aneurysm to prevent further bleeding. (Wright I. Cerebral aneurysm—treatment and perioperative nursing care. *AORN J.* 2007;85(6):1172–1186.)

DISPOSITION

Given the high mortality and necessity of specialized care, stroke patients should be admitted for close monitoring to dedicated stroke units or neurologic intensive care units. For free-standing EDs or hospitals without a specialized stroke unit, the patients may be transferred to a regional stroke center. The EDT should ensure close monitoring until patients are transported to their specialized stroke unit and should facilitate rapid transfer of these patients.

Conclusion

Acute stroke (both ischemic and hemorrhagic) carries a significant risk of morbidity and mortality, and the EDT is instrumental in facilitating timely evaluation and management of this neurologic emergency. Some key points to keep in mind when caring for a potential stroke patient include the following:

- "Time is brain." Early diagnosis and initiation of treatment can make the difference between life, death, or long-term disability.
- Do not hesitate to escalate your concerns for a possible stroke to the nurses or providers.
- Rule out stroke mimics (such as hypoglycemia) as soon as possible.
- Transport the patient to CT as quickly as possible for brain imaging to differentiate between ischemic and hemorrhagic strokes.

References for Additional Reading

Albers GW, Marks MP, Kemp S, et al. Thrombectomy for stroke at 6 to 16 hours with selection by perfusion imaging. *N Engl J Med.* 2018;378(8):708–718.

Brott T, Bogousslavsky J. Treatment of acute ischemic stroke. *N Engl J Med.* 2000;343(10):710–722.

Campbell BCV. Thrombolysis and thrombectomy for acute ischemic stroke: strengths and synergies. *Semin Thromb Hemost.* 2017;43(2):185–190.

Guzik A, Bushnell C. Stroke epidemiology and risk factor management. *Continuum (Minneap Minn).* 2017;23 (1, Cerebrovascular Disease):15–39.

Hankey GJ. Stroke. *Lancet.* 2017;389(10069):641–654.

Hemphill JC, Greenberg S, Anderson CS, et al. Guidelines for the management of spontaneous intracerebral hemorrhage. *Stroke.* 2015;46(7):2032–2060.

Ko S, Choi H, Lee K. Clinical syndromes and management of intracerebral hemorrhage. *Curr Atheroscler Rep.* 2012;14(4):307–313.

Nogueira RG, Jadhav AP, Haussen DC, et al. Thrombectomy 6 to 24 hours after stroke with a mismatch between deficit and infarct. *N Engl J Med.* 2018;378(1):11–21.

Powers WJ. Acute ischemic stroke. *N Engl J Med.* 2020;383(3):252–260.

Ragoschke-Schumm A, Walter S. DAWN and DEFUSE-3 trials: is time still important? *Radiologe.* 2018;58 (suppl 1):20–23.

Tromp G, Weinsheimer S, Ronkainen A, Kuivaniemi H. Molecular basis and genetic predisposition to intracranial aneurysm. *Ann Med.* 2014;46(8):597–606.

Wechsler LR. Intravenous thrombolytic therapy for acute ischemic stroke. *N Engl J Med.* 2011;364(22): 2138–2146.

CHAPTER 15

Vascular Access

Michael West ▪ Natalia Monsalve ▪ Claudia Ranniger

Introduction

Peripheral vascular access is an important emergency department (ED) technician (EDT) responsibility that involves cannulation of a peripheral vein for blood sample collection or medication, fluid, or contrast administration. The placement of an indwelling venous catheter allows the clinician to obtain multiple blood samples over time, avoiding the need for repeat sticks. Butterfly needles are most frequently used for single-time blood draws where the likelihood of ongoing sample collection is low. The scope of practice for EDTs varies from hospital to hospital, with some hospitals allowing techs to draw blood only through a butterfly needle. EDT's should work within their scope of practice for their institution that will follow the regulations for their location.

Common sites to obtain intravenous (IV) access include the antecubital fossa (commonly called the AC), the back of the hand, the wrist, and the forearm. Knowing the anatomy of the arm and where larger vessels are expected to be located is helpful in identifying viable spots for access (Fig. 15.1).

Needle through catheter devices come in different diameters (gauges) and lengths. Most devices in adults are 19 to 45 mm long, with the length increasing as the gauge decreases. Larger gauges permit increased flow but may be hard to place in smaller veins. Catheter diameter decreases as its gauge number increases. In most practice settings, gauges range from 14 gauge (largest) to 24 gauge (smallest).

Various products are available for both indwelling needles and butterfly needles. The EDT should be familiar with their institution's products, as each product may have unique features, such as an autoretracting needle, a needle guard, or a permanent needle. All of the IV products will have universal color code for needle gauge (Fig. 15.2). Finally, some institutions allow for placement of IVs under ultrasound guidance after completing additional training. Consult Chapter 16 of this manual for details of ultrasound-guided IV access.

Patient Triage and Assessment

INDICATIONS

The most common indications in the ED for IV access are the need for medication administration and obtaining blood for lab testin. As a general rule, vascular access should be obtained more urgently in acutely ill patients with lower Emergency Severity Index scores.

When deciding on the size and location of an IV, an EDT should consider what the IV is going to be used for. For example, if a patient needs aggressive IV hydration, an 18-gauge needle or larger is preferred. Whereas if a patient is going to receive slow IV push medications, a 22-gauge IV in the hand will be fine. A patient who needs a massive transfusion of blood would benefit most from a 16- or 14-gauge IV, as these lines are the largest and will allow the fastest flow. For the majority of patients, a 20- or 18-gauge IV in the AC will suffice for blood draws, medication, fluids, and contrast for imaging. Always think about why and how the line is going to be used to ensure the best placement and size for the patient.

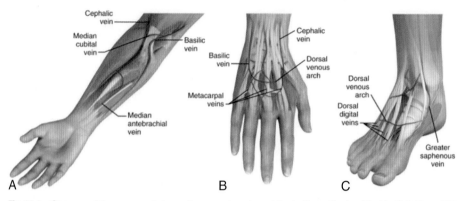

Fig. 15.1   Common IV access points on the arm, hand, and foot. (From Kaplan BL, Liu SW, Zane, RD. Peripheral intravenous access. In: Roberts JR, Custalow CB. *Roberts and Hedges' Clinical Procedures in Emergency Medicine and Acute Care*. 7th ed. Elsevier; 2019:394-404.e2.)

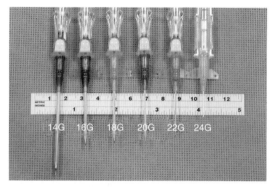

Fig. 15.2   Intravenous needle sizes ranging from 14 gauge to 24 gauge. (From Kaplan BL, Liu SW, Zane, RD. Peripheral intravenous access. In: Roberts JR, Custalow CB. *Roberts and Hedges' Clinical Procedures in Emergency Medicine and Acute Care*. 7th ed. Elsevier; 2019:394-404.e2.)

AREAS IN WHICH IV PLACEMENT SHOULD BE AVOIDED

The most common areas to avoid are areas that have been previously injured, have been operated on, or are near a dialysis fistula (Fig. 15.3). Ask the patient if there are any sites that IV placement should be avoided. Patients with contraindications to IVs will be aware that they should not receive an IV at a particular site or will wear a medical band on the affected side. Additionally, vascular access should be avoided in areas of skin with overlying infection or injury to underlying structures, such as broken or dislocated bones.

SPECIAL CONSIDERATIONS

A variety of clinical conditions can complicate vascular access. Patients who have a history of injecting drugs often have significant scaring to the peripheral veins they have repeatedly

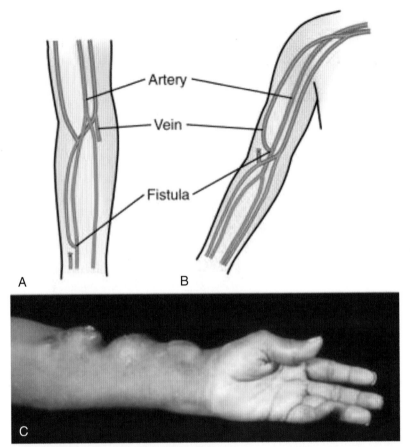

Fig. 15.3 Diagram showing fistula creation (A and B) as well as the external appearance of a hemodialysis fistula (C). (From Witt SH, Carr CM, Krywko DM. Indwelling vascular access devices: emergency access and management. In: Roberts JR, Custalow CB. *Roberts and Hedges' Clinical Procedures in Emergency Medicine and Acute Care.* 7th ed. Elsevier; 2019:447-460.e2. C, Adapted from Rutherford RB, ed. *Vascular Surgery.* 5th ed. Saunders; 2001.)

injected into. These patients may have veins that they have not injected into previously and can direct the EDT to areas where vascular access is more likely to be successful. Patients with sickle cell disease or other chronic medical conditions requiring numerous previous IV placements may also have significant vein scaring making cannulation more difficult. Ultrasound guidance, which may be needed to gain vascular access in this patient population, is discussed in Chapter 16 of this handbook. The ED technician may encounter other IV access challenges, such as the loss of skin elasticity and aging-related venous fragility in elderly patients or decreased venous pressure in dehydrated patients. Vascular access troubleshooting tips are reviewed later in this chapter.

If multiple attempts to obtain vascular access are unsuccessful, the EDT should inform the provider caring for the patient. It is possible that the provider will ask another staff member to attempt to place the IV, or the provider will place alternate forms of vascular access, such as a central line, or request an intraosseous (IO) line.

IV Peripheral Vascular Access

Before initiating any procedure, it is vital that the EDT practice good hand hygiene and follow Universal Precautions, including wearing gloves and disposing of needles in designated sharps containers.

EQUIPMENT NEEDED (FIG. 15.4)

- Tourniquet
- Chlorhexidine product or alcohol pad
- Tegaderm
- Tape
- Needle
- Extension set
- Vacutainer
- Tubes that correspond to labs ordered
- Gauze
- Saline flush

To start an IV line, begin by applying a tourniquet to the patient's arm and feel for an appropriate vein (Fig. 15.5, picture 1). The tourniquet should be sufficiently proximal on the arm so that the EDT has the whole arm to search for a suitable location, and tight enough to slow venous blood return to engorge the veins making them more easily palpable. The tourniquet should not be so tight that arterial flow to the limb is compromised. A vein that is a good candidate for an IV line will be large, "bouncy", and straight. These veins are most apparent in the antecubital space, forearm, wrist, or hands. It is important to feel for these veins and rely more on touch than visualization of a vein. A good place to start feeling is in the AC and then working down about an inch. Here the veins are still superficial, but the catheter is less likely to become bent with arm movement after successful placement.

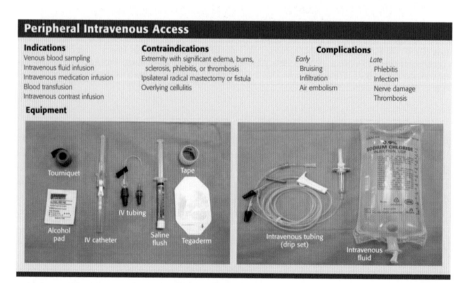

Fig. 15.4 Standard intravenous start kit supplies. (From Kaplan BL, Liu SW, Zane, RD. Peripheral Intravenous Access. In: Roberts JR, Custalow CB. *Roberts and Hedges' Clinical Procedures in Emergency Medicine and Acute Care.* 7th ed. Elsevier; 2019:394-404.e2.)

Peripheral Intravenous Access

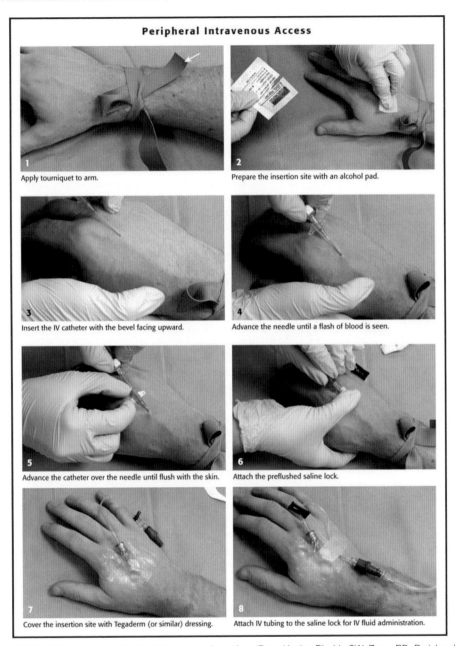

1. Apply tourniquet to arm.

2. Prepare the insertion site with an alcohol pad.

3. Insert the IV catheter with the bevel facing upward.

4. Advance the needle until a flash of blood is seen.

5. Advance the catheter over the needle until flush with the skin.

6. Attach the preflushed saline lock.

7. Cover the insertion site with Tegaderm (or similar) dressing.

8. Attach IV tubing to the saline lock for IV fluid administration.

Fig. 15.5 **Standard procedure for intravenous insertion.** (From Kaplan BL, Liu SW, Zane, RD. Peripheral intravenous access. In: Roberts JR, Custalow CB. *Roberts and Hedges' Clinical Procedures in Emergency Medicine and Acute Care*. 7th ed. Elsevier; 2019:394-404.e2.)

After a vein is chosen, clean the site with an alcohol swab or by scrubbing with chlorhexidine-based cleaning sponge for 30 seconds and letting the skin dry (Fig. 15.5, picture 2). At this point, ensure all equipment is open, set up, and readily available. Remember, once the needle is placed, the ED must have at least one hand stabilizing the catheter until the line is secured.

Take the needle, pull off the protective cap, and hold it bevel up. With the nondominant hand, hold the patient's skin taught to prevent movement of the vein. An easy way to do this is by wrapping the hand around the patient's arm and using the nondominant thumb to pull the skin directly below the vein down. This also helps straighten out veins that may be slightly curved.

Pierce the skin over the vein at a 30- to 60-degree angle along the direction of the vein (Fig. 15.5, picture 3). When blood appears in the needle's clear flash chamber (an area of the needle that allows a small amount of blood to enter), stop advancing, flatten the angle of the needle down closer to the skin, and advance the needle about 1 to 2 mm more (Fig. 15.5, picture 4). This step is important in making sure that not just the needle, but the needle and the catheter have sufficiently entered the vein before proceeding.

Keep the needle still and, using the dominant index finger, advance the catheter into the vein by gently pushing the base of the catheter (Fig. 15.5, picture 5). At this point, evaluate how well it is advancing: did it slide in easily, or are you encountering resistance? Do not force the catheter in if it is hard to do so, as this will likely damage the vein. With the catheter in place, remove the needle from within the catheter. Most modern IVs have a cap that will automatically slide over the needle's tip when removed. Nevertheless, this device should be carefully disposed of in a sharps container as soon as possible.

With the nondominant hand, hold pressure about an inch above the catheter to occlude the vein while placing the appropriate device on the catheter's proximal end (Fig. 15.5, picture 6).

If drawing blood, attach an extension set with a vaccuum tube collection holder (Vacutainer) connected. Press the cap side of the blood collection tube into the blunt tip inside the Vacutainer. Blood collection tubes are negatively pressureized creating a vaccum which pulls the blood into the tube. After all specified are filled, remove the tourniquet, attach a saline flush, and flush the blood out of the line by injecting the saline. The continued patency of the catheter can be assessed by the ease with which a 10-mL saline bolus can be administered or whether additional blood can be easily withdrawn from the catheter. Difficulty in administering the bolus or subcutaneous swelling suggests misplacement.

Secure the catheter by placing a commercial dressing such as Tegaderm or other appropriate securing device over the proximal end of the catheter, including the device to which it is connected (Fig. 15.5, picture 7). Alternative types of medical tape are used if the patient has particularly fragile skin.

If unsuccessful in placing an IV, remove the needle and safely dispose of the sharp in a safe container or location. Apply pressure to the puncture site with gauze and hold pressure for 1 to 2 minutes to prevent any bleeding or bruise formation. A compression dressing can be placed after initial hemostasis is obtained.

BUTTERFLIES

Butterfly needles are needles used for single venipuncture blood draws. They are also commonly used when obtaining blood cultures, which are less likely to become contaminated if a single draw needle is used. Butterfly needles are typically smaller gauges than most needle through catheter devices and can access shorter venous segments. To use a butterfly needle, begin by placing a tourniquet and finding a suitable vein, and clean the area. Open the butterfly needle kit, which may or may not already have a Vacutainer connected at the end, and ensure that the equipment is open and available. Unsheath the needle, and with the bevel up, hold the "wings" on either side of the needle. Enter the vein at a 30-degree angle and look for a flash of blood into the tubing located just under the needle. With one hand, hold the needle in place so that it does not fall out of the vein or move. With the other hand, use the Vacutainer to fill your tubes. When finished collecting blood, remove the tourniquet, remove the needle and hold pressure with gauze, and push the protective cap up over the butterfly needle.

COMPLICATIONS

The most common complication with peripheral venous access is the development of a hematoma around the vein ("blowing" the vein). This occurs when the needle perforates both sides of the vein, and does not remain within the veinous lumen. When this occurs, immediate swelling and bruising ensues. This site is no longer be suitable for IV insertion and the needle should be removed and local pressure applied. Clinical experience suggests that the veins of older patients are more fragile, making hematoma development more likely.

Another complication of improperly placed IV lines is the infiltration of fluids or medications into the tissues surrounding the vein. Infiltration may be apparent during the final step of the IV insertion when flushing saline through the line to ensure patency. If infiltrated, the line may flow slowly and swelling will appear around the access site. This IV line should also be removed, as it is not suitable for medication or blood draws and can cause damage to the surrounding tissue. If more than a few milliliters of fluid have infiltrated, offer the patient a heat pad as this may help the infiltrate disperse and be reabsorbed by the surrounding tissue more quickly.

If an IV remains in place for several days, it can serve as an entry point for bacteria, leading to a skin infection, or irritate and inflame the vein (phlebitis). Phlebitis, in turn, can lead to blood clot formation (thrombosis). The clinical findings of both infection and phlebitis are similar and include redness, tenderness, or warmth around the IV site.

DIFFICULT IV ACCESS

Over time, experienced EDTs develop a series of strategies to enable successful venous access. Some common strategies include:

- *Double tourniquet:* Place the first tourniquet high and tight on the patient's arm and begin looking for a vein. If there is a vein that is present but not "engorged" with blood, consider applying a second tourniquet to "plump" the vessel up. The second tourniquet should be place peripheraly to the first, either on the bicep or the forearm depending on the preferred access site. This additional pressure should make the veins easier to feel. Likewise, when looking for a hand vein, place one tourniquet on the forearm and another one a few inches above the wrist.
- *Heat:* Consider using a heat pack on a patient's AC or the back of their hand to make veins easier to find. Heat dilates the veins and will make vessels larger where applied.
- *Gravity:* In many instances the EDT can position a patient's arm on the rail of the bed or table parallel to the ground so that they are working on a flat surface. If veins are difficult to find, ask the patient to hang their arm off the side of the bed after applying the tourniquet. Gravity may make some veins, especially the more distal hand veins, more palpable.
- *Flicking or scrubbing:* A light flick on the skin over a vein can make it stand out. The EDT can use the chlorhexidine applicator or alcohol pad to vigorously scrub the site, which will also result in better visualization of the vein.
- *Vein pumping:* Have the patient squeeze something or open and close their fist, as this movement increases blood flow to the area.
- Try alternate access sites:

■ The basilic vein runs around the back of the forearm and can be quite large. This vein is not accessed as often as the veins on the anterior side of the forearm because of the dorsal positioning of this vessel—the EDT may need to ask the patient to bend their arm and present their elbow to the examiner who stands beside them to get the proper angle to cannulate the vein.

■ Feel both sides of the wrist. The cephalic vein can hide on the thumb (radial) side, and occasionally a vein can be seen on the outer (ulnar) side of the wrist below the fifth digit.

■ If the tourniquet is placed around the shoulder and the axilla, the EDT may be able to gain IV access through the cephalic or other superficial veins in the upper arm. The EDT should also look posteriorly above the elbow to feel for veins that are seldom used.

If after using all of these tips, the EDT is still unable to feel a vein suitable for IV access, they can use a vein finder device or ultrasound machine to locate an acceptable access site.

USING AN ESTABLISHED LINE

EDTs may be tasked with collecting blood samples from existing IV lines. This most commonly occurs when taking repeat venous samples. To take a blood sample from an existing line, ensure that any medication or fluid that is being administered through the line is stopped several minutes before the line is accessed. Begin by cleaning the hub of the extension set with an alcohol pad and flush the line with a saline flush to assess patency: the ease of flow into the vein will help predict of the flow out of the vein. Attach a 3-mL syringe and draw a minimum of 1 mL of "waste blood"
from the line. The EDT will be able to see how the initial blood removed is diluted by the saline in the extension set, and the undiluted blood will appear darker. Remove the waste syringe and attach a Vacutainer, and then use tubes to collect blood. Finish by disconnecting the Vacutainer and flushing line with saline once again.

TROUBLESHOOTING SAMPLE COLLECTION FROM EXISTING LINES

If unable to draw a blood from an existing line, there are several steps the EDT can take. Begin by flushing a full 10 mL of saline through the line. Have the tourniquet well above the access point, and then let the patient's arm hang down, as gravity may help. Using 3-mL syringes, begin by pulling several samples of "waste blood." If this is difficult, first try exerting less negative pressure on the catheter. Too much negative pressure from the syringe may be collapsing the vein or causing the venous wall to occlude the mouth of the catheter. Similarly, the catheter's position may have been secured so that the tip is against a valve, the wall, or at a venous bifurcation. Therefore, pulling the catheter out slightly might help backflow resume. If blood cannot be obtained from an existing line but the line can still be easily flushed with saline, the EDT may leave that IV in and insert an additional IV. Assess whether the patient needs another line or a blood draw with a butterfly needle will suffice. If the existing line does not flush with saline, remove it and start a new line.

FLUIDS

EDT's generally do not administer IV fluids, as this function is reserved for a nurse. Normal saline and lactated Ringer solution are commonly used in the ED for hydration and resuscitation.

Note that on the bottom of the bag of IV fluid bag there are two ports labeled "in" and "out." The "in" port is for adding medication to the fluids, and the "out" port is for attaching the IV tubing that in turn is connected to the venous access catheter (Fig. 15.4).

Laboratory Sample Acquisition

Blood collection tubes contain a variety of additives that prepare the samples for diffrent types of blood tests. Some additives excelerate blood cloting, while others inhibit clotting. Tubes may also have a separating gel that separates out serum when centrifuged. Blood collection tubes and their additives (or lack of) are differentiated by the color of their caps which indicate the type of blood tests that can be run from that tube. Be aware that tube colors may differ among different hospitals. Certain types of tubes may require specific handling measures (such as cooling) during lab transport. It is important to know hospital protocols when choosing and handling blood collection tubes.

Blood cultures are collected glass bottles containing nutrient broth and other additives to prevent clotting and inhibit the antimicrobial action of blood components. Blood cultures are always drawn in a set of two bottles, one for aerobic bacteria and the other for anaerobic bacteria. To prevent bacterial contamination while acquiring a sample, the venous access punture sight is prepared with chlorhexidine solution. Scrub the site back and forth for 30 seconds using a sponge-tipped chlohexidine applicator and allow it to dry completely. Do not touch the sight after preparation. Prepare the tops of the blood cutures bottles by wiping them with an alcohol wipe and allow them to dry fully. The aerobic culture bottle should be drawn first, before any other tube, as any air within the IV tubing can contaminate the anaerobic bottle. Follow with the aerobic bottle and then blood collection tubes. A blood culture bottle typically requires 10ml of blood and are marked with a 'fill line' as a guide. A provider may request two sets of blood cultures. In this case, a second set must be drawn from a different site and should be drawn 15 minutes after the first set is drawn. This second set of blood cultures will increase the chances of detecting a bacteria if present a=s well as help differentiate infectious organisms from contaminants.

IO Access

Interosseous (IO) access involves placing a needle into the bone marrow of a long bone, usually the tibia or humerus to access to the blood vessels within the bone to obtain blood and deliver medications and IV fluids (Fig. 15.6). With few exceptions, medicines that can be administered through a peripheral IV can be administered through an IO. Laboratory examinations can be acquired from the bone marrow, except for a complete blood count as the values from the study will reflect the bone marrow environment rather than the venous environment. IO access is often obtained if multiple peripheral IV attempts have failed. IO use is particularly common in pediatric patients and adults in cardiac arrest as it provides rapid vascular access. IO access through a previously used insertion site, areas of infection or injury should be avoided.

The most common form of IO access in the United States is an electric drill-based insertion set, which is a handheld device similar to a small low-speed construction drill. Placement sites for an adult IO are the proximal tibia, proximal humerus, and distal tibia. Pediatric IO sites also include the distal femur. Check manufacturer needle size guidelines according to patient size and application site. IO kits typically contain everything needed for an IO insertion.

Common complications of IO placement include overpenetration of the needle past the marrow space and leaking of fluids outside of the marrow cavity. If the line is not functioning due to overpenetration, pull back the IO line 1 to 2 mm while aspirating the line. Once bone marrow, blood, or fluid is aspirated, then resecure the device and continue use. If the area surrounding the IO shows signs of swelling or redness, discontinue use of the line and remove it.

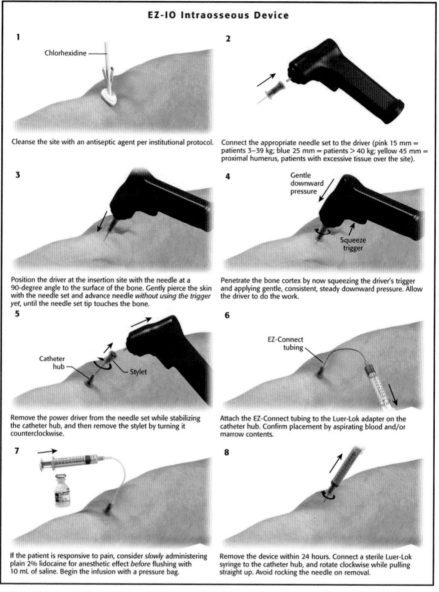

Fig. 15.6   Placement of an IO line using an electric drill-based insertion set. (From Deitch K. Intraosseous infusion. In: Roberts JR, Custalow CB. *Roberts and Hedges' Clinical Procedures in Emergency Medicine and Acute Care.* 7th ed. Elsevier; 2019:461-475.e3.)

Arterial Blood Gas Sampling

A provider may request an arterial blood gas (ABG) sample to evaluate the patient's pH and arterial levels of oxygen and carbon dioxide. Some EDT's will be permitted to perform this procedure, but some hospitals will limit the procedure to nurses or respiratory technicians. ABG sampling (also referred to as ABG) is performed using a small gauge needle attached to a syringe containing the anticoagulant heparin. The majority of ABGs are drawn from the radial artery. One should not attempt an ABG if there is damage to the area one is trying to access or the area has signs of infection.

To perform an ABG, gather the needed supplies including cleansing solution, arterial blood gas syringe, end cap, gauze, and a cup of ice. Some of these supplies may come in a prepackaged ABG kit. Before performing an ABG, feel for the radial artery, which is on the lateral side of the distal forearm. Then feel for the ulnar artery, which is medial to the radial artery. An Allen test (Fig. 15.7) should be performed to assure the hand has collateral blood flow from the ulnar artery.

If the Allen test is normal, feel the radial artery once more. Isolate the area of arterial pulsation with the index and middle fingers. Once the area of pulsation is isolated, indent the skin using the cap of the needle so as to mark the radial artery's path. Once marked, clean the wrist with chlorhexidine. Arterial puncture is best achieved by holding the syringe as if it is a dart with the bevel of the needle facing upward (or an approximately 30-degree angle to the skin). Slowly advance the needle through the marked area of pulsation until a flash of blood is seen. As the needle enters the artery, allow the plunger of the syringe to rise with each pulsation until you have captured at least 1 to 2 mL of arterial blood. After obtaining the blood, cap the needle using the hinged capping device attached to the needle. Remove the needle from the syringe and place the provided end cap over the end of the syringe. Place the sample on ice. Hold firm, focused pressure on the puncture site for 3 to 5 minutes. If pressure is not held after completing an ABG, significant injury can result. Uncontrolled bleeding can cause a large bruise or cause a malformation of the blood vessel called a pseudoaneurysm.

If the radial artery is difficult to locate, place the patient's wrist on a rolled towel to extend the wrist and reattempt palpation. Occasionally, the needle will penetrate through the back wall of the artery as evidenced by an initial flash of blood, but no continued return. In this case, gently retract the needle until flow is achieved. Accidental puncture into a vein of the wrist may also occur. Suspect accidental venous cannulation if the ABG syringe does not fill spontaneously with each pulsation. If this occurs, remove the ABG needle and attempt again with a new ABG setup. For difficult ABGs, consider using ultrasound guidance utilizing similar techniques to ultrasound-guided peripheral IV placement.

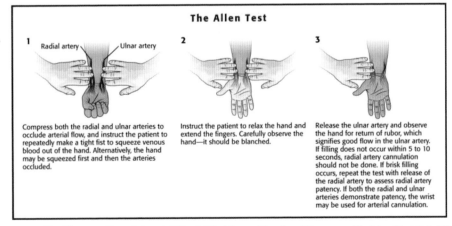

The Allen Test

1 Radial artery   Ulnar artery

Compress both the radial and ulnar arteries to occlude arterial flow, and instruct the patient to repeatedly make a tight fist to squeeze venous blood out of the hand. Alternatively, the hand may be squeezed first and then the arteries occluded.

2

Instruct the patient to relax the hand and extend the fingers. Carefully observe the hand—it should be blanched.

3

Release the ulnar artery and observe the hand for return of rubor, which signifies good flow in the ulnar artery. If filling does not occur within 5 to 10 seconds, radial artery cannulation should not be done. If brisk filling occurs, repeat the test with release of the radial artery to assess radial artery patency. If both the radial and ulnar arteries demonstrate patency, the wrist may be used for arterial cannulation.

Fig. 15.7   **The Allen test.** (From Schwartz GR, ed. *Principles and Practice of Emergency Medicine*. Saunders, 1978.)

Reference for Additional Reading

Baker RB, Summer SS, Lawrence M, Shova A, McGraw CA, Khoury J. Determining optimal waste volume from an intravenous catheter. *J Infus Nurs*. 2013;36(2):92–96. https://doi.org/10.1097/NAN.0b013e318282a4c2.

CHAPTER 16

Ultrasound-Guided IV Access

Carin Gannon ▓ Keith Boniface

Introduction

Ultrasound-guided insertion of an intravenous catheter (US IV) uses ultrasound (US) imaging to search for suitable peripheral veins that will support intravenous (IV) catheter placement, as well as visualize the IV needle approach and cannulation in real time. This procedure can be done on patients with difficult access due to obesity, burns, IV drug use, chronic illness such as sickle cell disease, or in patients with limited access to one arm, such as dialysis patients and breast cancer survivors. This procedure may be used when veins are not visible or palpable from the surface. Emergency department (ED) technicians (EDTs) who are trained in IV access can be trained to place US IVs.

Benefits to US IV insertion include access to veins that are not accessible to conventional (landmark) technique; decreasing time to diagnostic testing; and administration of IV therapy, such as fluids, medications, and blood transfusion. US IV placement in difficult-access patients also significantly decreases the number of central lines placed in the ED and in doing so decreases the risk of associated mechanical central line complications, such as pneumothorax and hematomas, as well as blood clots, and central line–associated bloodstream infections.

Equipment

The items necessary for placement of US IV are a US machine with a vascular probe, disinfectant for the machine, sterile US gel, and all the equipment typically used for landmark-based IV placement (Fig. 16.1).

ULTRASOUND MACHINE

US equipment has evolved rapidly in recent years, and clinicians have a wide range of options that are suitable for US-guided vascular access. From cart-based systems, to compact US systems, to hand-carried devices that connect to tablets and smartphones, a wide range of options exist to fit needs and budgets. New developments include handheld devices that display both long- and short-axis views simultaneously, avoiding a long-running debate over the best approach to US IV visualization (https://www.butterflynetwork.com/iq). The most important feature to consider when choosing US equipment for needle guidance is the resolution of superficial structures. A high-frequency probe capable of identifying the needle tip, vasculature, nerves, tendons, and soft tissue with a high degree of resolution is essential to successful US IV placement (Fig. 16.2).

IV CATHETERS

Veins identified on US can be superficial or deep. If a patient has superficial veins visualized, these may be cannulated by a standard IV catheter. When cannulating deeper veins (such as in the medial upper arm), a longer catheter may be necessary in order to have sufficient catheter left in the vessel after transiting the soft tissues, in order to prevent dislodgement and infiltration. In our practice, we use 1.75- and 2-in angiocatheters for deeper vessels (Fig. 16.3).

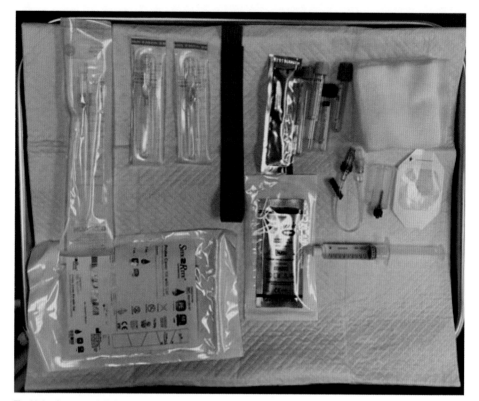

Fig. 16.1 A setup of all the equipment necessary to start an ultrasound intravenous line: needles, tourniquet, skin disinfectant, tubes corresponding to labs ordered, gauze to clean up gel and/or blood, occlusive dressing, Vacutainer, extension set, saline flush, sterile ultrasound gel, and the optional sterile probe cover.

For smaller, difficult-to-access veins, some operators prefer to use an IV catheter that contains a wire that works as a guide. These catheters are more commonly utilized for arterial access. Once the IV catheter pierces the vessel and there is a flash in the hub, the wire can be advanced, and then the catheter itself can be easily advanced over the wire as a guide.

STERILE PROBE COVER

US IV placement is a sterile procedure, and as the probe will be moving back and forth across the area of access, it is important to have a sterile barrier between the probe and the patient, taking care to avoid the inclusion of air bubbles at the probe face, which would disrupt the image. This sterile barrier can be a sterile glove, a sterile US probe cover, or an occlusive dressing. To use a sterile glove, first place gel inside the glove, insert the probe into the glove, then fold the fingers out of the way. The first and fifth digits of the glove can be tied together to keep the other three fingers of the glove folded back. Sterile probe covers are commercially available, typically prepackaged with sterile gel, and are most commonly used for US-guided central line placement. Occlusive dressings (e.g., Tegaderm), most commonly used to secure an IV cannula in place, have been used to cover the face of the probe as a sterile barrier. However, these are not approved by the United States Food and Drug Administration, and many manufacturers in the United States recommend against this, citing concerns of damaging the probe.

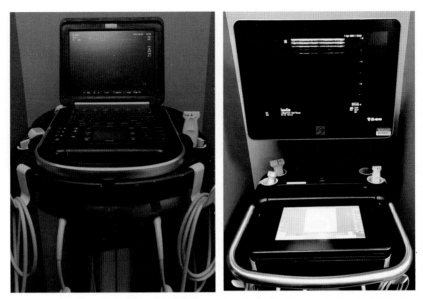

Fig. 16.2 Two examples of common ultrasound machines: *(left)* the Sonosite Edge; *(right)* the Sonosite Xporte.

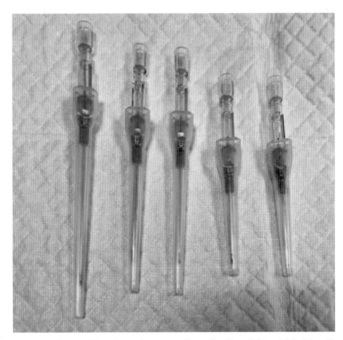

Fig. 16.3 A comparison of several lengths and gauges of needles (from left to right): 2 in, 18 gauge; 1.75 in, 18 gauge; 1.75 in, 20 gauge; 1.25 in, 18 gauge; and 1.25 in, 20 gauge.

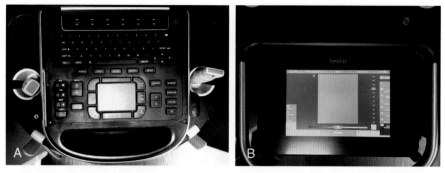

Fig. 16.4 (A) Control buttons on the Sonosite Edge. (B) The touch screen on the Sonosite Xporte. Both machines have buttons in the top right corner to power on.

Knobology

Although high-end US machines can have a bewildering array of controls, the controls necessary for guidance of insertion of IV catheters are relatively few: power, probe select, orientation marker, depth, gain, color Doppler, and center guideline.

1. *Power:* Finding the power button is an essential first step. If pressing the power button does not turn the machine on, check to see if the power cord is plugged in and securely seated into the machine, and that the battery is charging. (Fig. 16.4A and B).

2. *Probe (also known as "transducer"):* If the US machine has multiple probes attached to it, identify the linear probe (also known as a "vascular" or "high frequency" probe) (Fig. 16.5). Controls to select the probe vary by machine manufacturer and can be a button to select the probe, a touch-screen selection, or a manual connection of the probe. Once the linear probe is active, a rectangular imaging window will appear on the screen (as opposed to the pie-shaped sector from the phased array or curvilinear) (Fig. 16.6).

3. *Orientation indicator:* The probe has an indicator (raised ridge, groove, dot, or light) that corresponds to the orientation mark on the screen of the display. For transverse views, this orientation indicator should point to the *operator's* left side in order to line up with the orientation mark on the left of the display screen (Fig. 16.7).

4. *Depth:* The vessels targeted for IV access are superficial, so bringing the depth up to a minimum setting (usually ~2 cm) can make your target vessel appear larger while removing inaccessible vessels from the screen (Fig. 16.8A and B).

5. *Gain:* The default gain setting (overall brightness of the screen) is adequate the majority of the time; however, fine-tuning the gain may make it easier to visualize the bright, echogenic needle tip.

6. *Color Doppler ("color flow"):* Activating this mode places a box on the screen. Any movement inside that box is highlighted by blue or red to indicate speed of flow along with direction of flow relative to the probe face (use the mnemonic BART: *B*lue *A*way, *R*ed *T*oward). This feature is occasionally helpful in determining patency of the target vein and distinguishing arteries from veins, although it is not necessary in most cases (Fig. 16.9A and B).

7. *Center guideline:* This vertical center line, often with depth markers corresponding to the scale to the side of the image, helps the operator align the center of the probe over the center of the vessel, providing a landmark for needle placement (see Fig. 16.9B).

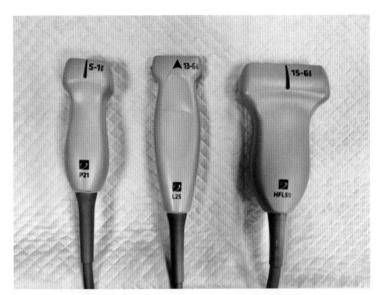

Fig. 16.5   **Probes commonly found in portable ultrasound machines in the emergency department.** From left to right: phased array for cardiac and abdominal scans; small linear for vasculature and musculoskeletal scans; a wider linear probe also for vasculature, nerves, and other small structures. Each probe is labeled with its operating frequency, with the phased array probe at 1 to 5 mHz and the linear probes from 6 to 16 mHz. The higher frequency of the linear probes allows better resolution when looking for a vein or needle tip.

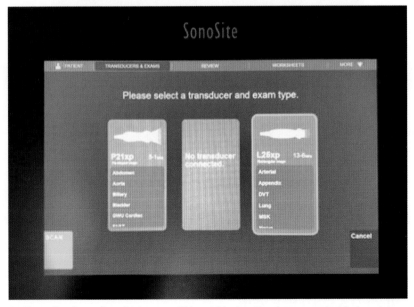

Fig. 16.6   **Example of a probe select screen.** This machine has 2 probes connected, but can have up to 3. Here we need to choose a probe and preset exam type settings.

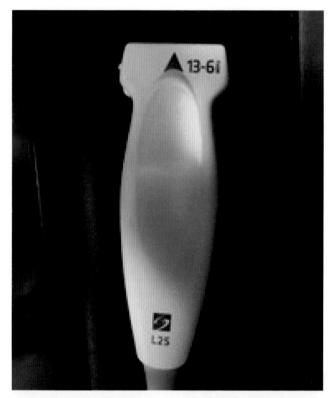

Fig. 16.7   Linear probe with raised indicator in the left side of probe at the top.

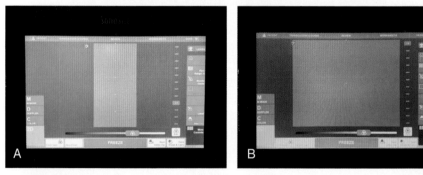

Fig. 16.8   (A) The display of the Sonosite Xporte control screen when the depth of 4.9 cm is selected. (B) The same control screen when the depth of 2 cm is selected. This machine uses a blue sliding bar on the right side of the screen that the operator can move up or down as needed. Other machines may have physical up or down arrow buttons to change the selected depth.

IDENTIFYING A SUITABLE VEIN

When approaching a patient to place an US IV, first ensure that both you and your patient are comfortable. The machine should be positioned directly in front of you so that there is no need to turn your head to see the screen. The patient's arm should be outstretched and relaxed in front of you at a comfortable height. This may mean raising the stretcher or putting their arm on an arm board, bedside table, or pillow.

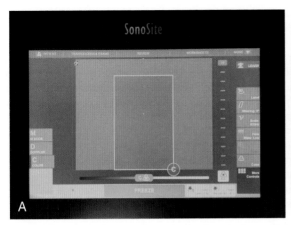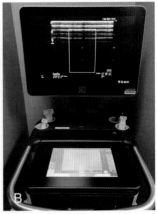

Fig. 16.9 (A) The control screen when selecting the color flow setting on the lower left side. A box will appear on the screen that can be moved to isolate just the area of interest if needed. (B) The ultrasound display when color flow is selected. The boxed area in the center of the screen will light up with color corresponding to blood flow inside the selected area. Here we can also see the needle guide (the three dots running down the center of the screen denoting the center of the probe).

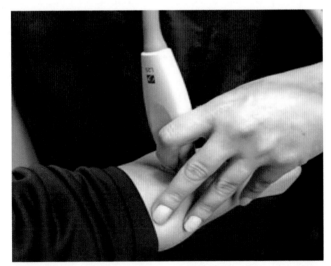

Fig. 16.10 Nondominant hand holds near the base of the probe with thumb and index finger while middle, ring, and pinky fingers brace the arm. This is a slight variation of the described "tripod grip," but the important components are still stability on the patient and maneuverability with the probe.

Hold the probe in the nondominant hand, as the dominant hand will be placing the needle. The probe should be held in a "tripod grip," with the probe held with the thumb, index, and middle fingers (Fig. 16.10). This frees up the ring and pinky fingers and the side of the hand to brace against the patient's arm for stability.

For the transverse view, the orientation marker on the probe should be to the left of the operator. An initial scan to identify prospective veins is done with nonsterile gel. Once the probe is placed against the skin, the image displayed at the top of the screen is where the probe is touching the skin, and deeper areas will be displayed toward the bottom of the screen. Decrease the depth to ~2 cm to maximize size of needle and selected vessel on the screen, essentially cropping and zooming into the area of interest.

A good place to start looking for vessels is at the level of the elbow crease, the antecubital fossa, commonly referred to as the AC. If a vessel is identified there, attempt to trace it distally down into the forearm so that the subsequently placed IV will not kink and occlude if the patient bends their arm. Another site, infrequently used for landmark IVs, is in the medial upper arm. Place the probe 2 to 3 cm proximal to the elbow crease, above the medial epicondyle of the elbow, where the deep brachial artery, paired deep brachial veins, and basilic vein can be visualized.

On the transverse view, both veins and arteries will appear as anechoic (black) circles. Nerves will appear as a honeycomb cluster of small circular black bundles surrounded by white connective tissue. Muscles will appear as striated tissue enveloped in bright white fascia. There are several ways of distinguishing arteries from veins. Arteries have thicker, more echogenic walls, and with gentle compression they will be seen to pulsate. Veins have thin walls and are collapsible with gentle compression (Video 16.1).

Another way of distinguishing an artery from a vein is to use color Doppler. Color Doppler flow mapping uses color to indicate velocity and general direction of flow relative to the probe face. It is important to understand that color Doppler will *not* necessarily show arteries as red and veins blue, but rather will assign color based on directional flow toward or away from the probe face, with flow toward the probe demonstrated as red and flow away as blue. Angulation of the probe away from perpendicular can change whether blood is moving toward the probe face or away. If the flow is perpendicular to the probe face, there may be mixed or minimal Doppler signal; angling the probe to shine the beam toward the patient's head will demonstrate red arterial flow moving toward the probe face, while angling the probe to shine toward the patient's hand will demonstrate blue arterial flow moving away from the probe face (Fig. 16.11) (Video 16.2).

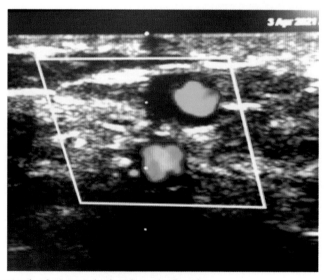

Fig. 16.11 An example of artery and vein using color Doppler.

Needle Guidance

STATIC VERSUS DYNAMIC

Static or indirect US guidance utilizes US to identify the vessel, to measure depth and angle of approach, and can be used to plan the procedure. US is not used for the procedure itself, so no probe cover or sterile gel is necessary. We do not recommend this procedure, and we advocate the dynamic method, using direct US guidance of the needle as it moves through the tissue and toward the vein, with either a transverse or longitudinal plane view of the vein.

For dynamic or direct US guidance, after an appropriate vein is identified, the gel is wiped off the patient and the probe. The skin site is then cleaned with a disinfectant such as chlorhexidine, the probe disinfected with manufacturer-approved disinfectant, and a sterile probe cover is applied. A tourniquet is placed and sterile gel (either US gel or a sterile packet of lubricant) is used to reacquire the image of the vein. This may be done in the transverse or longitudinal planes of view, but the transverse approach is usually easier for new US users to understand and successfully utilize than the longitudinal approach.

TRANSVERSE APPROACH ("OUT OF PLANE")

In this view the vein is visualized in the short axis as a black (anechoic) circle, and because the needle is denser than the surrounding tissue, it will be seen as a bright (echogenic) dot. Position your probe perpendicular to the length of vein, which should look like a circle and not an ellipse if positioned correctly, and make sure the needle guideline of the US is lined up with the center of the vein. The needle is then inserted into the skin at a 30- to 45-degree angle approximately 1 cm behind the probe, which is centered directly overlying the vein using the center of the probe as a marker for the center of the vessel. After inserting the needle, stop the needle advance as superficially as possible, just after penetrating the skin. Then slide the probe toward your needle to identify the needle tip before slowly sliding the probe away from your needle to the point where it just disappears from the screen. Then advance the needle slowly until it breaks the plane of the probe and is seen again. Repeat this "inchworm" process of alternating needle advancement with sliding the probe back and forth to ensure that the needle tip is visualized until the needle enters the vein. If the needle tip is unable to be visualized, a tiny movement of the needle up and down, almost like a tiny tremor, can shake the surrounding tissue and may enable it to be identified.

When the needle tip enters the vein, it will appear as a bright white dot inside a black circle. To ensure the catheter is appropriately threaded into the vein, use the "train in the tunnel" technique. This approach is to imagine the vein as a tunnel and the bright spot of the tip of the needle as the light of an approaching train. Slide the probe up the patient's arm until you lose sight of the needle, then advance the needle through the "tunnel" until it is visible once more, keeping the needle tip as centered as possible and away from the vessel walls. This "train in the tunnel" technique places the catheter deeper into the vein and will prevent its movement out of the vein, reduce the risk of infiltration, and eliminate the problem of being unable to thread the cannula. This technique should be continued until the tip of the needle can no longer be kept in the middle of the vein or until the entirety of the needle is in the vein. At that point, the catheter can easily be advanced off the needle and secured.
(Video 16.3 – Out-of-plane insertion technique.)

LONGITUDINAL APPROACH ("IN PLANE")

The longitudinal view of the desired vein will show the length of the vein as a horizontal, anechoic tube across the US screen and the needle as a linear, brightly echogenic structure. This view of the vein is helpful to visualize the entire length to be cannulated and potentially not having to move the probe during the entirety of the cannulation procedure, but many users find it hard to keep the vein, probe, and needle parallel throughout the procedure. It is also more challenging to get back on track once you get out of plane, and it can be difficult to see surrounding structures such as a neighboring artery in this view. Many find this approach useful after using the transverse (out-of-plane) approach for the beginning and middle of the procedure, switching to the long axis to finish the procedure once well on track, and identifying the needle tip clearly entering the vein.

SECURING THE IV CATHETER

After the catheter is advanced to the hub, use gauze to wipe away any blood or US gel. Use a Vacutainer to draw any labs necessary. Disconnect the tourniquet and connect the pre-flushed extension tubing connected to a saline-filled syringe and flush the IV, observing and palpating for signs of infiltration. Place an occlusive dressing over the site and use multiple pieces of tape to secure the catheter and extension tubing to the patient.

EVALUATING FOR COMPLICATIONS

If there is a question of whether the catheter is inside the vein or not, a long axis view of the catheter can be obtained showing the location of the cannula. Flushing the catheter will distend the vein transiently, and applying color Doppler before flushing will give a color indication inside the vein if there is IV placement.

Starting a Program

Our ED has been using US to guide IV placement for almost 20 years. We began to train our nurses and EDTs in US IV placement in 2007, and it is now a requirement that our technicians become certified in this procedure within 6 months of being hired. Training sessions are 2 hours, with a half hour of didactics covering basics of the US machine, US anatomy, guidance of the needle toward the target, and infection control, and 1.5 hours of hands-on time identifying arteries and veins with US, then guiding IVs toward a target in a commercial US phantom. After completing training and passing a test, technicians and nurses need to successfully place 10 US IVs under the observation of a "superuser" technician with more extensive experience before being allowed to place them independently.

Dedication

We would like to dedicate this chapter to the memory of Russ Eggleton, EDT at George Washington University Hospital. Russ was instrumental in creating the US IV program for our EDTs; taught a generation of technicians, nurses, and physicians; and provided exceptional care for the patients of the GWUH ED.

References for Additional Reading

Duran-Gehring P, Bryant L, Reynolds JA, Aldridge P, Kalynych CJ, Guirgis FW. Ultrasound-guided periph-eral intravenous catheter training results in physician-level success for emergency department technicians. *J Ultrasound Med.* 2016;35(11):2343–2352. https://doi.org/10.7863/ultra.15.11059.

McGee DC, Gould MK. Preventing complications of central venous catheterization. *N Engl J Med.* 2003;348 (12):1123–1133. https://doi.org/10.1056/NEJMra011883.

Shokoohi H, Boniface K, McCarthy M, et al. Ultrasound-guided peripheral intravenous access program is associated with a marked reduction in central venous catheter use in noncritically ill emergency department patients. *Ann Emerg Med.* 2013;61(2):198–203. https://doi.org/10.1016/j.annemergmed.2012.09.016.

Wound Management

Ryan Strauss ▪ Amy Keim ▪ Sara Feeley ▪ Madeleine Rosenstein

Acute Traumatic Wounds

Acute traumatic wounds such as lacerations (Fig. 17.1) and crush injuries are frequent presenting complaints to emergency and urgent care settings. Acute wounds can be broadly classified as puncture, laceration, avulsion, amputation, or a combination of the aforementioned. A puncture is a wound that is deeper into the tissue than it is long across the tissue, whereas a laceration is longer than it is deep. An avulsion involves loss of soft tissue, whereas an amputation involves loss of bone.

The goal of acute wound care is to improve outcomes and reduce complications such as functional deficits and infection. Acute wound management is much more than simply suturing lacerations. Although suturing a wound decreases tension and improves cosmesis, it can also increase the risk of infection as wounds need to drain cellular debris and bacteria while healing. The "tighter" (meaning the closer together the sutures are placed as well as the number of tissue layers sutured) the wound is closed, the less it is able to drain, thereby increasing the risk of infection. Wound infections can put patients at risk of serious complications, including side effects from then required antibiotics, need for hospitalization and/or surgical interventions, significant scarring, decreased function of affected area, and even loss of limb or life. As such, proper wound care is essential to ensuring good outcomes.

Acute wounds can be managed in three general ways. Primary closure is the reapproximation of tissue using sutures, staples, skin adhesive, or surgical tape to close the wound at the time of injury. This is a common approach to relatively low-risk wounds to help improve cosmesis and healing time. Secondary intention occurs when the wound is cleaned and dressed but is not closed, allowing the wound to heal on its own. This approach is more commonly used in high-risk wounds where a potential infection is likely to worsen the outcome. A tertiary or delayed primary closure technique can be used for wounds that ,are too contaminated or present outside the time frame for primary closure. On initial presentation, the wound is cleaned and a wet-to-dry dressing applied. Over the next 72- to 96 hours, host immune defenses will lower the bacterial load in the wound an enable a primary closure, either in the ED or by a specialist. This approach is an excellant option for high-risk wounds that cannot be closed at the time of injury but require primary closure to maintain function or cosmesis, such as a dog bite to the hand (function) or face (cosmesis).

To provide proper wound care, one should obtain a brief history, perform a good physical examination, and formulate an appropriate management plan specific to the patient and their injury. A brief patient history should include the location of the wound, patient risk factors, mechanism of injury, time of injury, and treatments rendered prior to arrival. The anatomic location of the wound must be considered, as highly vascularized wounds, such as those on the head, tend to heal faster with a lower risk of infection compared with wounds with poor vascularity, such as a wound on the foot. Diabetes, obesity, malnutrition, chronic renal failure, immunosuppression, anticoagulation, larger wounds, and extremes of age are also associated with impaired wound healing and increased risk of infection.

Time between injury and wound care also effects outcomes as bacterial load in the wound increases significantly around the 6-8 hour mark. The time frame in which primary closure of

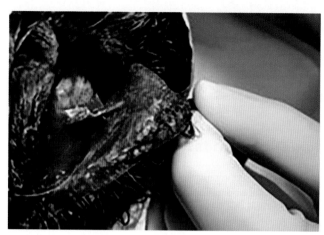

Fig. 17.1   Scalp laceration involving periosteum. (Photo by Amy Keim.)

laceration is optimal is not well supported by research. Traditionally, closure times for low-risk wounds have been 24 hours for the face, 12 hours for upper extremities and 8 hours for lower extremities. Ultimately, the provider will dertermine the appropriagte timing and closure method based on the risk-factors of the patient and the wound as well as evidence-based best practices.

Understanding the mechanism of injury will provide insight concerning the type of wound, as well as additional factors associated with poor outcomes. Bites and other crush injuries can lead to devitalized and necrotic tissue, open fractures, and bacterial contamination. Conversely, a laceration from a clean knife may have less contamination risk, however, it can be associated with significant injury to blood vessels or tendons. The mechanism of injury can also provide insight as to the presence of a foreign body, a significant source of infection, and possibly even litigation if overlooked.

Once patient and wound factors have been considered, a physical examination should be performed. Appropriate evaluation requires adequate lighting and hemostasis. Wounds should be evaluated for devitalized tissue, involvement of deeper structures (Fig. 17.2), and foreign bodies. A physical examination should include assessment of sensation, vascular involvement, range of motion, and strength. Anesthesia may be necessary for proper wound evaluation but should only be completed following a sensory examination. Specialist evaluation should generally be considered for all wounds involving sensory deficits, significant vascular injury, tendon injury, involvement of a joint space, or wounds communicating with fractures (termed *open fracture*). Once a wound has been examined, always reapproximate the tissue as best possible and cover with slightly moistened gauze followed by a dry dressing in order to optimize vascular support and prevent desiccation and resultant necrosis of tissue while awaiting definitive care.

Preparing a Wound for Laceration Repair

Proper wound care can be performed following the patient and wound evaluation. Vasovagal syncope is a potential response to seeing blood and injuries. Always protect your patient by placing them in the supine position before performing wound care. Limit the number of people in the room and ensure that visitors remain seated. The ED technician should work in an ergonomic position to maintain comfort and efficiency. Proper personal protective equipment includes eye protection and gloves and should be used at all times. Any needed supplies should be ready at the bedside on a clean mayo stand.

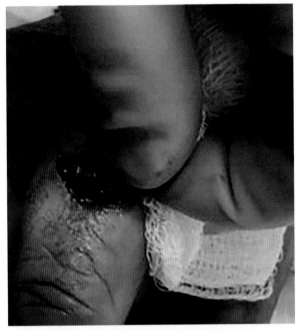

Fig. 17.2 Finger laceration with exposed tendon. (Photo by Amy Keim.)

Preparation for closure begins with skin preparation, including the removal of any debris and cleaning of the skin surrounding the wound. Any area of skin that will be part of the aseptic field should be prepped so as to prevent cross-contamination. Common skin preparation agents include iodine and chlorhexidine-based agents. These should only be used to cleanse intact skin, as they are cytotoxic. Soaking wounds in antiseptic solutions should be avoided. Hydrogen peroxide is also cytotoxic; however, it can be used to break up stubborn dried blood around the wound. Never use hydrogen peroxide in or on a wound.

Wound preparation is achieved through irrigation under pressure. When done properly, irrigation mechanically debrides contaminates and dilutes bacteria concentrations to levels not associated with infection. Wounds should ideally be irrigated with sterile saline or sterile water. Sterile saline is used more frequently than sterile water as it is more physiologically similar to human tissue and does not damage healing tissue. Research suggests that tap water irrigation and wound cleaning does not necessarily increase infection rates and may be an acceptable alternative for wounds that are at very low risk for infection or complicated wound healing. A pressure of 5 to 8 psi is required to achieve adequate cleaning without causing tissue destruction. This can be achieved using a 30- to 60-mL syringe with commercially available products (Fig. 17.3) that also prevent splashing of the technician or by using an 18- or 20-gauge angiocath with a medicine cup used as a splash guard. Wounds with little to no contamination should be irrigated with a minimum of 50 to 100 mL/cm of wound. Use at least twice that amount for contaminated or higher-risk wounds. Wounds involving open bone or tendons require 1 to 2 L of irrigation. Open joints typically require washouts with high volumes in the operating room. After cleaning, wounds can be prepped for closure or dressed appropriately if no closure is indicated.

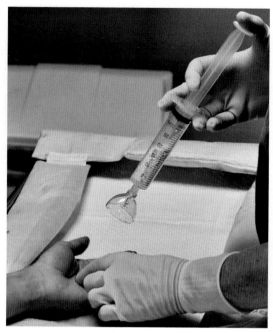

Fig. 17.3 Irrigation set up using a commercially available splash guard on a 30-mL syringe. (Photo by Amy Keim.)

Aseptic Technique

Wounds that are closed in the ED should be done so using aseptic technique to limit risk of infection. Aseptic technique involves the use of special processes, sterile materials, and sterile barriers to prevent transmission of microorganisms from the environment and provider to the patient during a procedure.

Aseptic wound closure is achieved by:
- Reducing microorganism load on the skin with an antiseptic skin preparation
- Reducing microorganism load within the wound with irrigation
- Creating a dry sterile field around the wound using sterile drapes
- Using sterile equipment and materials placed only on a sterile surface, including:
  - Sterile gloves
  - Sterile instruments
  - Sterile supplies
- Avoiding contamination while performing the procedure, including:
  - Maintaining a sterile field between the wound and sterile procedure tray
  - Minimizing traffic, visitors, and personnel around the procedure area
  - Allowing only sterile-to-sterile contact during procedure (e.g., only sterile gloves touch sterile instruments)

Sterile procedure trays are typically set up on a mayo stand that is placed near the patient in such a way as to limit the space between the patient and procedural supplies while optimizing the provider's position during the procedure (Fig. 17.4). Always wipe down the mayo stand with an antimicrobial product according to the product's instructions, and allow it to dry before use.

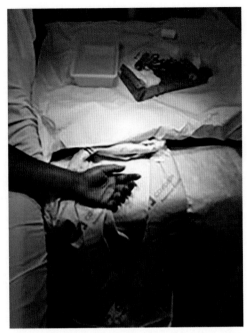

Fig. 17.4 Setup for irrigation followed by laceration repair of hand wound. (Photo by Amy Keim.)

Equipment and supplies commonly used for a laceration repair that should be included on the sterile tray include (Fig. 17.5):
- Laceration tray
  - These typically include sterile drapes and instruments but may also include a plastic tray for irrigation solution, a splash guard, a syringe for irrigation or injection, needles of varying size, plastic cups that can be used for skin preparation product, and gauze.
  - The sterile wrapping around the tray is often used as the sterile drape that covers the mayo stand, thereby creating the sterile field that all additional supplies can be placed on.
- Irrigation solution (sterile saline or water poured into plastic tray using aseptic technique)
- Skin preparation product
- Suture material
- Bacitracin or emollient-impregnated dressing
- Gauze wrap (2 in for digits, 3 in or 4 in for extremities)

If not already included in the laceration tray, add:
- Sterile instruments including Webster needle driver, Adson 1 × 2 teeth forceps, and Iris scissors
- Sterile 4-in × 4-in gauze (can use the container to hold sterile irrigation solution off the field if needed)
- Splash guard
- 30- to 60-mL syringe for irrigation

Always ask the provider performing the procedure if they have any specific needs, including suture type, size and needle, scalpel (commonly #10, #11, or #15), as well as postprocedural dressing, which may include antibiotic ointment, impregnated gauze (such as Xeroform), nonstick

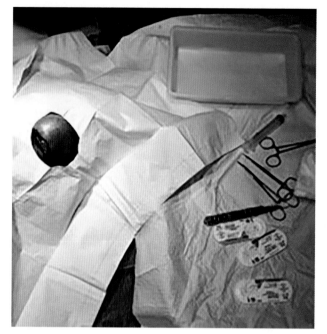

Fig. 17.5 **Setup for aseptic closure of a facial laceration.** (Photo by Amy Keim.)

gauze (such as Telfa) and nonsterile items such as elastic bandage or splint. Remember, only sterile items should be placed on the sterile field. Once the technician has prepared a wound for closure, it is important that the wound and field be kept aseptic and that the wound be closed by the provider as soon as possible.

Acute Wound Dressings

Although multiple specialized dressings are available, most sutured and open acute wounds can be dressed with an application of a thin layer of antibiotic ointment or other emollient, such as petroleum jelly, followed by a nonadherent bandage and then wrapped in gauze. If the wound was closed primarily, this is done using aseptic technique. The dressing acts to both maintain moisture balance and to protect the wound from contamination. Facial wounds typically do not require a gauze covering because the face is highly vascular and fast healing, which inherently decreases risk for infection. Always ask a patient about allergies before using antibiotic ointment. If they do have an allergy or if it is unknown whether they do, use petroleum jelly. Wounds susceptible to hematoma formation should be covered with a gentle pressure dressing. Circumferential dressings should not impede circulation; always check for good capillary refill (<2 seconds) and distal pulses after a dressing is applied. Extremity wounds, particularly those on the hand and/or fingers, should be elevated whenever possible to help decrease swelling. Wounds that occur on or near joints should be splinted, typically in the position of comfort, to decrease tension on the wound as it is healing.

Follow-up and aftercare are crucial aspects of proper acute wound management. Patients should be instructed to observe wounds for signs of infection, such as redness, warmth, drainage, and/or swelling, and to be cognizant of symptoms such as fever and increased pain. They should be advised to seek immediate medical attention for these or other concerning symptoms. Wounds at higher risk for infection, such as bites, punctures, crush injuries, highly contaminated wounds and wounds involving deeper structures such as tendons or bone, should be reevaluated in the ED in 24 to 48 hours.

Patients with wounds closed with sutures or staples should return for removal after adequate time has passed to allow healing, but before the inflammatory reaction from the suture becomes problematic. A general guideline is 7 days for scalp wounds, 5 days for facial wounds, 7 to 10 days for extremity and trunk wounds, and 12 to 14 days for wounds over joints or in areas of high tension.

Suture and Staple Removal

When a patient returns for suture or staple removal, the wound must be evaluated for appropriate healing prior to removal. Factors that may complicate the healing process include:

- *Foreign body reaction:* Look for nontenderness, redness without tissue warmth, occasionally with swelling, localized to wound edges or suture sites.
- *Infection:* Look for erythema spreading out around the wound edges; feel for increased tissue warmth, induration, fluctuance, and tenderness.
- *Dehiscence:* Look for well-approximated wound edges versus overlapping or rolled-in edges. Edges that rolled in or overlapped without notice during wound closure tend not to heal properly. In such cases, leaving the sutures or staples in longer will not improve healing; they will need to be removed and the wound be allowed to heal secondarily.

Always have a medical provider evaluate a wound prior to removing sutures or staples. Once they are removed, apply a clean wound dressing. For the face and scalp, an emollient dressing like bacitracin or petroleum jelly alone can be used.

CHRONIC WOUND

When a wound fails to heal by normal healing processes, it is considered a chronic wound. Common medical conditions associated with poor wound healing or development of chronic wounds include diabetes mellitus, infection, malignancy, peripheral vascular disease, poor mobility, and venous hypertension. Other contributing factors include foreign bodies, poor nutritional status, medications, focal pressure, and a history of radiation. Based on the causative etiologies, the Wound Healing Society classifies chronic wounds into four categories: pressure ulcers, diabetic ulcers, venous ulcers, and arterial insufficiency ulcers. Patients may also present with poorly healing traumatic or surgical wounds resulting from significant tissue loss, infections, poor wound care, or limited access to appropriate resources.

Assessment

A detailed wound history helps determine causative factors and guides treatment. This includes underlying medical conditions, inciting or contributing factors, progression of the wound (changes in size, drainage, or other symptoms), current wound care regimen, previous treatment, and prior wounds. Physical examination includes evaluation for signs of infection, including blanching erythema surrounding the wound, increased warmth of tissue, edema, lymphangitis (red streaking proximally), foul odor, warmth, fever, increasing tenderness, and purulent drainage. Additionally, the provider will look for the presence and quality of peripheral pulses and evaluate sensation in the surrounding area and distal to any wound.

Chronic Wound Types

ARTERIAL INSUFFICIENCY ULCERS

In patients with arterial insufficiency, arterial blood flow to the tissue is diminished, leading to a decrease in the delivery of oxygen and nutrients to the wound. Patients may present with claudication and/or pain at rest depending on the severity. The locations of the ulcers are typically in the most distal part of the toes where there is the least blood flow or in areas of pressure or repetitive trauma, such as contact points with footwear or between toes. The ulcers usually have sharply demarcated, punched-out margins with minimal drainage (Fig. 17.6). Due to the insufficient blood flow, the wound bed of the ulcers is usually pale, gray, or yellow with very little evidence of granulation tissue growth. Gangrene may be present. Pulses may be diminished or absent. Chronic ischemia makes the skin of the foot appear thin, dry, shiny, and hairless, and the nail beds appear brittle, hypertrophic, and ridged.

VENOUS ULCERS

Venous ulcers are typically located between the knee and the ankle, with the medial and lateral malleolus being the most common sites. The patients generally describe a dull ache and swelling that improve with elevation. Venous ulcers are generally shallow and irregular with a wound bed lined with beefy red granulation tissue (Fig. 17.7). There can be scaling, weeping, crusting, and pruritus of the skin surrounding the ulcer. The leg is usually edematous, firm, and warm with reddish-brown hyperpigmentation.

DIABETIC ULCERS

Chronic ulceration in diabetic patients can result from neuropathy, ischemia, or both combined. They commonly occur in locations that experience repeated trauma or contact with footwear. About half of all diabetic foot ulcers occur on the plantar surface and are mainly caused by elevated pressure during ambulation. Thick callus formation in the area of the ulcer with associated undermining of the borders (punched-out appearance) may be present (Fig. 17.8). The loss of pressure or pain sensation is indicative of peripheral neuropathy.

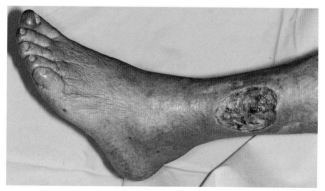

Fig. 17.6 Arterial insufficiency ulcer. (From Hafner A, Sprecher E. Ulcers. In: Bolognia JL, Schaffer JV, Cerroni L, eds. *Dermatology.* 4th ed. Elsevier; 2018:1828-1846.e1.)

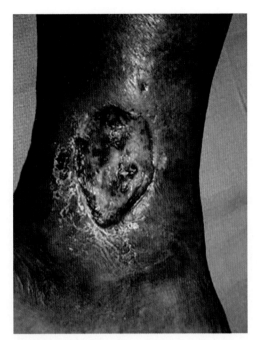

Fig. 17.7 Venous stasis ulcer. (From Bello Y, Charles CA, Falabella AF, Fernández-Obregón AC. Leg ulcer management. In: Robinson JK, Hanke CW, Siegel DM, Fratila A, eds. *Surgery of the Skin Procedural Dermatology*. 3rd ed. Elsevier; 2015:729-754.)

PRESSURE ULCERS

Pressure ulcers are more prevalent in bedridden hospitalized patients and patients living in nursing homes. Pressure ulcers usually develop in skin and soft tissue overlying bony prominences. Some common areas are the sacrum (Fig. 17.9), ischial tuberosities, calcaneum, medial and lateral metatarsal heads, and fibula head. Pressure injury can present as intact skin or as an open ulcer. The most used staging system in the United States is the National Pressure Ulcer Advisory Panel classification system (Fig. 17.10).

Wound Care Principles

For proper wound healing, the wounds need to be clear of infections, free of necrotic tissue, adequately perfused, and moist. Wound debridement removes infected or devitalized tissue, pathogens, contaminants, and foreign materials in order to prepare the wound bed for optimal healing and closure. Wound irrigation should be performed routinely to debride loose necrotic material and reduce bacterial load. For most chronic wounds, irrigation with saline or water using a bulb syringe is adequate. Moisture level is another key component of wound healing. Studies have shown that moist wounds heal faster than dry wounds. The primary purpose of wound dressings is to regulate the moisture level on and around the wound, which keeps the wound moist while removing any excess fluid (wound exudate or serous drainage) to prevent maceration of healthy tissue. Choosing the correct dressing (Table 17.1) for the wound is extremely important to preventing wound progression and facilitating healing.

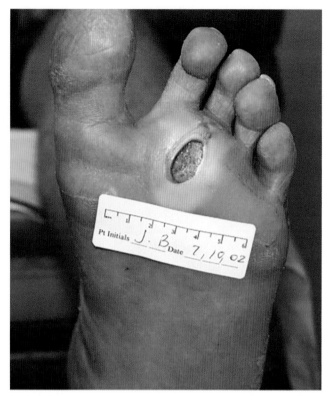

Fig. 17.8 **Diabetic foot ulcer.** (From Marston WA. Wound care. In: Sidawy AN, Perler BA, eds. *Rutherford's Vascular Surgery and Endovascular Therapy*. 9th ed. Elsevier; 2019:1536-1556.e3.)

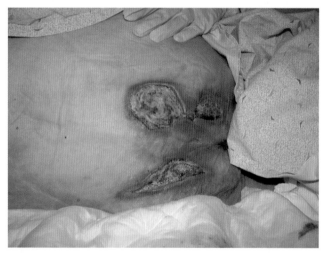

Fig. 17.9 **Pressure ulcers of the sacrum.** (From Bauer C. Pressure ulcer update for primary care. *J Nurse Pract*. 2012;8(9):729-735.)

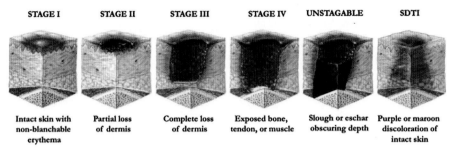

STAGE I	STAGE II	STAGE III	STAGE IV	UNSTAGABLE	SDTI
Intact skin with non-blanchable erythema	Partial loss of dermis	Complete loss of dermis	Exposed bone, tendon, or muscle	Slough or eschar obscuring depth	Purple or maroon discoloration of intact skin

Fig. 17.10 Ulcer staging guidelines. (From Geller CM, Seng SS. How to keep patients un-HAPI: cardiac surgery and sacral pressure injuries: invited expert opinion: hospital-acquired pressure injuries. *J Thorac Cardiovasc Surg.* 2020;160(1):158-163.)

Burn Wounds

Every year in the United States, over 450,000 burn injuries require medical attention. At the receiving medical facility, the medical provider will determine whether the injuries can be treated within the ED or if it is necessary to transfer the patient to a designated burn center after stabilization. Burn centers are equipped to treat unstable, life-threatening injuries and provide emergent surgery, skin grafting, and ongoing specialized care. Specific burn center transfer criteria as established by the American Burn Association include:

- Second- or third-degree burn of 10% of the body in patients older than 10 or less than 50 years
- Second- or third-degree burn over more than 20% of the body in all other ages
- All second- or third-degree burns to face, hands, feet, genitalia, perineum, or major joints
- All electrical, chemical, or inhalation burns
- Circumferential burns of extremities or chest
- Burns on patients with preexisting medical conditions or associated traumatic injuries that may complicate recovery time or affect mortality

Burn care encompasses total patient care including airway management, carbon monoxide or cyanide toxicity management, fluid resuscitation, management of physiologic responses to burn injury, and wound care. This section is focused on wound care in non–burn center settings.

To properly provide burn care, an EDT must understand how to assess burn type and severity, properly irrigate and debride the site, and appropriately dress the burn injury.

TYPES OF BURNS

- Thermal: Flames, scalds, steam, flash burn (explosions or lightning), inhalation
- Chemical: Caustic or acidic substances (bleach, battery acid, ammonia)
- Electrical: Flash (no electrical current past the skin), flame (flash ignites clothing with minimal current through skin), lightning (short but high voltage through entire body), and true (patient becoming part of an electrical circuit with an entrance and exit site)
- Radiation: Ultraviolet exposure, medical treatment radiation, welding exposures

CLASSIFYING BURN SEVERITY

Burns are classified by the depth of skin injury. Skin appendages such as hair follicles, sweat glands and oil glands, as well as vascular supply, play a critical role in reepithelization and wound healing.

TABLE 17.1 ■ **Common Chronic Wound Dressings**

Dressing	Wound Indications	Characteristics	Technique
Woven Gauze	• Infected and/ or exudative wounds requiring debridement with dressing changes • Deeper wounds that require packing to cover exposed surfaces	• Moist gauze dries out • Wound debris adheres to the dried gauze and comes off with the gauze when removed (mechanical debridement)	• Moisten (don't soak) gauze with saline or water and place within wound edges • Pack into deeper wounds • Cover with absorbent pad and tape into place or wrap with gauze
Impregnated Gauze • Adaptic • Xeroform	• Partial thickness wounds requiring protection from drying out	• Fine mesh gauze impregnated with petrolatum or antimicrobial (3% bismuth-tribromphenate) • Maintains moist wound environment • Non-adherent	• Apply single layer over wound • Cover with absorbent pad and tape into place or wrap with gauze
Hydrogels • Solosite • Skintegrity	• Non-infected dry wounds or dehydrated wounds	• Re-hydrates wound bed by donating moisture to wound	• Apply directly to wound and cover with occlusive film or sponge • Some are in the form of impregnated gauze or sponges with adherent borders and film backing and do not require additional gauze cover
Silver Dressings	• Infected wounds	• Antimicrobial • Additive in multiple types of dressings (often identified with 'Ag')	• Apply according to dressing type
Alginate Dressings • Aquacel • Maxsorb • Algisite	• Partial thickness and full thickness moderately to heavily exudative wounds	• Highly absorbent fiber that converts to gel when in contact with exudate. • Maintains wound moisture	• Cut to size/shape with at least 1cm border on all sides. • Apply to wound bed • Cover with absorbent pad and tape into place or wrap with gauze

Continued

TABLE 17.1 ■ **Common Chronic Wound Dressings—Cont'd**

Dressing	Wound Indications	Characteristics	Technique
Foam Dressing • Mepilex • Allevyn	• Partial thickness and full thickness moderately to heavily exudative wounds	• Highly absorbent sponge removes exudate from wound bed • Maintains wound moisture • May have silicone adhesive contact layer • Non-adherent	• Cut to size/shape with at least 1 cm border on all sides • Apply to wound bed • Cover with absorbent pad and tape into place or wrap with gauze • Some have adherent borders with film backing and do not require additional gauze cover
Hydrocolloid Dressings • Duoderm	• Partial thickness and full thickness non-infected minimally or moderately exudative wounds	• Absorbs wound fluid • Promotes autolytic debridement • Forms gel against wound bed • Maintains wound moisture	• Cut to size/shape with at least 1 cm border on all sides. • Apply to wound bed • Cover with absorbent pad and tape into place or wrap with gauze • Some have adherent borders and film backing and do not require additional gauze cover
Transparent Films • Tegaderm film	• Partial thickness non-infected wounds with low or no exudate	• Occlusive semi-permeable membrane • Allows oxygen exchange but is waterproof • Promotes epithelialization	• Self-adhesive • Apply over wound

Thus the deeper the injury, the less likely it will heal spontaneously (Fig. 17.11). Classifying a burn correctly guides appropriate management and allocation of resources to best meet the needs of the patient (Table 17.2).

IDENTIFYING HIGH-RISK BURNS

Total body surface area percentage (TBSA%) is an assessment of the extent of burn injury. The *Rule of Nines* is the standardized method to approximate the total body surface area of a burn (Fig. 17.17). In conjunction with varying degrees of burn depth, a high TBSA% can be life-threatening. This calculation is critical in determining whether a patient needs care by a designated burn center, as well as the volume of fluid resuscitation required within the first 24 hours of patient care. TBSA% is used to measure partial-thickness or full-thickness burns only. TBSA% non–burn center ED classification criteria for adult, pediatric (<10 years old), and geriatric patients (>50 years old) include:

- Minor burn injury can be managed in outpatient care for adults: less than 15% body surface area (BSA%); younger than 10 years and older than 50 years with BSA 10%.
- Moderate burn injuries may require hospitalization for adults: 15% to 25%; younger than 10 years and older than 50 years with BSA 10% to 20%.

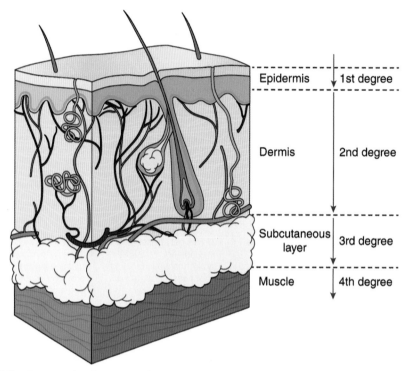

Fig. 17.11 Cross-sectional representation of normal layers of skin and subcutaneous tissue *(left)* and representative degrees of burn injury based on depth of burn *(right)*. (From Shiland B. *Mastering Health Care Terminology*. 2nd ed. Elsevier; 2006.)

- Major burn injuries should be transferred to a burn center for further care for adults: more than 25%; younger than 10 years and older than 50 years with BSA greater than 20%.

Age of a patient is a major factor in determining the severity of a burn, patient survivability, and healing duration. Children younger than age 5 and adults older than age 55 have less tolerance to burn injuries and are at higher risk of succumbing to injuries compared with mid-range adults.

Circumferential full-thickness burns around an extremity can be limb threatening. As the injured tissues lose elasticity and edema develops as a response to injury, blood vessels become compressed, leading to progressive extremity ischemia. Significant burns across the torso can decrease chest wall mobility and interfere with ventilation and can also compress the abdomen and result in visceral hypoperfusion. In such cases, a procedure called an escharotomy will be performed to decrease compartment pressures and improve mobility (Fig. 17.18).

Facial burns may damage various delicate tissues. Burns of cartilaginous areas, sweat and sebaceous glands, and of the cornea, eyelids, and lips may result in irreversible loss of function and cosmesis and require specialized burn care. Singed facial hair or mucosal burns or swelling suggest airway involvement, requiring emergent evaluation and invention. Burns on the *hands, feet, genitalia, perineum, and major joints* are at risk of sepsis, scarring and contractures during the healing process, and require specialized burn care.

TABLE 17.2 ■ **Burn Classification and Interventions**

Burn Type	Physical Findings	Management
First-degree (superficial) burn (Fig. 17.12)	Involves epidermis layer only Skin intact and erythematous May be painful, as underlying dermis receptors are still intact.	Does not require extensive medical attention; no wound dressing needed, but optional antimicrobial ointment or cold compress for pain relief during brief healing duration (3–6 d).

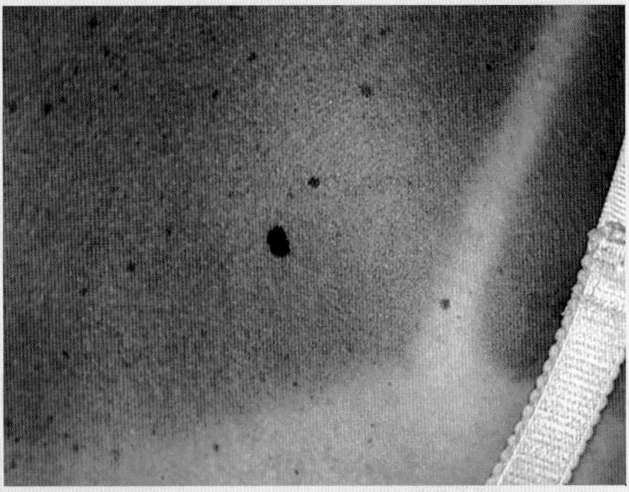

Fig. 17.12 First-degree (superficial) burn. (From Ferri FF. Diseases and disorders. In: Ferri, FF. *Ferri's Fast Facts in Dermatology.* 2nd ed. Elsevier; 2019:89, Fig 3-58.)

Second-degree (partial thickness) burn	Violates the epidermis to involve portions of the dermis *Superficial partial-thickness* burns present as blanchable reddened skin with thin-walled blisters. *Deep partial-thickness* burns present as wet or waxy, dry, and blanchable, with thick-walled blisters. Hair is not firmly attached. May have decreased sensation due to superficial nerve injury May not bleed as easily due to capillary bed injury	Requires appropriate wound dressings to protect the wound and promote healing during prolonged healing process *Superficial partial-thickness* burns usually heal in 7–21 d (Fig. 17.13). *Deep partial thickness* burns may require surgical intervention to heal (>21 d) (Fig. 17.14).

Continued

TABLE 17.2 ■ **Burn Classification and Interventions—Cont'd**

Burn Type	Physical Findings	Management

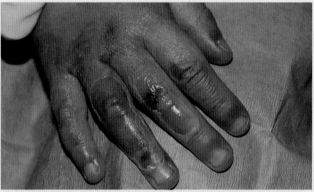

Fig. 17.13 **Superficial partial thickness burn.** (From Romanelli T. Anesthesia for burn injuries. In: Davis PJ, et al., eds. *Smith's Anesthesia for Infants and Children*. 8th ed. Mosby; 2011:1003–1022, Fig. 31-1.)

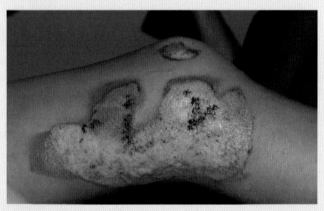

Fig. 17.14 **Deep partial thickness burn.** (From Romanelli T. Anesthesia for burn injuries. In: Davis PJ, et al., eds. *Smith's Anesthesia for Infants and Children*. 8th ed. Mosby; 2011:1003-1022, Fig. 31-1.)

TABLE 17.2 ■ **Burn Classification and Interventions**—Cont'd

Burn Type	Physical Findings	Management
Third-degree (full-thickness) burn (Fig. 17.15)	Epidermis and dermis are destroyed. Tissue is white and nonblanching, or dark necrotic tissue (eschar). Does not bleed No pain receptors are left intact (although surrounding tissue with varying degrees of burn may be quite painful).	Requires surgical intervention, including skin grafting Tissue reconstruction reduces contracture and scar formation.

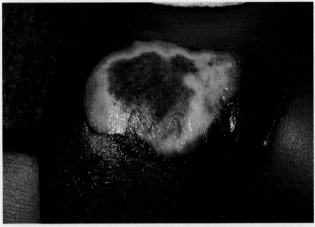

Fig. 17.15 Deep partial thickness burn. (From Romanelli T. Anesthesia for burn injuries. In: Davis PJ, et al., eds. *Smith's Anesthesia for Infants and Children.* 8th ed. Mosby; 2011:1003-1022, Fig. 31-1.)

Fourth-degree burn (Fig. 17.16)	Epidermis and dermis are destroyed. Involves eschar and damage to exposed muscle or bone Does not bleed No pain receptors are left intact.	Life-threatening, multisystem injuries May cause permanent damage to affected area, requiring surgical invention or amputation.

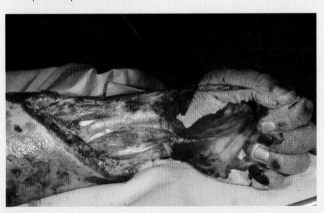

Fig. 17.16 Fourth-degree burn. (From Romanelli T. Anesthesia for burn injuries. In: Davis PJ, et al., eds. *Smith's Anesthesia for Infants and Children*. 8th ed. Mosby; 2011:1003-1022, Fig. 31-1.)

EMERGENT BURN INJURY PROTOCOL

The goal of burn care is to slow progression of injury and restore the integrity and barrier function of the skin while minimizing infection, scarring, and contracture. EDTs play an important role in providing immediate interventions to mitigate burn injury.

- Remove hot or burned clothing or debris immediately. Remove any jewelry on the affected limb, face, or torso.
- If the burn occurred just before arrival, immediately cool the wound area to slow heat-related injury to the tissue. Place room temperature or slightly cool (around 54 °F) saline-moistened sterile gauze directly on the wound. To prevent hypothermia, do not use cold water or ice. Do not rub or wipe the burn.
- Prompt pain management should be used to ensure patient comfort and to allow for burn care.
- Remove gauze once the area has cooled and gently irrigate the wound of foreign bodies and large contaminants.
  - Ensure the patient is in a position of comfort.

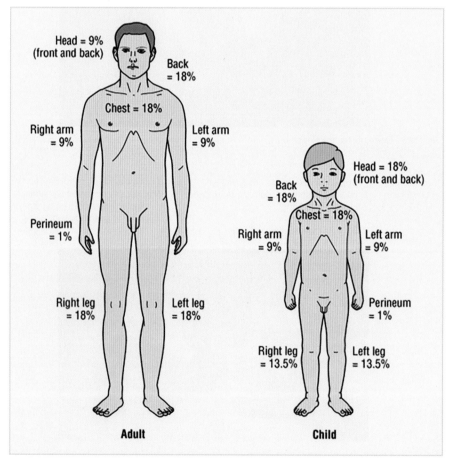

Fig. 17.17   Rule of nines for adult and pediatric patients. (From Suman A, Owen J. Update on the management of burns in paediatrics. *BJA Educ.* 2020;20(3):103-110.)

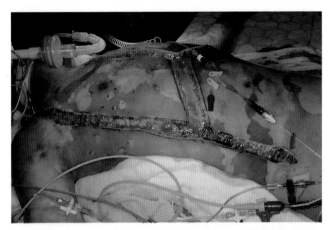

Fig. 17.18 Escharotomy of chest wall to allow chest wall movement during breathing. (From McCann C, Watson A, Barnes D. Major burns: Part 1. Epidemiology, pathophysiology and initial management. *BJA Educ.* 2022;22(3):94-103.)

- For facial burns, position the patient so as to protect the eyes, nasal passages, and mouth while irrigating. Have another provider assist in irrigation if any liquefied tissue, chemicals, soot, or large particulate matter are present around the eyes, nose, ears, or mouth.
- For torso and abdominal burns, cover the surrounding field under the affected site with an absorbent pad. Allow the washed runoff to absorb into the pad and change when saturated. Be cautious of the increased risk of hypothermic shock with large TBSA% burns, especially in areas around organ cavities. Maintain patient core warmth at all times.
- For extremity burns, place the hand or foot above a catch basin while washing out the wound. Remove any jewelry immediately.
- Sharp debridement with a scalpel or scissors facilitates wound healing by removing devascularized and necrotic tissue (Fig. 17.19). Consult the provider if the injury presents with blisters. Depending on the size and location, smaller blisters can potentially be left intact to aid in the healing process. However, large blisters may negatively impact wound healing and ruptured blisters may increase risk of wound bed desiccation and/or infection.
  - If indicated, gently debride necrotic tissue with forceps until the wound edge meets flat, uninjured skin. Irrigate to remove remaining debris as needed.
  - Depending on the depth of the burn, this process may be painful and distressing for the patient. The technician should perform this procedure in a gentle and considerate manner. Ultimately, anesthesia may be needed for proper burn care.

BURN DRESSINGS

The goals of a burn dressing are to provide a barrier to bacteria, prevent progression of the burn injury, absorb exudate, prevent wound desiccation, and promote healing. Dressings must contour and adhere well to the site, be easily removed and replaced, and allow for range of motion during the healing process. As burns heal, they require different types of dressings. The choice of burn dressing is highly dependent on the qualities of the wound, preferences of the provider, institutional standards of practice, and types of dressings available (Table 17.3). Always discuss the appropriate dressing with the provider before applying.

Each of the aforementioned dressings has its own indications, side effects, and complications and should be chosen by a provider trained in their use.

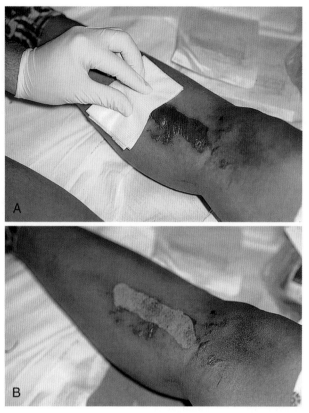

Fig. 17.19 Photo A: Intact second degree burn blister. Photo B: Burn wound after blister debridement. (From Mazzeo AS. Burn care procedures. In: Roberts JR, ed. *Roberts and Hedges' Clinical Procedures in Emergency Medicine and Acute Care*. 7th ed. Elsevier; 2019:774-805.e2, Fig. 38.14.)

TABLE 17.3 ■ Burn Dressings

Dressing Type	Dressing Qualities	Product Types
Initial inflammatory phase dressing (24–72 h)	Absorbent dressing for exudative wounds	Alginates Carboxymethylcellulose
Moisture-retentive dressings	Keeps the wound hydrated and prevents skin desiccation Kept on for up to 7 d to reduce disturbance of reepithelization, fibroblast proliferation and angiogenesis	Hydrocolloids Bismuth-impregnated petroleum-based gauze Hydrogels
Topical antimicrobials	Most are readily available Maintains a moist barrier Easily applied by the patient Requires frequent dressing changes, which may disrupt reepithelization	Antibiotic ointment (best for superficial burns) Silver sulfadiazine (no evidence to support reduced rates of infection) Mafenide (penetrates eschar)

(continued)

TABLE 17.3 ■ Burn Dressings—Cont'd

Dressing Type	Dressing Qualities	Product Types
Silver-impregnated dressings	Releases ionic silver into the wound Antimicrobial and potentially antiinflammatory action	Nanocrystalline dressings (decrease the need for frequent dressing changes) Silver sulfadiazine (should not be used once reepithelization occurs) Silver nitrate

Ensure that the patient understands outpatient instructions, including location for follow-up wound care clinics or manageable at-home care. If possible, provide the patient with the instruction and resources to remove, clean, and redress their injury as appropriate for the time between ED discharge and follow-up care.

References for Additional Reading

ACS/ASE medical student core curriculum: non-healing wounds. Accessed June 11, 2022. https://www.facs.org/-/media/files/education/core-curriculum/nonhealing_wounds.ashx

American Burn Association: burn center referral criteria. Accessed June 11, 2022. https://ameriburn.org/public-resources/burn-center-referral-criteria/

American Burn Association: burn incidence report in the United States. Accessed June 11, 2022. https://ameriburn.org/who-we-are/media/burn-incidence-fact-sheet/

American College of Emergency Physicians: clinical policy for the initial approach to patients presenting with penetrating extremity trauma. *Ann Emerg Med*. 1999;33(5):612–636.

Edlich RF, Rodeheaver GT, Morgan RF, Berman DE, Thacker JG. Principles of emergency wound management. *Ann Emerg Med*. 1988;17(12):1284.

Edsberg LE, Black JM, Goldberg M, McNichol L, Moore L, Sieggreen M. Revised National Pressure Ulcer Advisory Panel Pressure Injury Staging System: Revised Pressure Injury Staging System. *J Wound Ostomy Continence Nurs*. 2016;43(6):585–597.

Fernandez R, Griffiths R. Water for wound cleansing. *Cochrane Database Syst Rev*. 2012;(2):CD003861.

Lammers RL, Hudson DL, Seaman ME. Prediction of traumatic wound infection with a neural network-derived decision model. *Am J Emerg Med*. 2003;21(1):1–7.

Mazzeo Anthony S. Burn care procedures. In: Roberts JR, ed. *Roberts and Hedges' Clinical Procedures in Emergency Medicine and Acute Care*. 7th ed. Elsevier; 2019:774–805.

Moore R. A., Waheed A., Burns B. 10). *Rule of Nines*. National Center for Biotechnology Information; 2020, July. https://www.ncbi.nlm.nih.gov/books/NBK513287/.

National Hospital Ambulatory Medical Care survey: 2017 emergency department. Accessed June 11, 2022. https://www.cdc.gov/nchs/data/nhamcs/web_tables/2017_ed_web_tables-508.pdf

Schaefer T. Burn evaluation and management. National Center for Biotechnology Information. August 10, 2020. Accessed June 11, 2022. https://www.ncbi.nlm.nih.gov/books/NBK430741/

Svensjö T, Pomahac B, Yao F, Slama J, Eriksson E. Accelerated healing of full-thickness skin wounds in a wet environment. *Plast Reconstr Surg*. 2000;106(3):602–612; discussion 613-614.

Vogt PM, Andree C, Breuing K, et al. Dry, moist, and wet skin wound repair. *Ann Plast Surg*. 1995;34(5):493–499; discussion 499-500.

Warby R. *Burn Classification*. National Center for Biotechnology Information. September 5, 2020. Accessed June 11, 2022. https://pubmed.ncbi.nlm.nih.gov/30969595/

CHAPTER 18

Musculoskeletal Injuries

Jesús Treviño ▪ Joseph Kunic ▪ Jason Gray

Emergent General Assessment

The initial evaluation of musculoskeletal (MSK) injuries is dictated by the severity of the injury and risk to limb or life. Presentations of significant mechanisms of injury, such as a fall from 20 feet, are approached using the Advanced Trauma Life Support algorithms to ensure life-threatening injuries are prioritized and stabilized before proceeding to non–life-threatening injuries. See Chapter 20 for an approach to trauma evaluations.

After determining that the patient is stable, a focused MSK examination starts with the visual inspection for gross limb deformities, soft-tissue edema, soft-tissue defects, passive positioning of limbs, limb length discrepancies, and skin tone. Vasculature is assessed by palpating peripheral pulses and checking capillary refill and distal extremity warmth. Loss of a pulse is an orthopedic emergency, and immediate intervention is essential to limb survival. Joints are evaluated for impairments in active and passive range of motion (ROM). Bones are palpated for tenderness or step-offs, and ligamentous laxity is assessed by provocative maneuvers. It is important to thoroughly evaluate injuries at least one joint above and below the site of injury to avoid missing adjacent injuries. Neurologic function is assessed by evaluating strength and sensation.

Immediate General Interventions

Always make sure that a patient is fully undressed and placed in a gown so that they can be thoroughly examined. Remove any jewelry or accessories on or near injured body parts. As the injured region becomes more edematous, circumferential accessories may inadvertently become tourniquets. Jewelry and clothing can also interfere with the interpretation of radiographic imaging by overlying fractures or appearing as foreign bodies.

Immobilization is an essential intervention for MSK injuries, especially those with high risk of nerve or vascular injury. Patients with a high-energy mechanism of injury with midline cervical and/or thoracolumbar vertebral tenderness require a cervical collar and/or logroll precautions, respectively. Fractures, dislocations, and soft-tissue injuries potentially involving bone are commonly immobilized in the prehospital setting, but if not, they should be immobilized as soon as possible in the emergency department (ED). ED technicians (EDTs) can use readily available supplies in the ED including rolled blankets, intravenous (IV) arm boards, or preformed fiberglass/aluminum splints to carefully support the injury while the patient is awaiting a medical provider. Care should be taken to ensure that the extremity remains vascularly intact during movement and immobilization. When possible, elevate the injured body part with 1 or 2 pillows, and place ice packs to reduce edema and pain.

Common Musculoskeletal Injuries

SPRAINS AND STRAINS

Tendons and ligaments are collagenous connective tissues that are inelastic and can withstand high tension. A tendon attaches muscle to bone, whereas a ligament attaches bone to bone. A sprain involves an injury of ligaments that join two or more bones (e.g., ankle sprain). A strain involves an injury of muscle or tendon (e.g., lumbar strain). Either can result from traumatic or atraumatic etiologies (e.g., overuse injury).

ANKLE SPRAINS

The most common mechanisms of injury of ankle sprains are inversion (foot rolls inward) and eversion (foot rolls outward) at the ankle joint. Tenderness of the lateral aspect of the ankle suggests injury to the anterior tibiofibular ligament and/or calcaneofibular ligament, whereas medial aspect tenderness suggests injury to the deltoid ligament. Plain films (i.e., x-rays) are often used to differentiate an ankle sprain from an ankle fracture.

The Ottawa Ankle Rules (Fig. 18.1) is an evidence-based clinical decision-making tool that helps clinicians to determine whether an x-ray is appropriate and to minimize unnecessary costs and exposure to radiation.

Management of most MSK injuries, including sprains, includes RICE therapy (i.e., rest, ice/immobilize, compression, and elevation).

Rest: Limited weight bearing initially followed by progressive weight bearing as tolerated. Crutches or a cane may be required for weight support.

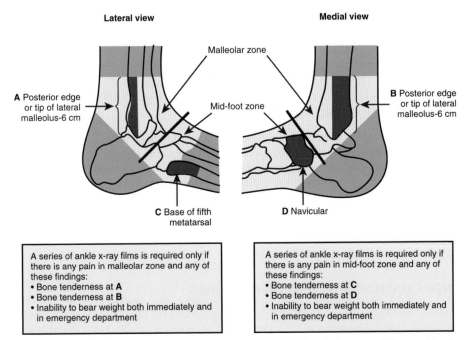

Fig. 18.1 **Ottawa ankle rules.** (From Bachmann LM, Kolb E, Koller MT, et al. Accuracy of Ottawa ankle rules to exclude fractures of the ankle and mid-foot; systematic review. *BMJ*. 2003;326:417–419.)

Ice/Immobilization: Ice over cloth or a cold compress for 10 to 20 minutes three or more times per day for 48 to 72 hours.

Compression: All-cotton elastic (ACE) wrap or premade pneumatic ankle splints.

Elevation: Elevate the area of injury above the level of the heart as often as possible until swelling resolves.

WRIST SPRAINS

A fall on outstretched hand (FOOSH) is the most common mechanism of wrist sprains. Other common mechanisms include hyperflexion/extension at the wrist and overuse injuries stemming from poor ergonomics at work. Plain films may be performed depending on the mechanism or injury. Management of wrist sprain includes RICE therapy. Immobilization is achieved with premade wrist splints (e.g., cock-up wrist, thumb spica splints). Chapter 19 covers splints in detail.

KNEE SPRAINS

Minor trauma of the knee involving hyperflexion/extension or varus/valgus may result in knee sprain. Initial assessment includes looking for obvious deformity, patellar displacement, weakness, joint laxity, and effusion. ROM assessment is done through a series of specific examinations in which the provider assesses individual ligaments, as well as possible injury to the joint cartilage. Redness or erythema of the joint and warmth to touch suggest an inflammatory response requiring evaluation, potentially including blood work and analysis of joint fluid obtained by arthrocentesis, to evaluate for potential infection (septic joint).

In the case of significant knee strains and sprains, immobilization of the knee joint may be required. This is accomplished with an elastic bandage or a premade knee immobilizer and accompanying crutches. Patients should implement RICE therapy and may bear weight as tolerated.

TENDON AND LIGAMENT RUPTURES

More serious injuries can result in the complete disruption of tendons and ligaments or avulsion of the bone where a tendon or ligament inserts.

ACHILLES TENDON RUPTURE

The Achilles tendon has the primary function of plantar flexion. The mechanism of injury commonly involves sudden and forceful ankle dorsiflexion (e.g., landing after a jump shot). Risk factors for Achilles tendon rupture include chronic steroid use, fluoroquinolones, male gender, and chronic high heel use. The examination may reveal a palpable defect along the Achilles tendon, and diagnosis is supported by inability to plantarflex and a positive Thompson test (i.e., no passive plantarflexion with calf squeeze by examiner) (Fig. 18.2). Management includes RICE, immobilization with a short posterior mold splint with the ankle at 110 degrees plantarflexion to reapproximate the separated tendon, crutch walking with no weight bearing, and referral to orthopedics for nonoperative versus surgical repair for the tendon.

KNEE LIGAMENT AND TENDON RUPTURES

There are four ligaments responsible for maintaining the stability of the knee joint: the medial and lateral collateral ligaments and the anterior and posterior cruciate ligaments (Fig. 18.3). As mentioned earlier, each knee ligament and tendon is tested by specific maneuvers that challenge the integrity of the structures. Any perceived laxity or instability suggests a ligamentous injury, which can be confirmed by magnetic resonance (MR) imaging, typically on outpatient follow-up.

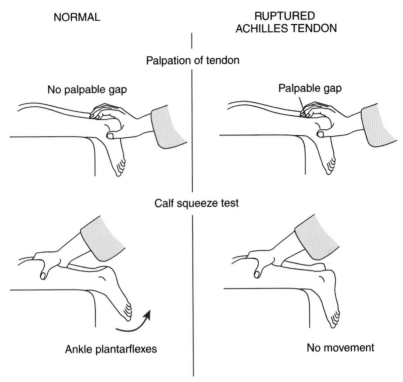

Fig. 18.2 Tests for rupture of the Achilles tendon. (From McGee S. Examination of the musculoskeletal system. In: McGee S, ed. *Evidence-Based Physical Diagnosis*. 5th ed. Elsevier; 2022:467-495.)

The quadriceps tendon, inserting at the proximal patella, and the patellar tendon, inserting at the distal patella, are responsible for leg extension. Ruptures to either of these structures may result in a palpable defect and inability to lift and extend at the knee. Partial and complete tendon ruptures can be confirmed by ultrasound or MR imaging.

Ligament and tendon ruptures of the knee require orthopedic evaluation, which may occur in the ED, and follow-up. Acute management includes RICE, knee immobilization, and crutch walking.

FRACTURES

Fractures involve a break in the cortex of the bone and are categorized as follows (Fig. 18.4):

Nondisplaced: There is no disruption of bone alignment.

Displaced: The bone alignment is disrupted.

Angulated: The distal portion of the bone is tilted away from the axis of the proximal portion of the bone.

Intraarticular: The fracture extends through the articular surface.

Comminuted: The bone is fragmented into three or more pieces.

Avulsion: There is separation of bone at the site of tendon insertion.

Pathologic: The fracture occurs with a low-energy mechanism and is accompanied by an underlying condition that predisposes to fracture (e.g., osteoporosis, bone metastasis).

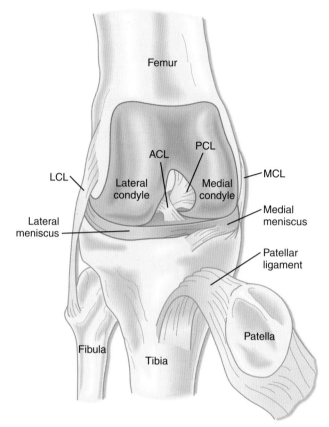

Fig. 18.3   Knee anatomy. (From Adams JG. *Emergency Medicine: Clinical Essentials*. 2nd ed. Saunders; 2013:731-744.e1, Fig. 84.1.)

Open: There is a soft-tissue defect overlying the fracture, thereby exposing the fractured bone to contamination and infection. Almost all open fractures require copious sterile irrigation, IV antibiotics, and ED orthopedic consult.

Pediatric fractures can occur along growth plates, thereby affecting bone growth. These types of fractures are categorized by the Salter-Harris classification system (Fig. 18.5). Other fractures common in children include greenstick fractures, which involve a rupture of one side of bone with intact periosteum of the opposite aspect of the bone, and buckle fractures, which involve a compaction mechanism resulting in flaring out of unilateral or bilateral aspects of the bony cortex on plain films.

Common Fractures

HAND FRACTURES

Hand fractures are commonly due to blunt trauma, including crush injuries. Assessment includes thorough evaluation, in comparison to the contralateral hand, of sensation (two-point discrimination of 5 mm), motor, capillary refill (<2 seconds), ROM, and strength. Keep in mind that dominant hand strength is greater and flexion strength is greater than extension.

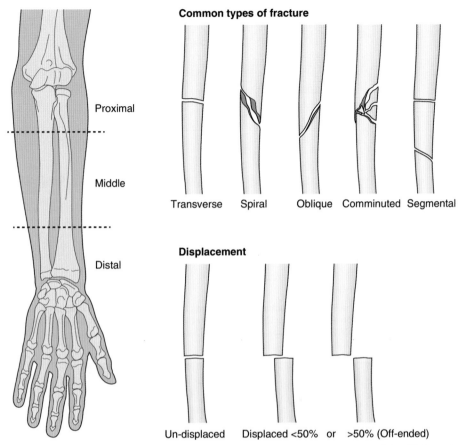

Fig. 18.4 **The location and description of many common fracture types.** (From McKinley JC, Issaq A. Orthopaedic surgery. In: Garden OJ, Parks RW, eds. *Principles and Practice of Surgery*. 7th ed. Elsevier; 2018:528-547, Fig. 27.28.)

Phalanx fractures that are not significantly displaced or angulated can managed with RICE and immobilized by aluminum foam splint or buddy taping. Significantly displaced and angulated phalanx fractures may require reduction (anatomic realignment) and/or orthopedic intervention.

The most common metacarpal fracture involves the head and/or neck of the fourth or fifth digits, and these are usually due to axial loading of the area with a clenched fist (i.e., boxer's fracture) (Fig. 18.6). Nondisplaced fractures of the fourth or fifth metacarpal are immobilized with an ulnar-gutter splint or dorsal hand splint. Nondisplaced second or third metacarpal fractures require a radial-gutter splint or dorsal hand splint. Hand splints for metacarpal fractures should maintain 30-degree extension at the wrist and 90-degree flexion at the metacarpophalangeal joint, with proximal interphalangeal and distal interphalangeal joints in slight flexion. Based on their degree of angulation, displaced metacarpal fractures may require reduction by the ED provider or orthopedist before splinting.

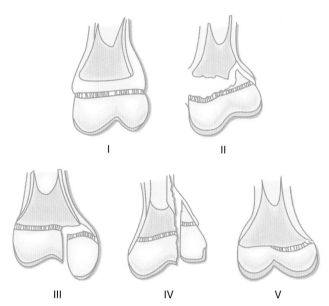

I   II

III   IV   V

Fig. 18.5 **Illustration of the 5 types of fractures (Salter-Harris I through V) involving the epiphysis in the Salter-Harris classification system.** (From Castillo J. Foot and ankle injuries. In: Adams JG, ed. *Emergency Medicine: Clinical Essentials*. 2nd ed. Saunders; 2013:745-755.e1.)

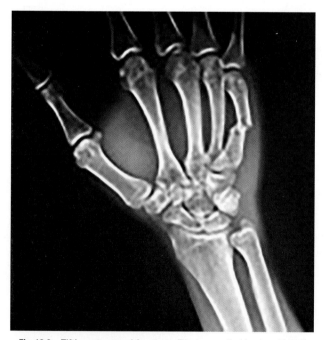

Fig. 18.6 **Fifth metacarpal fracture.** (Photo supplied by Amy Keim.)

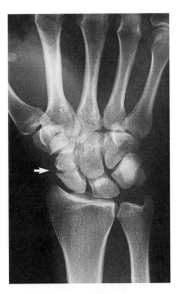

Fig. 18.7   Scaphoid bone fracture. (From Petering RC. Carpal fractures. In: Eiff MP, Hatch RL, eds. *Fracture Management for Primary Care and Emergency Medicine.* 4th ed. Elsevier; 2020:94-114.e1.)

WRIST FRACTURES

The mechanism of injury of wrist fractures commonly involves a FOOSH injury. Any of the carpal bones may be affected in a FOOSH; however, here we will focus on the more common scaphoid and distal radius fractures.

The scaphoid bone lies at the base of the thumb and receives retrograde (reverse) blood flow. Because of this, a fracture across this bone can interrupt that blood flow and put the bone at risk of avascular necrosis (bone death) (Fig. 18.7). Occult fractures may not be seen on plain films; therefore, if the patient is tender to palpation of the anatomic snuffbox (Fig. 18.8), the wrist and thumb should be immobilized with a thumb spica splint until the patient undergoes outpatient follow-up with orthopedics.

A Colles fracture is the most common distal radius fracture and is characterized by dorsal displacement of the fracture fragment (Fig. 18.9). Alternatively, volar displacement of the fracture fragment is known as a Smith's fracture; this deformity may cause median nerve impingement at the carpal tunnel (Fig. 18.10). Given the increased ROM at the wrist, enhanced immobilization is achieved with a sugar tong forearm splint.

HUMERUS FRACTURES

The most common fractures of the humerus occur proximally. The mechanism of injury typically consists of blunt trauma to the area often a result of a fall. The axillary nerve injury is assessed by testing sensation over the deltoid muscle. Proximal fractures are managed with arm slings and distal fractures with long posterior arm splints.

HIP FRACTURES

Hip fractures frequently occur in the elderly after falls from standing height. The patient may demonstrate a passive, externally rotated hip with a foreshortened limb compared with the

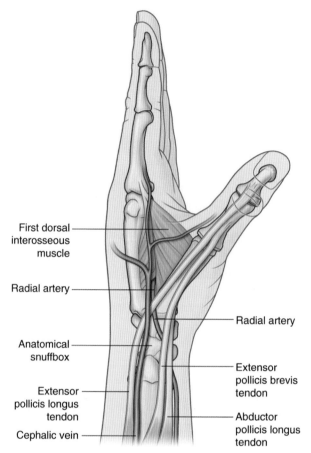

First dorsal interosseous muscle

Radial artery

Radial artery

Anatomical snuffbox

Extensor pollicis brevis tendon

Extensor pollicis longus tendon

Abductor pollicis longus tendon

Cephalic vein

Fig. 18.8 **Anatomic snuff box of the left hand.** (From Drake RL, Vogl AW, Mitchell AWM. Upper limb. In: Drake RL, Vogl AW, Mitchell AWM, eds. *Gray's Anatomy for Students*. 4th ed. Elsevier; 2020:671-821.e4.)

unaffected limb (Fig. 18.11). Examination maneuvers (i.e., palpation, logroll, axial loading) reveal significant tenderness and limited hip ROM. Plain films may be negative in 3% to 4% of encounters in the ED; therefore, when there is a high degree of suspicion for a hip fracture, definitive imaging such as computed tomography or MR imaging is warranted. Hip fractures require pain control, orthopedic consultation to determine operative treatment based on the type of fracture, and admission to the hospital.

ANKLE FRACTURES

Ankle fractures are categorized as stable versus unstable. Anatomy of the ankle involves the medial malleolus, lateral malleolus, and posterior malleolus. Fracture of a single malleolus is typically considered stable (Fig. 18.12). Bimalleolar and trimalleolar fractures also involve significant injury of the joint ligaments and are considered unstable fractures (Fig. 18.13). Unstable ankle fractures typically require surgical intervention. A lateral malleolar fracture (distal fibula) can often be managed with a controlled ankle motion (CAM) boot or sugar tong splint. All other

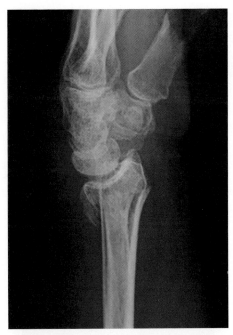

Fig. 18.9 **Colles fracture.** Dorsal displacement of the distal radius. (From Hughes PM, Davies A. Appendicular and pelvic trauma. In: Adam A, Dixon AK, Gillard JH, Schaefer-Prokop CM, eds. *Grainger & Allison's Diagnostic Radiology*. 7th ed. Elsevier; 2020:1142-1183.)

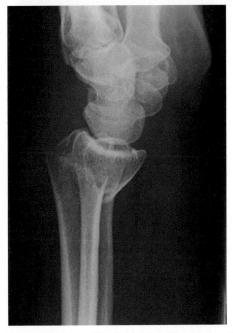

Fig. 18.10 **Smith fracture.** Volar displacement of the distal radius. (From Hughes PM, Davies A. Appendicular and pelvic trauma. In: Adam A, Dixon AK, Gillard JH, Schaefer-Prokop CM, eds. *Grainger & Allison's Diagnostic Radiology*. 7th ed. Elsevier; 2020:1142-1183.)

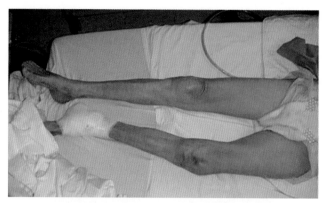

Fig. 18.11 A patient with a left intertrochanteric femur fracture lying in a typical position with a short-ened and externally rotated lower extremity. (From Huggins BS, Sridhar MS. Traumatic hip fractures. In: Miller MD, Hart JA, MacKnight JM, eds. *Essential Orthopaedics*. 2nd ed. Elsevier; 2020:500-504.)

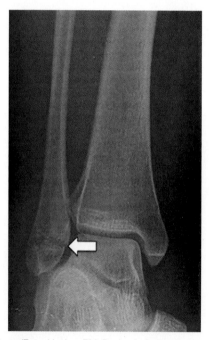

Fig. 18.12 Distal fibula fracture. (From Hughes PM, Davies A. Appendicular and pelvic trauma. In: Adam A, Dixon AK, Gillard JH, Schaefer-Prokop CM, eds. *Grainger & Allison's Diagnostic Radiology*. 7th ed. Elsevier; 2020:1142-1183.)

ankle fractures require immobilization with a short posterior splint combined with an overlying sugar tong splint. Additional management includes RICE and non–weight bearing crutch walk-ing for splinted patients. Patients who are discharged with CAM boots may also require crutches until they are fully comfortable weight bearing.

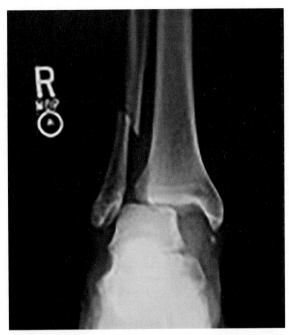

Fig. 18.13 Unstable ankle with fracture of fibula and ruptured ligaments resulting in complete joint disruption. (Photo provided by Amy Keim.)

TOE FRACTURES

Toe fractures commonly occur after stubbing the foot and present with edema and ecchymosis of the toe. RICE therapy, immobilization with buddy taping, and an orthopedic shoe for comfort care are routine. Minor toe fractures may be weight bearing as tolerated.

CLAVICLE FRACTURES

Clavicle injuries typically occur after falls directly on the shoulder. Plain films will show the fracture and should also be scrutinized for a pneumothorax (Fig. 18.14). An examination finding of tenting of the skin at the fracture site is an indication for emergent orthopedic evaluation. Minimally or nondisplaced clavicle fractures are treated conservatively with cold compresses, sling, shoulder ROM exercises, and instructions for outpatient orthopedic follow-up.

Dislocations

A dislocation refers to the separation of two articular surfaces of a joint that results in significant pain and loss of mobility. Dislocations are described in terms of the affected articular surfaces and the abnormal positioning of the distal articular surface relative to the proximal articular surface (e.g., a knee dislocation involving the tibia located anterior to the femur is called an anterior knee dislocation). It is important to also note the presence of a complication (i.e., fracture, open wound, neurovascular deficit).

Common joints involved in dislocations include the hand phalanges and shoulder. Phalangeal dislocations may occur with a hyperextension injury and tend to result in posterior dislocations at the metacarpophalangeal or interphalangeal joints. Plain films are routinely obtained to evaluate

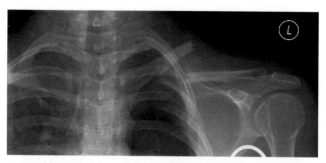

Fig. 18.14 An anterior chest radiograph reveals a displaced midshaft clavicle fracture in addition to multiple lateral displaced rib fractures and an underlying pneumothorax. (From McDonald D, Karodeh CR, McKee MD. Fractures of the clavicle. In: Parsons BO, Antuña S, Sperling JW, et al., eds. *Rockwood and Matsen's The Shoulder*. 14th ed. Elsevier; 2022:247-308.e10.)

for concomitant fractures. Management includes the application of ice, elevation, and a digital nerve block as anesthesia, and bedside reduction with a traction technique. After reduction, it is important to recheck for brisk capillary refill. The digit is then splinted, and postreduction x-rays are performed to confirm anatomic alignment and evaluate for fractures that may have been obscured by abnormal alignment previously or may have occurred during the reduction (Fig. 18.15).

Shoulder dislocations occur when the humeral head is fully rotated while force is applied. The most common type is an anterior dislocation, which results from abduction and forceful external rotation of the arm. Patients will present with the arm in abduction and internal rotation. Shoulder dislocations can result in brachial plexus or axillary nerve and vascular injury and require prompt evaluation. Injuries with evidence of vascular involvement require emergent intervention. Plain films of the shoulder should include axillary and scapular views, which will show the relationship of the humeral head to the glenoid (Fig. 18.16). Inferior dislocations (patient will present with arm raised above their head) are particularly concerning, as the humeral head may enter the chest cavity, requiring emergency surgical intervention. Anterior dislocations without significant fracture can be reduced in the ED by a variety of reduction techniques (e.g., traction–countertraction, Stimson, Cunningham, scapular massage, Kocher). Procedural pain control includes an intraarticular injection of local anesthetic and muscle relaxers; however, difficult reductions may require procedural sedation. Following reduction, distal pulses are rechecked, and patients are carefully placed in a shoulder immobilizer (sling and swathe), so as not to re-create the injury, and are taken for postreduction imaging. Patients are discharged with instructions to follow up with orthopedics.

Contusions

A contusion is an injury sustained by blunt trauma that results in only a soft-tissue injury. Contusions present as focal soft-tissue swelling, overlying ecchymosis without laceration, and mild local tenderness. Presentations with high-energy mechanisms, substantial edema, gross deformity, and/or significant tenderness warrant consideration for plain films to evaluate for underlying fracture. Any motor, neurologic, or vascular compromise warrants additional evaluation for underlying injury, which may include more comprehensive imaging.

Management of contusions is mainly supportive and includes RICE and over-the-counter analgesia.

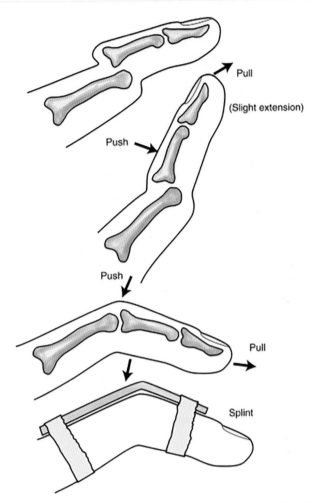

Fig. 18.15 **Reduction maneuver for dorsal proximal interphalangeal dislocation.** Gentle traction and slight exaggeration of deformity followed by volar pressure to slide the joint back into place. (From Kite A, Isaacs JE. Finger dislocations. In: Miller MD, Hart JA, Macknight JM, eds. *Essential Orthopaedics*. 2nd ed. Elsevier; 2020:391-395.)

Amputations

Amputation is loss of an appendage through the bone, whereas disarticulation is the loss of an appendage through the joint. For major injuries, initial assessment and stabilization occurs according to Advanced Cardiac Life Support (ACLS) protocols. Immediate methods of hemorrhage control of the injury site include direct pressure over the artery just proximal to the wound or on the wound itself. If this is not effective or practical, a tourniquet may need to be applied. Additional methods of hemorrhage control include arterial ligation, pressure dressing, hemostatic agent dressing (e.g., chitosan, kaolin), and medications designed to support blood clotting (e.g., topical thrombin, tranexamic acid). Partially amputated/disarticulated parts should be placed back in anatomic alignment and covered with saline-soaked gauze. Completely amputated parts should be wrapped in saline-soaked gauze and cooled.

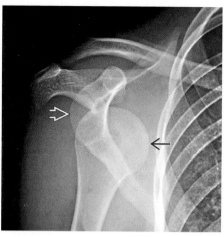

Fig. 18.16 **Anterior shoulder location.** (From Buttaravoli PM, Leffler S, Herrington RR. Shoulder dislocation. In: Buttaravoli PM, Leffler S, Herrington RR, eds. *Minor Emergencies.* 4th ed. Elsevier; 2022:562-570.)

Amputated or disarticulated appendages that have undergone cooling (permissible *cold ischemia*) have a higher salvage rate.

The initial management of digit amputations focuses on hemostasis and tissue preservation. As it is not always clear if the amputated digit is amenable to reimplantation, every effort must be made to keep the amputated part clean and cooled while awaiting prompt orthopedic consult. Once bleeding is controlled and wound is covered in clean moistened gauze, the patient should be taken for x-ray. Expect that the patient will require IV antibiotics. Distal tip amputations are frequently managed in the ED, whereas injuries amenable to reattachment are managed in the operating room.

Compartment Syndrome

Compartment syndrome is a limb-threatening condition that occurs when a tissue injury leads to swelling and increased pressures of an anatomic compartment (groups of muscles, vasculature, and nerves wrapped in fascia) resulting in decreased local perfusion pressure and tissue ischemia. The potential for compartment syndrome should be anticipated with the following mechanisms of injury: long-bone fractures (particularly the tibia), crush injuries, snakebites, circumferential thermal burns, electrical injuries, deep venous thrombosis, reperfusion (e.g., release of a tourniquet after prolonged application), and iatrogenic (e.g., overly constrictive splint or cast application, spontaneous hematoma in setting of anticoagulation).

Classically, compartment syndrome presents with pain, pallor, paresthesia, paralysis, and pulselessness (the 5 P's). Compartment pressures of extremities are measured using a device that is inserted percutaneously into the anatomic compartment of concern (Fig. 18.17).

An absolute pressure of 30 mm Hg or more or a perfusion pressure of 20 mm Hg or less (i.e., diastolic pressure less compartment pressure) warrants an emergent surgical consult to consider a fasciotomy. Patients must also be monitored for complications of tissue ischemia, including electrolyte derangements, dysrhythmias, rhabdomyolysis, and acute kidney injury.

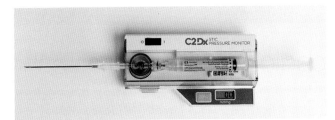

Fig. 18.17 **Stryker handheld compartment pressure monitor.** (Courtesy C2Dx, Inc, Kalamazoo, MI.)

Back Pain

Back pain is one of the most common complaints seen in the ED and is commonly attributable to MSK strain. However, a careful history and examination is paramount to identifying more serious causes of back pain including infection (associated fever, history of IV drug use), fracture (history of trauma, cancer, or osteoporosis), nerve injury (weakness, numbness in extremities or "saddle anesthesia," bladder or bowel incontinence).

Features of mechanical back pain include localized pain that is nonradiating and reproducible with movement and abates with rest, and lack of significant mechanism of injury. Mechanical back pain also lacks the "red flag" signs and symptoms associated with serious causes of back pain as listed above.

A majority of patients that lack any red flag symptoms or signs can be effectively treated with topical warm compresses, acetaminophen, nonsteroidal antiinflammatory drugs, and topical anesthetic patches.

References for Additional Reading

Bengtzen R, Daya M. Shoulder. In: Walls R, ed. *Rosen's Emergency Medicine: Concepts and Clinical Practice*. 9th ed. Elsevier; 2019:549–568.

Cannon J, Silvestri S, Munro M. Imaging choices in occult hip fracture. *J Emerg Med*. 2009;37(2):144–152.

Geiderman JM, Katz D. General principles of orthopedic injuries. In: Walls R, Hockberger R, Gausche-Hill M, eds. *Rosen's Emergency Medicine: Concepts and Clinical Practice*. 9th ed. Elsevier; 2018:445–463.

Khiami F, Gérometta A, Loriaut P. Management of recent first-time anterior shoulder dislocations. *Orthop Traumatol Surg Res*. 2015;101(1):S51–S57.

Kobayashi L, Inaba K, Barmparas G, et al. Traumatic limb amputations at a level I trauma center. *Eur J Trauma Emerg Surg*. 2011;37(1):67–72.

Noback PC, Jang ES, Cuellar DO, et al. Risk factors for Achilles tendon rupture: a matched case control study. *Injury*. 2017;48(10):2342–2347.

Reid DBC, Shah KN, Eltorai AEM, Got CC, Daniels AH. Epidemiology of finger amputations in the United States from 1997 to 2016. *J Hand Surg Glob Online*. 2019;1(2):45–51.

CHAPTER 19

Orthopedic Immobilization Techniques

Amy Keim ■ Jason Gray ■ Jesús Treviño ■ Joseph Kunic

Immobilization techniques are implemented in the emergency setting to:
- Reduce swelling
- Decrease pain
- Decrease tension on soft tissue injuries such as lacerations to skin, nerves, ligaments or tendons during healing
- Maintain anatomic alignment of fractures during healing

Immobilization is achieved through splinting or casting. Acutely injured tissue tends to swell, sometimes even more so in the days following an injury. It is important to reduce the risk of injury to soft tissue structures secondary to tissue compression from swelling with proper immobilization technique. Casts provide rigid circumferential immobilization, however they do not stretch or expand in response to swelling. As such, casts are typically reserved for definitive fracture management (after the swelling has resolved) or to stabilize complex fracture reductions (anatomic realignment of the bone). Splints provide rigid support that is noncircumferential and can accommodate tissue swelling. Because of this quality, splints are more commonly the preferred initial method of immobilization in the emergency setting and will be the focus of this chapter.

Although immobilization is an important adjunct to care, it is not without risk. Improper technique or excessive or prolonged immobilization can lead to skin breakdown (pressure ulcers) and associated infection, peripheral nerve injury, vascular compromise, joint stiffness, muscle atrophy, deep vein thrombosis, and chronic pain disorders. Choosing an appropriate method of immobilization based on the type, acuity, anatomic location, and stability of the injury, combined with good technique, is essential to ensuring the best outcomes for your patients. Additionally, all patients who are immobilized require close monitoring and follow-up to help decrease the liklihood of developing complications.

Prefabricated Immobilization Products

Splinting materials may be preformed to provide a specific anatomic alignment or made from malleable materials that are manipulated to conform to the extremity in the desired position (Table 19.1).

FINGER IMMOBILIZATION

Finger splints are commonly supplied as prefabricated aluminum with attached foam padding. These can be preformed or come in strips of varying widths and lengths that can be cut and molded to customize the splint. These splints are then held in place by adhesive tape, elastic wrap, or self-adherent wrap (Table 19.2).

TABLE 19.1 ■ Common Prefabricated Immobilization Products

Type	Characteristics	Common Applications	Image
Stack splint (Fig. 19.1)	Plastic, positions finger with slight extension at DIPJ, multiple sizes	Avulsion of extensor tendon at DIPJ (mallet finger)	Fig. 19.1 Stack splint. (Photo by Amy Keim.)
Aluminum with foam pad (Fig. 19.2)	May be preshaped or come in moldable strips, multiple lengths and widths	Finger sprain, dislocation, simple fracture, tendon injury	Fig. 19.2 Volar aluminum splint. (Photo by Amy Keim.)
Velcro wrist splint (Fig. 19.3)	Semirigid, holds wrist in 30-degree extension, universal as well	Wrist sprain, carpal tunnel syndrome, arthritis	Fig. 19.3 Velcro wrist splint. (Photo by Amy Keim.)

(Continued)

TABLE 19.1 ■ **Common Prefabricated Immobilization Products—Cont'd**

Type	Characteristics	Common Applications	Image
Velcro thumb spica (Fig. 19.4)	Semirigid, holds wrist in 30-degree extension and thumb aligned with radius	Tenosynovitis; thumb ligamentous injury, arthritis	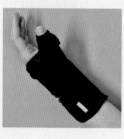 **Fig. 19.4** Velcro thumb-spica wrist splint. (Photo by Amy Keim.)
Sling/sling and swathe (Figs. 19.5 and 19.6)	Sling (fabric or foam) holds elbow at 90 degrees and arm adducted against body and extends past the wrist to support the hand. The swathe wraps around the adducted arm and under the unaffected arm to keep the shoulder adducted	Sling: clavicle fracture, proximal humerus fracture, radial head fracture, to support splinted extremity Sling and swathe: reduced shoulder dislocation	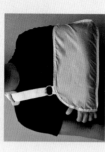 **Fig. 19.5** Sling. (Photo by Amy Keim.) 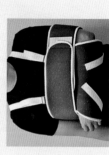 **Fig. 19.6** Sling and swathe. (Photo by Amy Keim.)

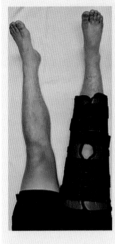

Fig. 19.7 Three-panel knee immobilizer. (Photo by Amy Keim.)

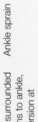

Fig. 19.8 Ankle stirrup splint. (Photo by Amy Keim.)

(Continued)

| Knee immobilizer (Fig. 19.7) | Foam wrap with embedded bilateral and posterior rigid stabilizers; may be hinged to allow range of movement or hold knee in locked position; may have patella stabilizer "cut-out" | Cruciate ligament injury, patella or quadriceps tendon rupture, patella fracture or dislocation, arthritis, effusion |
| Ankle stirrup (Fig. 19.8) | Outer plastic shell with foam surrounded by air bladder that conforms to ankle, prevents inversion and eversion at ankle, ambulatory, can be worn with shoes | Ankle sprain |

TABLE 19.1 ■ Common Prefabricated Immobilization Products—Cont'd

Type	Characteristics	Common Applications	Image
Walking boot/ CAM (controlled ankle motion) boot (Fig. 19.9)	Rigid posterior lower leg and foot shell with a flexible padded liner, ambulatory	Foot and/or ankle sprain, some stable fractures of foot and ankle	Fig. 19.9 Controlled ankle motion boot. (Photo by Amy Keim.)
Orthopedic shoe (Fig. 19.10)	Hard-soled, open-toed shoe	Toe fracture, gout, some simple foot fractures	Fig. 19.10 Orthopedic shoe. Photo by Amy Keim.

DIPJ, Distal interphalangeal joint.

| Dorsal finger splint (Fig. 19.11A) | * Middle or distal phalanx fracture
* Dislocation | * Typically in extension
* Volar plate injuries/avulsion fractures in slight flexion
* Reduced dorsal dislocation in 20- to 30-degree flexion (Fig. 19.11B)
* Reduced volar dislocation in extension | 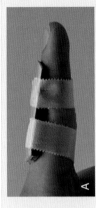
Fig. 19.11A Dorsal PIPJ splint. (Photo by Amy Keim.)
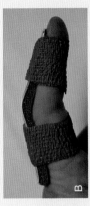
Fig. 19.11B Dorsal PIPJ splint in 30-degree flexion. (Photo by Amy Keim.) |
| Mallet finger | * Mallet finger injury (avulsion fracture or rupture of extensor tendon) | * Aluminum foam applied over dorsal DIPJ with DIPJ in slight hyperextension
* Stack splint (Fig. 19.12) | **Fig. 19.12** Stack splint. (From Chudnofsky CR, Chudnofsky AS. Splinting techniques. In: Roberts JR, Custalow CB, eds. *Roberts and Hedges' Clinical Procedures in Emergency Medicine and Acute Care.* 7th ed. Elsevier; 2019:1027-1056.e1.) |

DIPJ, Distal interphalangeal joint.

Buddy Taping

Buddy taping is a form of dynamic splinting that binds the injured digit to an adjacent digit. This method provides stabilization of the injured digit while allowing for some continued mobility. Dynamic splinting is commonly for toe fractures and dislocations, as well as stable finger dislocations and some nondisplaced/nonintraarticular phalanx fractures (Fig. 19.13).

Custom Made Splints

Most emergency departments will have plaster and fiberglass splinting material. Plaster, also known as gypsum, comes in rolls of 2-, 3-, 4-, and 6-inch widths of mesh impregnated with plaster. Plaster splinting material is layered to give it more strength. Use 8 layers for upper extremities and 12 to 15 layers for lower extremities. The layers are moistened, and the plaster takes on a paste-like consistency that is held into place by the mesh. In this form, the plaster is highly moldable and hardens as molded via exothermic reaction (note that the more layers of plaster, the hotter it gets). The plaster is sandwiched between layers of synthetic or cotton roll padding before applying to the extremity. Sufficient undercast padding is essential to help prevent thermal injury to tissue. Once the plaster is applied and while it is hardening, an elastic bandage is applied directly over the plaster to hold the splint in place in its final form. Hardening times typically range from 2 to 10 minutes, and complete cure time can take up to 48 hours depending on the brand, ambient temperature, and humidity.

Fiberglass splinting material typically comes in prepadded splint rolls (whereas cast fiberglass comes in nonpadded rolls) in 2-, 3-, 4-, and 6-inch widths. There are multiple brands of this type of splinting material. Most consist of a long foil-wrapped roll of malleable fiberglass mesh enclosed in a sleeve of thick synthetic padding on one side and a thinner material on the other side. The fiberglass can be cut to the length required for individual splints. Although this form of fiberglass splinting material provides some padding, it is still important to apply stockinette and several layers of undercast padding, as fiberglass also cures by exothermic reaction. Additionally, extra padding helps to prevent pressure points and skin breakdown. Fiberglass will harden with

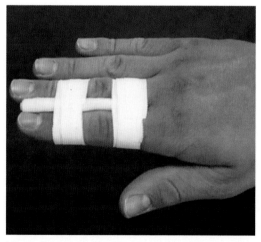

Fig. 19.13 Buddy-taped fingers. Note gauze between the digits to absorb moisture and deter skin breakdown. (From Richards G. Taping and bandaging. In: Auerbach P, Cushing TA, Harris NS, eds. *Auerbach's Wilderness Medicine.* 7th ed. Elsevier; 2017:517-532.e1.)

exposure to air (so always make sure to seal the foil closed after you cut off the amount you are using!) but hardens faster when moistened with water. Once in place, the splint is secured by an elastic bandage and molded into the desired position while it hardens. Fiberglass becomes firm within several minutes (depending on type and conditions) and hardens completely within several hours. Although more expensive than plaster, prefabricated rolls of fiberglass save time and are far less messy than plaster, making prefabricated fiberglass the material of choice in most EDs.

GENERAL SETUP

- Pain medication should be administered by the nurse before any painful manipulation.
- Place the patient in a position that is safe and comfortable for them while facilitating good splint positioning and access to your materials.
- Expose the extremity completely. Keep in mind that any clothing proximal to the injury may not fit over the splint once done, which can be problematic for the patient.
- Make sure that all open wounds are appropriately treated and dressed.
- Have all your supplies bedside before starting the procedure.
  - Trauma shears (better cutting ergonomics)
  - Water and paper or cloth towels
  - Splinting material
  - Stockinette
  - Splint padding
  - Elastic bandages (2-, 3-, 4-, and 6-inch widths should be available)

GENERAL TECHNIQUE

- Check sensation and pulses/capillary refill before applying the splint. This will give you a baseline to which you can compare your post splint exam. It may also identify any concerning changes that may have occurred since the patient's initial evaluation.
- For most fractures, the splint should immobilize the joint proximal to *and* the joint distal to the site of injury.
- For most dislocations, the splint should immobilize the bone proximal to *and* the bone distal to the site of injury.
- Leave the tips of the fingers or toes exposed to allow for your post splint assessment of sensation, color, and capillary refill.
  1. Choose the right splint width.
     - Children: the width of the material should cover one-half of the circumference of the extremity
     - Adult finger: 2 inches
     - Adult upper extremity: 3 or 4 inches
     - Adult lower extremity: 4, 5, or 6 inches
  2. Provide sufficient padding to relieve pressure points and prevent skin breakdown.
     - First apply stockinette that extends slightly past the length of the planned splint so that it can be rolled back over the ends of the splinting material and provide added protection from the fiberglass edges.
     - Stockinette can be cut out over the flexor surfaces of joints to prevent bunching.
     - Padding comes in cotton and synthetic materials in a variety of widths.
     - Choose a padding width that can easily be rolled over the extremity without bulky folds and bumps.

- Apply 2 to 3 layers of undercast padding with the extremity in the position of splinting.
- When rolling the undercast padding, wrap distal to proximal and overlap 50% of the prior layer as you continue to wrap proximally.
- Apply extra padding to elbows, heels, bony prominences, and over the fracture site.
- Smooth out any lumps or folds that may produce pressure points against the skin.
- Apply padding between digits to absorb moisture and prevent maceration.
3. Moisten and apply your splinting material.
4. Apply an elastic bandage to hold the splinting material in place.
5. Mold the splint into proper form and hold in place until it hardens.

Correct Anatomic Positioning

The resting hand position (i.e., the position of comfort) is used for upper extremities not involving the hand.

- Wrist in 10- to 20-degree extension
- Metacarpophalangeal joints (MCPJs) in 50-degree flexion
- Proximal interphalangeal joints (PIPJs) and distal interphalangeal joints (DIPJs) in 5- to 10-degree flexion

The intrinsic-plus hand position (i.e., position of safe immobilization) is used for hand and finger injuries (Fig. 19.14).

- Wrist in 20- to 30-degree extension
- MCPJs in 70- to 90-degree flexion (which pulls the collateral ligaments taut, thereby adding stability)
- PIPJs and DIPJs in full extension (which helps prevent stiffness from contracted ligaments and joint capsule)
- Thumb in adduction such that the index finger, first webspace, and thumb form a "C" shape.

Tables 19.3 and 19.4 provide details on the indication, application, and position of common extremity splints.

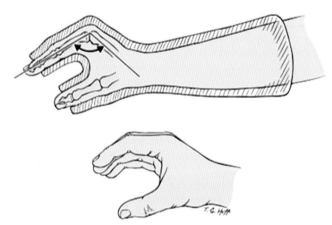

Fig. 19.14   Intrinsic-plus position. (From Browner BD, Jupiter JB, Levine AM, et al, eds. *Skeletal Trauma: Basic Science, Management, and Reconstruction.* 4th ed. Saunders; 2008.)

TABLE 19.3 ■ Common Upper Extremity Splints

Splint Type	Indication	Description	Position	Anatomic Positioning
Dorsal hand (Fig. 19.15)	* Boxer's fracture * Hand and finger injuries	* 3-inch width * Starts at dorsal fingertips and extends over dorsal hand and wrist to mid-forearm * Secure with 2- to 3-inch elastic bandage	* Forearm in thumbs-up position * DIPJ and PIPJs in full extension * MCPJs in 90-degree flexion * Wrist extended 20 to 30 degrees	**Fig. 19.15** Dorsal hand splint. (Photo by Amy Keim.)
Ulnar gutter (Fig. 19.16)	* Fourth and fifth metacarpal fractures * Injuries to the ring and small finger	* 3-inch width * Starts at ulnar aspect small finger folding over to incorporate ring finger as well, extends over ulnar aspect of hand and wrist to mid-forearm * Secure with 2- to 3-inch elastic bandage	* Forearm in thumbs-up position * DIPJ and PIPJs 5- to 10-degree flexion * MCPJs in 50-degree flexion * Wrist extended 10 to 20 degrees ** If boxer's fracture or hand injury, MCPJs in 90-degree flexion and DIPJ and PIPJ in extension	**Fig. 19.16** Ulnar gutter splint. (Photo by Amy Keim.)
Radial gutter (Fig. 19.17)	* Second and third metacarpal fractures * Injuries to index and middle fingers	* 3-inch width * Starts at fingertips and extends along radial forearm to mid-forearm * Secure with 2- to 3-inch elastic bandage	* Forearm in thumbs-up position * DIPJ and PIPJs 5- to 10-degree flexion * MCPJs in 50-degree flexion * Wrist extended 10 to 20 degrees	**Fig. 19.17** Radial gutter splint. (Photo by Amy Keim.)

TABLE 19.3 ■ Common Upper Extremity Splints—Cont'd

Splint Type	Indication	Description	Position	Anatomic Positioning
Volar wrist (Fig. 19.18)	* Carpal bone fractures * Second through fifth metacarpal head fractures	* 3-inch wide * Starts at volar MCPJ and extends over volar wrist to mid-forearm * Secure with 3-inch elastic bandage	* Forearm in thumbs-up position * Wrist extended 10 to 20 degrees	Fig. 19.18 Volar splint. (Photo by Amy Keim.)
Sugar tong (Fig. 19.19)	* Distal radius and ulna fractures	* 3- to 4-inch width * Starts at volar MCPJs, extends along anterior forearm, around elbow, and back down posterior * Secure with 3-inch elastic bandage arm to end at dorsal MCPJs	* Elbow at 90 degrees * Forearm in thumbs-up position * Wrist extended 10 to 20 degrees	Fig. 19.19 Upper extremity sugar tong splint. (Photo by Amy Keim.)

Continued

TABLE 19.3 ■ Common Upper Extremity Splints—Cont'd

Splint Type	Indication	Description	Position	Anatomic Positioning
Posterior long arm (Fig. 19.20)	Humerus fractures *Olecranon fractures * Radial head fractures	* 4- to 6-inch width * Starts at posterior upper arm, extends over elbow, along ulnar forearm to MCPJ * Secure with 3-inch elastic bandage	* Elbow at 90 degrees * Forearm in thumbs-up position * Wrist extended 10 to 20 degrees	 **Fig. 19.20** Posterior long arm splint. (Photo by Amy Keim.)
Thumb spica— triple-S (Fig. 19.21)	* Scaphoid and lunate fractures * Suspected occult scaphoid fractures * Injuries to first metacarpal and thumb * De Quervain tenosynovitis * Triple-S splint technique avoids compression over the anatomic snuffbox and radial nerve	* 3-inch width * Starts along dorsal ulnar thumb tip, wraps over dorsal thumb and wrist (avoid pressure point on the anatomic snuffbox), continue to wrap around ulnar aspect of forearm in a spiral shape ending on volar mid-forearm * Secure with 2- to 3-inch elastic bandage	* Forearm in thumbs-up position * Thumb abducted and in line with radius with slight flexion at the MCPJ and IPJ ("wineglass position") * Wrist extended 20 to 30 degrees	 **Fig. 19.21** Thumb spica splint. (Photo by Amy Keim.)

DIPJ, Distal interphalangeal joint; *MCPJ*, metacarpophalangeal joint; *PIPJ*, proximal interphalangeal joint.

TABLE 19.4 ■ Common Lower Extremity Splints

Splint Type	Indication	Description	Position	Finished Splint
Posterior ankle (Fig. 19.22)	* High-grade ankle sprains * Foot fractures	* 4-inch width * Starts at toes and extends over plantar foot to posterior mid-calf * Secure with 3- to 4-inch elastic bandage	* Patient in prone position with knee 90-degree flexion * Ankle at 90 degrees ** Ankle should be splinted in plantar flexion for Achilles tendon rupture	Fig. 19.22 Posterior ankle splint. (Photo by Amy Keim.)
Stirrup (U-splint, sugar tong) (Fig. 19.23)	* Ankle injuries	* 4-inch width * Start 4 cm distal to fibular head, extend under plantar foot and then medial leg to level of starting point * Secure with 3- to 4-inch elastic bandage	* Patient in prone position with knee 90-degree flexion * Ankle at 90 degrees	Fig. 19.23 Ankle stirrup splint. (Photo by Amy Keim.)
Posterior ankle with stirrup (Fig. 19.24)	* Complex ankle fractures * Ankle reductions * Unstable ankle injuries	* 4-inch width * Starts with posterior ankle slab fixed into place with web roll followed by sugar tong slab * Secure with 3- to 4-inch elastic bandage	* Patient in prone position with knee 90-degree flexion * Ankle at 90 degrees	Fig. 19.24 Posterior ankle with stirrup splint. (Photo by Amy Keim.)

After Splinting

After splinting, it is crucial to assess the splint for excessive tightness, pressure points, and shaping. Patient feedback plays a significant role in this assessment (e.g., "Does the splint feel too tight?" "Are you experiencing numbness or tingling sensations?"). All patients should receive a postsplint neurovascular exam.

A normal postsplint exam includes:

- Capillary refill less than 2 seconds
- Sensation to light touch intact and equal to the nonsplinted extremity (unless a nerve injury is present)
- Motor function of digits outside of the splint grossly intact

Any issues should be addressed immediately and may require resplinting. Issues not resolved with proper re-splinting should be brought to the attention of the medical provider.

Patient Counseling

Patients should receive counseling on splint care, including the following:

- Keep the splint in place until otherwise directed by provider.
- Keep the splint clean and dry.
- Return to the ED if the splint becomes wet, as it will need to be replaced.
- Do not insert objects into the splint.
- Elevate the affected limb above the level of the heart whenever possible, or as directed by the provider, to help decrease swelling and pain.

Patients must also be counseled on concerning symptoms that warrant a return visit to the ED, including the following:

- Dusky skin tone
- Coolness or blue hue to extremity distal to splint
- Numbness of affected limb
- Worsening pain
- Increased swelling
- Redness, foul odor or drainage from splinted area, or fever

Finally, review adjunct therapies for the care of any soft tissue injury (i.e., RICE [rest, ice, compression, elevation]).

Ambulatory Assist Devices

Ambulatory assist devices, such as crutches and walkers, should be provided to patients who receive lower extremity immobilization devices and are instructed to be non–weight bearing or partial weight bearing. Weight bearing patients can be given a cane for added stability. Instruct the patient on the proper use of their walking assist device, and provide training before discharge.

CRUTCHES

- Adjust the length of the crutches such that the arm rests are 2 to 3 inches below the level of the axilla.
- Adjust the handles of the crutches to the level of the wrist when the arm is held straight (this will create a slight bend at the elbow when the hand grips the handle).
- Instruct the patient to bear weight with hands only and avoid direct pressure on axilla.
- The bottom ends of the crutches should be positioned wider than the shoulders.
- Instruct the patient on how to use the crutches on stairs and standing from a sitting position.

CANE

- Adjust the handle of the cane to the level of the wrist when the arm is held straight.
- The cane should be held on the side opposite of the injured side and adjacent to the body.
- Instruct the patient to move the cane in concert with the injured limb.
- Instruct the patient on how use the cane on stairs and standing from a sitting position.

WALKER

- Adjust the handles of the walker to the level of the wrists when the arms are held straight.
- Instruct the patient on how use the walker on a step or curb and standing from a sitting position.
- Walkers should not be used on steps or escalators.

Conclusion

Immobilization and ambulatory assist devices play a major role in emergency care and are a vital skill set for ED technicians. Proper technique takes attention to detail, practice, and patience. When well done, it can make the difference between a poor patient outcome and an excellent one.

References for Additional Reading

Azar FM, Canale ST, Beaty JH. *Campbell's Operative Orthopedics*. 14th ed. Elsevier; 2022.

Miller M, Hart J, MacKnight J. *Essential Orthopedics*. 2nd ed. Elsevier; 2020.

Roberts JR, Custalow CB, Thomsen TW. *Roberts and Hedges' Clinical Procedures in Emergency Medicine and Acute Care*. 7th ed. Elsevier; 2019.

Stracciolini, A. Basic techniques for splinting of musculoskeletal injuries. UpToDate. 2022. Last updated June 3, 2021. Accessed July 6, 2022. https://www.uptodate.com/contents/basic-techniques-for-splinting-of-musculoskeletal-injuries#H17439119.

Tintinalli JE, Stapczynski J, Ma OJ, et al. *Tintinalli's Emergency Medicine: A Comprehensive Study Guide*. 8th ed. McGraw-Hill Education; 2016.

CHAPTER 20

The Major Trauma Patient

Matthew Pyle ■ Jason S. McKay ■ Sara Lenard

Introduction

Every year 35 million people visit an emergency department (ED) because of an injury. Trauma is the leading cause of death in the United States for people under the age of 44. Tragically, trauma accounts for a disproportionate percentage of deaths in younger people, causing 31.8% of all deaths for people aged 1 to 9 years, 40.6% for those aged 10 to 24, and 34.6% for those aged 25 to 44. Because the care of trauma patients can be resource-intensive and trauma resuscitation is often a fluid enterprise, it is crucial that trauma care be delivered by a team of providers who are all familiar with their specific roles but are also able to perform any of a core set of skills described in this chapter.

Trauma Activation

The purpose of a trauma activation system is to alert the relevant personnel, gather equipment, and mobilize resources necessary to care for complex trauma patients. Ideally, this activation occurs before the patient arrives, based on emergency medical services (EMS) information from the scene of the trauma. This additional time before patient arrival allows the team to prebrief regarding the impending patient encounter, tailor their preparations to the clinical scenario, and don the appropriate personal protective equipment (PPE).

As prearrival notification does not always occur, it is important for the ED always to have a baseline level of readiness. Critical equipment (e.g., material to start peripheral intravenous [IV] lines, secure the airway, control bleeding) should be kept in the trauma bay or other designated area in a clear and organized fashion. ED staff that will care for trauma patients should be pre-designated and their other duties adjusted to allow for the fact that they may need to respond at a moment's notice.

Because the care of trauma patients is multidisciplinary, trauma activations tend to involve resources and personnel from multiple services in the hospital. Trauma protocols are institution specific, but in general they may include the following:

- General/trauma surgery team to come to the ED to be part of the team assessing the patient
- Anesthesiology to either come to the ED to help manage the patient's airway or to stand by in the operating room (OR) in case the patient is taken to surgery
- Radiology technicians to come to the ED with a portable x-ray machine to take whatever images are required immediately (a chest x-ray is part of the standard trauma patient evaluation)
- Radiology department to hold a computed tomography (CT) scanner open
- OR team to standby to open an OR as needed
- Blood bank to prepare to send blood products to the ED quickly (some blood products require a period to thaw before use)
- Chaplain services to come to the ED to attend to spiritual needs of the patient and their family

- Security services to come to the ED to ensure a safe environment for staff and patients
- An administrative team member (e.g., nursing administrator, trauma coordinator) to help coordinate the logistical needs of the team

Many trauma centers will have at least two levels of trauma activation to better align the resources expended to the patient severity. Based on patient characteristics and mechanisms of injury the goal is to identify "major" or "level I" traumas who are likely to require any/all of the resources described and "minor" or Level II" traumas who will still require more resources than the average patient, but less than a major trauma. These criteria are institution specific, but some common examples are included in Table 20.1:

TABLE 20.1 ■ Simplified Trauma activation criteria in the emergency department (Trauma center)

Level I Trauma activation	Level II Trauma activation
Critically ill patient with unstable vital signs: • Sign of shock, blood pressure less than 90 • Gunshot wound or stab wound (Head, neck, chest, abdomen, thigh, elbow) • Glasgow Coma Scale less than 9 • Active arterial bleeding requires blood transfusion • Any traumatic injuries require intubation • Multi-organ involvement with unstable vital signs	Patient with stable vital signs: • Motor vehicle crash with significant mechanism • Older adult on anticoagulant and Head injury • Penetrating injuries distal to knee and elbow • Fall more than 20 feet • Open long bone fracture

Initial Assessment

Initial assessment of the trauma patient is crucial for identification of life-threatening injuries and rapid application of life-saving therapies. Preparation is key. Once a trauma patient is identified, coordinating with prehospital agencies and obtaining necessary equipment ensures a smooth transition from the prehospital to the hospital phase. The ED technician (EDT) assist in the preparation by listening to the prehospital report, noting the patient age, the type of injury, any specific patient history, and any special considerations.

After the prehospital information is received, the role of the EDT is often to prepare the resuscitation room, gather needed equipment, and don the appropriate PPE to await the arrival of the trauma patient.

When the patient arrives, multiple team members have individual assignments that occur simultaneously. These actions include:

- Disrobing the patient, often by cutting off their clothes (nurse or tech)
- Obtaining IV access with one or two large-bore IV catheters (nurse or tech)
- Taking vital signs (nurse or tech)
- Placing the patient on a cardiac monitor (nurse or tech)
- Obtaining a brief history, focusing on underlying medical problems, medications, and allergies (nurse)
- Beginning the primary survey (provider)

The provider begins the primary survey, which is focused on identifying and prioritizing all the patient's injuries. The team leader makes a visual assessment, noting any areas of trauma or hemorrhage. By looking at the chest, abdomen, pelvis, and the floor, the team leader may reprioritize hemorrhage control prior to continuing with the initial assessment.

If no excessive bleeding is noted in the trauma patient, the team leader will proceed with the initial assessment (ABCDE). These ABCDEs of trauma include the following:

A: Airway maintenance with cervical spine precautions

B: Breathing and ventilation

C: Circulation with hemorrhage control

D: Disability (neurologic evaluation)

E: Exposure and environmental control

If concerns are discovered at any point during the primary survey, the team will pause and try to correct the issue. For example, if the team discovers an airway issue, they may suction the airway, insert an oropharyngeal airway, or even perform rapid-sequence intubation to establish a secure airway. It is important to note that once an intervention is completed, the team will reassess the effectiveness of that intervention before moving to the next stage of the trauma process.

Once the primary survey is complete and any life-threatening injuries are addressed, the team will complete any adjuncts to the primary survey and begin the secondary survey. These include the following:

F – Full set of vital signs

G – Get necessary adjunct measures, and give comfort measures (pharmacologic and nonpharmacologic)

H – Head-to-toe assessment and complete history

I – Inspect posterior surfaces

Adjunct measures may include electrocardiogram monitoring, urinary and nasogastric suction catheters, arterial blood gases, and diagnostic studies such as CT scans or x-rays. The role of the EDT in trauma resuscitation may include direct patient care, patient transport to imaging, and continued communication with the trauma team regarding the patient's progress. Depending on the institution, at this time the patient may be prepared for transport to a higher level of care.

After the primary and secondary surveys are complete, the trauma patient will require constant reevaluation. Trauma patients can quickly deteriorate, and reassessment of both the primary and secondary surveys, as well as specific findings identified during those surveys, can prevent the trauma patient from decompensating.

VASCULAR ACCESS

Reliable vascular access is critical, as it allows the trauma team to administer medications, IV fluids, blood products, and to draw blood for diagnostic testing. Because many of these functions are time-sensitive, vascular access should be obtained during the primary survey.

The ideal site for vascular access depends on a number of factors, including patient habitus, injury pattern, and preexisting medical conditions (e.g., dialysis access, prior surgeries that preclude using that limb). Because vascular access in trauma patients is often used for rapid administration of high volumes of resuscitative fluids, it is preferred to obtain large-bore access (18 gauge), usually in the upper extremities. In patients where rapid administration or multiple simultaneous products are anticipated, two IVs are often placed simultaneously, one in each arm. In choosing a site for IV access, you should consider the length and gauge of the intended catheter and select a site where the vein is both large enough and travels in a straight line long enough to accommodate the catheter.

Traditional peripheral IV placement using anatomic landmark and palpation is not always possible, particularly in patients with challenging anatomy, obesity, or a history of IV drug use. In those situations an ultrasound-guided or ultrasound-assisted peripheral IV may be employed (see Chapter 16). Because ultrasound allows for direct visualization of the vessel, it enables the user to access deeper vessels that cannot be palpated, identify tortuous or branching vessels, and directly visualize placement of the catheter in the vein. Ultrasound-guided peripheral IVs have also been shown to decrease complication rates and central line utilization, and to have a higher success rate than the traditional approach.

INTRAOSSEOUS ACCESS

Intraosseous (IO) access is another form of vascular access, which can be used either when traditional IV access cannot be obtained or as a first-line technique in patients where difficulty with vascular access is anticipated (e.g., pediatric patients, morbidly obese patients). IO access involves using a specially designed, commercially available drill to insert a metal catheter through the cortex and into the medullary space of a long bone. Because the medullary space is supported by rigid bone, it does not collapse or become harder to access in hypotensive patients the way peripheral veins do. Studies have shown that IOs can be placed as quickly, but with much higher rates of success, than peripheral IVs in hypotensive patients.

The preferred sites for IO access in adults are the humeral head (2 cm above the surgical neck, into the greater tubercle) and proximal tibia (2 cm inferior and medial to the tibial tuberosity). In pediatric patients, only the tibia should be used (1 cm below the tibial tuberosity), and care must be taken to avoid the epiphyseal plate.

Contraindications to IO placement include prior attempt at IO placement in that bone, fracture of the bone, overlying cellulitis or infection, or adequate venous access having already been established. Once obtained, IO access can be used to infuse any medication that can be given intravenously, and studies have shown that routine laboratory tests run on blood aspirated from an IO will yield similar results to blood drawn from a vein (though formal blood work should be obtained to ensure accuracy).

Blood Products

In resuscitating a trauma patient, four simultaneous objectives are pursued: improve blood pressure to reverse or reduce hypoperfusion of tissues, maintain oxygen delivery to tissues, reduce or halt ongoing blood loss, and avoid coagulopathy. Transfusing blood products with different physiologic properties is the best way to accomplish all of these objectives.

PACKED RED BLOOD CELLS

Red blood cells are responsible for oxygen delivery, so transfusing them in traumatic patients is logical. However, as they have no hemostatic properties (will not enhance coagulation) transfusing them alone is insufficient, as they will not prevent further blood loss. Transfusion of packed red blood cells (PRBCs) will also improve the volume status of the patient, raising blood pressure and improving hypoperfusion; however, this increased hydrostatic pressure at the site of injured tissue could increase the rate of blood loss.

There are four major blood types: A, B, AB, and O. When transfusing PRBCs, it is important to administer compatible blood. If incompatible blood is administered, the patient could have a severe transfusion reaction leading to shock and kidney damage. Patients with blood type A, AB, and B must be given either their blood type or type O, which is known as the "universal donor." It takes the blood bank some time to determine the patient's blood type and perform a crossmatch, by which the donor blood of the patient's blood type is mixed with the patient's blood to confirm their compatibility. In the meantime, the clinician has two alternatives to obtain blood rapidly for unstable patients. The first is to administer type O blood, and the second is to administer type-specific blood without having done the crossmatch.

This process is further complicated by the additional need to determine the presence of the Rh factor, another genetically determined protein located on the outside of red cells that influences the compatibility of blood to be used for transfusion. Rh-negative blood is safe to administer to both Rh-negative and Rh-positive patients, so it should be safe to administer type O, Rh-negative blood to any patient without knowing their blood type in advance.

FRESH FROZEN PLASMA

Trauma patients who are bleeding will deplete their own plasma proteins that are needed to form clots in damaged blood vessels. Fresh frozen plasma (FFP) is a product that, when administered, will replace the patient's own procoagulant proteins that are depleted by the trauma. FFP is separated from whole blood and stored frozen in units of 200 to 250 mL. FFP requires time to defrost before use, so providers must notify the blood bank early if they anticipate needing it. Some facilities (particularly trauma centers) will keep a small amount of FFP defrosted and ready for use at all times.

PLATELETS

Platelets are the cellular components of blood that are responsible for triggering the coagulation cascade by adhering to the lining of damaged blood vessels and clumping together, forming a clot. They are generally pooled from multiple donors and concentrated into a unit of platelets, which will raise the patient's platelet count by roughly 50,000/μL.

Transfusion Protocols

The ratios of blood products given in trauma resuscitation has been long debated, but currently a 1:1:1 ratio of PRBCs, FFP, and platelets is most commonly used. There is growing interest in the use of whole blood in the resuscitation of trauma patients, as it would seem to be the ideal resuscitative product in terms of addressing physiologic derangements.

Massive transfusion is generally defined as more than 10 units of PRBCs in the first 24 hours, but protocols for how the blood products are released, in what ratios, and under what circumstances are institution specific. It is important to obtain samples for crossmatching prior to initiating massive transfusion, as it will be difficult to perform the test on samples drawn after the patient has received large volumes of donor blood.

Tourniquet

A tourniquet is an external hemorrhage control device that obtains hemostasis by applying circumferential compressive force proximal to the wound. By applying enough force to halt blood flow to the injured area, the tourniquet prevents further blood loss from the wound. Although they are often thought of as prehospital/EMS devices, tourniquets are frequently used in the OR during limb surgeries in order to maintain a bloodless surgical field. Because they can be applied quickly and easily (in some cases with one hand) and can improve the survival of bleeding patients, they are an invaluable tool in the care of trauma patients. Commercially available combat-style tourniquets are now commonly used in urban trauma centers (Fig. 20.1), and instructions for their specific application should be consulted before use.

Tourniquets should be applied 2 inches proximal to the wound and tightened until they are applying more force than the blood pressure in the underlying arteries. Operators will know that point has been reached when the distal pulses are no longer felt. In larger vessels, this amount of force will likely require a windlass. If one tourniquet alone cannot control the bleeding, a second tourniquet should be applied proximal to the first. Tourniquet application is not definitive management of a bleeding wound, but rather should be used in conjunction with other hemostatic therapies (e.g., compression bandage, sutures). Once those other measures are in place, the tourniquet should be loosened (but not removed) and the wound observed to see if hemostasis has been achieved. If not, the tourniquet can be retightened and additional dressings and direct pressure applied.

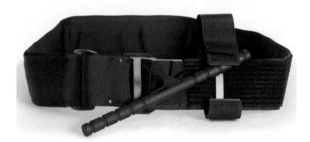

Fig. 20.1 Example of a tourniquet. (Samuel PC, Nathan TM, Shayn MR, Wayne MJ. Management of acute trauma. In: *Sabiston Textbook of Surgery: The Biological Basis of Modern Surgical Practice*, 21st ed. St Louis: Elsevier; 2022:386-428.)

Because a properly applied tourniquet cuts off arterial flow, and that ischemia will damage tissues over time, it is important to make note of the time that a tourniquet is applied, either in the medical record or written directly on the limb. A general recommendation is that tourniquets *not* be kept in place for more than 2 hours. The compressive force of the tourniquet itself may also damage underlying tissues or cause discomfort for the patient. Use of a wider tourniquet will minimize both of these issues. Finally, as a patient is resuscitated and their blood pressure increases, wounds with tourniquets in place should be reassessed to ensure that additional tightening is not necessary.

Cervical Spine Stabilization

In the United States, there are approximately 18,000 new spinal cord injuries documented annually. The majority of spinal injuries (55%) documented in the United States involve the cervical spine (C-spine). The remaining spinal injuries are divided equally among the thoracic, lumbar and sacral vertebrae. Of the spinal injuries treated annually, 5% of cases present with initial or worsening neurologic symptoms. Common causes of worsening or secondary injury include excessive movement, uncontrolled ischemia, and spinal cord edema. Protecting the spacing inside the descending spinal canal can prevent or limit additional injury.

Most blunt trauma and certain penetrating trauma patients must be assumed to have a C-spine injury, and the team should stabilize and splint the trauma patient's neck upon arrival until their actual situation can be determined. This will prevent exacerbation of any vertebral or spinal cord injury sustained in the field. Excessive extension, flexion, or rotation can create an opportunity for secondary injury. Stabilization of the C-spine requires achieving neutral alignment of the vertebral anatomy and reduces range of motion (ROM). The most expedient method for attaining this alignment is to perform manual C-spine immobilization (Fig. 20.2).

Although manual C-spine immobilization can be obtained from an anterior or lateral approach, a coronal orientation by the provider is usually preferred and allows for assisting personnel to approach the patient from the lateral sides. Direct pressure to the midline or lateral soft tissues of the neck should be avoided to prevent compression of the patient's airway or carotid vessels. When possible, obstruction of the auricular canal should be avoided in the conscious patient to preserve their ability to respond to verbal communication.

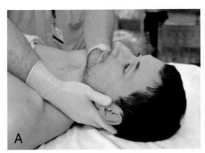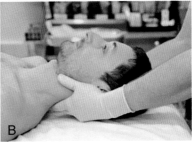

Fig. 20.2 Manual inline stabilization of the cervical spine demonstrated in the inferior (A) and superior (B) approaches. (Grissom TE, Stephens C. Airway management in the trauma patient. In: *Hagberg and Benumof's Airway Management*. 4th ed. Philadelphia: Elsevier; 2018:584–599.)

C-spine Immobilization

In order to sustain C-spine immobilization while the patient undergoes evaluation and treatment, a cervical collar is often employed. When properly sized and applied, these collars may help maintain neutral alignment of the neck. Selection of the proper cervical collar should be based on the desired effect. The majority of cervical collars deployed are classified as either rigid or soft. Soft collars are rarely deployed in the emergency setting due to their failure to restrict a large degree of ROM. Rigid cervical collar types applied include extrication cervical collars and Philadelphia cervical collars.

The extrication cervical collar is most often employed by the EMS provider to sustain C-spine immobilization during the extrication and transport phase of care. This type of collar, which is stored flat as a linear piece, has adjustable components and locks to allow for sizing and support of the chin to reduce ROM. Hook-and-loop tape is used to join the ends of the collar on the lateral side of the neck after being threaded underneath the posterior C-spine and wrapped back toward the midline. An anterior window is built in to allow for direct visualization of the patient's trachea. Sizing of extrication collars should be performed prior to application using the manufacturers' specifications. Specifically, the height from the patient's proximal trapezius muscle to the chin line is compared with the size gradations on the device. Although effective, this device can create uncomfortable pressure points or damage to the skin, especially the longer it is left in place (Fig. 20.3).

The Philadelphia cervical collar is a rigid foam collar that also affixes anterior and posterior pieces bilaterally. The size options include medium (13- to 16-inch circumference), large (16 to 19 inches) and extra large (>19 inches), which also precludes usage on the majority of smaller pediatric patients. The top of the anterior piece should cup the chin and rise almost to the level of the lower lip. The posterior should thread underneath or inside the anterior section before being secured bilaterally with hook-and-loop tape.

Failure to properly size or apply a cervical collar may allow for increasing degrees of ROM after application. Additionally, a paradoxical extension forcing articulation at the C1–C2 area may also be caused by improper sizing. Even when properly applied, a cervical collar rarely affords 100% motion restriction, and it does not effectively immobilize areas of the spine inferior to C7. Therefore application of a collar does not necessarily alleviate the need to dedicate clinical staff to manual stabilization at the bedside without additional immobilization devices (Fig. 20.4).

Cervical Collar Application

A Posterior-First Method

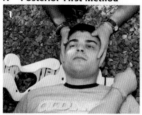 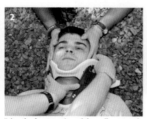 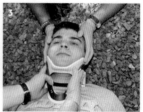

While one provider applies in-line stabilization (*not* traction!), slide the posterior portion of the collar behind the patient's neck. Maintain in-line stabilization in the neutral position until the patient is fully immobilized.

Bring the front portion of the collar around, under the patient's chin. Ensure that the chin is well supported by the chin piece. Difficulty positioning the chin piece may indicate the need for a shorter collar.

Attach the loop Velcro from the posterior portion of the collar to the hook Velcro on the anterior portion. Recheck the position of the patient's head for proper alignment. Tighten the collar as needed until proper support is obtained.

B Anterior-First Method

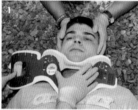 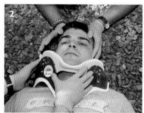 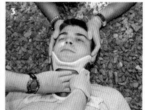

While in-line stabilization is provided, position the chin piece under the patient's chin.

Slide the posterior portion of the collar behind the patient's neck.

Secure the collar and assess proper placement as described above.

Fig. 20.3 Cervical collar application.

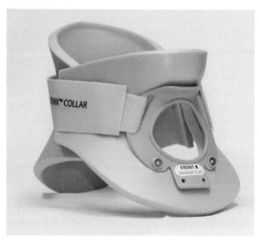

Fig. 20.4 Philadelphia cervical collar for cervical immobilization.

References for Additional Reading

American College of Surgeons. (2018). Advanced trauma life support: student course manual. 10th ed. https://www.academia.edu/39781997/Student_Course_Manual_ATLS_Advanced_Trauma_Life_Support.

Baker D, Keller, IV AP, Knight RM, et al. Military medicine. In: Tintinalli JE, Ma O, Yealy DM, Meckler GD, Stapczynski J, Cline DM, Thomas SH. eds. Tintinalli's Emergency Medicine: A Comprehensive Study Guide. 9th ed. McGraw-Hill; Accessed March 07, 2021. https://accessmedicine-mhmedical-com.proxygw.wrlc.org/content.aspx?bookid=2353&sectionid=226636519.

Bogdan Y, Helfet DL. Use of tourniquets in limb trauma surgery. *Orthop Clin North Am.* 2018;49(2):157–165. https://doi.org/10.1016/j.ocl.2017.11.004.

Brannam L, Blaivas M, Lyon M, Flake M. Emergency nurses' utilization of ultrasound guidance for placement of peripheral intravenous lines in difficult-access patients. *Acad Emerg Med.* 2004;11(12):1361–1363. https://doi.org/10.1197/j.aem.2004.08.027.

Centers for Disease Control and Prevention. National Vital Statistics Reports, Vol. 68, No. 6, June 24, 2019.

Chreiman KM, Dumas RP, Seamon MJ, et al. The intraosseous have it: a prospective observational study of vascular access success rates in patients in extremis using video review. *J Trauma Acute Care Surg.* 2018;84(4):558–563. https://doi.org/10.1097/TA.0000000000001795.

Gazendam A, Wood TJ. Cochrane in CORR®: tourniquet use for knee replacement surgery. *Clin Orthop Relat Res.* 2021;479(3):445–451. https://doi.org/10.1097/CORR.0000000000001668.

Jousi M, Björkman J, Nurmi J. Point-of-care analyses of blood samples from intraosseous access in pre-hospital critical care. *Acta Anaesthesiol Scand.* 2019;63(10):1419–1425. https://doi.org/10.1111/aas.13443.

Kragh Jr JF, Walters TJ, Baer DG, et al. Survival with emergency tourniquet use to stop bleeding in major limb trauma. *Ann Surg.* 2009;249(1):1–7. https://doi.org/10.1097/SLA.0b013e31818842ba.

Lasfargues JE, Custis D, Morrone F, Carswell J, Nguyen T. A model for estimating spinal cord injury prevalence in the United States. *Paraplegia.* 1995;33(2):62–68. https://doi.org/10.1038/sc.1995.16.

McQuilten ZK, Crighton G, Brunskill S, et al. Optimal dose, timing and ratio of blood products in massive transfusion: results from a systematic review. *Transfus Med Rev.* 2018;32(1):6–15. https://doi.org/10.1016/j.tmrv.2017.06.003.

National Center for Health Statistics. Health, United States, 2019: Table 037. Hyattsville, MD. 2021. Available from: https://www.cdc.gov/nchs/hus/contents2019.htm

Petitpas F, Guenezan J, Vendeuvre T, Scepi M, Oriot D, Mimoz O. Use of intra-osseous access in adults: a systematic review. *Crit Care.* 2016;20:102 https://doi.org/10.1186/s13054-016-1277-6.

Whitcroft KL, Massouh L, Amirfeyz R, Bannister GC. A comparison of neck movement in the soft cervical collar and rigid cervical brace in healthy subjects. *J Manipulative Physiol Ther.* 2011;34(2):119–122. https://doi.org/10.1016/j.jmpt.2010.12.007.

CHAPTER 21

Behavioral Health and Toxicologic Emergencies

Leah Steckler ■ Zeina Saliba ■ Aileen Chowdhury

Introduction

Nearly one out of every eight emergency department (ED) visits in the United States is related to mental illness or substance use. ED visits for mental health issues have been rising by over 20% during the period 2006 to 2018. Acute behavioral disturbances in the ED are both common and potentially dangerous. They are most frequently caused by some combination of acute intoxication, substance withdrawal, and underlying mental illness. Knowledge of common causes of agitation and recognition of signs of escalation are vital to provide effective, patient-centered treatment.

ED technicians (EDTs) play an integral role in the care of patients with mental health disorders. Many resources are often required to effectively care for patients with acute mental health complaints and to avoid an unnecessarily prolonged length of stay in the ED. Thus a streamlined, individualized, and efficient approach to care of this population is vital. Safety of staff and other patients is always paramount.

TERMINOLOGY

Mental health professionals have a rich vocabulary to describe the symptoms and behavior of their patients; key mental health terms and their definitions follow:

- *Bipolar disorder:* A condition characterized by manic or hypomanic episodes alternating with depressive episodes, with periods of normal mood between episodes.
- *Catatonia:* A dramatic reduction of psychomotor activity, may present with rigidity, mutism, failure to eat, use the bathroom, or perform other necessary functions.
- *Delirium:* An acute, transient, usually reversible, fluctuating disturbance in attention, cognition, and consciousness level. Causes include almost any serious illness or medication. Diagnosis is clinical, with laboratory and usually imaging tests to identify the cause. Treatment is correction of the cause and supportive measures.
- *Delusions:* Firmly held false beliefs.
- *Hallucinations:* False perceptions, often auditory or visual.
- *Hypomania:* Similar to mania (see below); however, symptoms are to a lesser degree.
- *Mania:* May include euphoric or irritable mood, impulsivity, pressured speech, hypersexuality, inflated self-esteem or grandiosity, flight of ideas, or loosely connected thoughts.
- *Psychosis:* Hallucinations or delusions that are caused by an underlying psychiatric, medical, neurologic, drug, or other etiology.
- *Schizophrenia:* A condition characterized by psychosis, hallucinations, delusions, disorganized speech and behavior, flattened affect (restricted range of emotions), impaired reasoning and problem-solving, and often occupational and social dysfunction.

Initial Patient Assessment and Room Assignment

Patients presenting to the ED with abnormal behavior must be rapidly assessed. There are several medical conditions that can mimic psychiatric symptoms, and patients must be screened for these medical problems. Hypoglycemia (low blood sugar), hypoxia (low oxygen), drug or medication overdose, infection, and brain tumors can all masquerade as acute psychiatric illness.

Room assignment is one of the early and critical decision points in the care of a patient experiencing what appears to be an acute psychiatric emergency. The patient should be rapidly evaluated and *not* be placed in a general waiting area. The individual should be escorted to a special behavioral health room or area with minimal medical equipment and minimal moveable furniture. This type of room most often has a plastered ceiling and walls, a door that can be locked from the outside, and an observation window in the door. Limiting noise and other distractions can help create a more therapeutic physical environment. A 1:1 patient observer (sitter) should be assigned to continually visually monitor the patient to ensure safety. In some institutions, there may be a "tele-sitter" assigned to the patient.

A clinical staff member should assist the patient to completely disrobe, don a special hospital gown that is used specifically for patients with suspected mental illness, and secure the patient's belongings. This allows for early recognition of a patient who has surreptitiously brought a weapon or other dangerous object into the ED; it also allows easier patient identification if the patient were to elope from the ED. All belongings, including cell phones, are typically removed from the patient, placed in a belongings bag, and locked in a designated belongings area.

Medical evaluation of all patients (especially those presenting with agitation or intoxication) is necessary, as is looking for organic (physical illnesses) causes of abnormal behavior. Although not always possible, it is preferable to obtain vital signs and an electrocardiogram prior to medication administration. The technician may be asked to help with both of these tasks, as well as to obtain bloodwork and a urine specimen for laboratory studies.

Signs of psychiatric illness are not always immediately identified upon patient presentation to the ED. Likewise, a patient may not initially share symptoms such as suicidal thoughts or thoughts of harming others with ED staff. The EDT may be the first staff member aware of such thoughts, and it is important that they alert/inform a nurse or other higher-level provider. If the technician is with the patient and not able to quickly maintain a safe environment or prevent the patient from absconding, the technician should escalate the situation immediately.

If the EDT begins the evaluation on a patient who seems angry or whose potential for violence has not yet been assessed by the physician, they should always stay between the patient and the door or exit. The EDT should keep a safe distance from the patient to avoid physical harm when managing a patient with the potential for aggressive behavior. It is also recommended to avoid wearing a badge or badge clip, jewelry, stethoscope, or a hair style (e.g., a ponytail) that can be used by a patient to cause harm. If the EDT feels threatened at any time during their interaction with the patient, they should call for help, leave the patient's bedside, and seek assistance immediately.

Techniques for Verbal De-escalation

It is vital to develop a rapport with the patient by introducing oneself with a smile and using a calm tone of voice. If the technician is not sure how to respond to a patient concern, an effective technique can be to repeat terms that the patient used to describe their condition. Initially, use open-ended questions while talking with a patient, and transition to more specific, detailed questions. Many institutions also offer specific training or coursework, including simulation sessions, to practice these techniques in a protected environment. Practice and training in managing patients experiencing psychiatric emergencies is essential to success in caring for this particular population. Table 21.1 describes the elements of verbal de-escalation.

TABLE 21.1 ■ Elements of Verbal De-escalation

Maintain a distance of two arm's length when possible. Respect personal space.
Keep hands relaxed. Do not stare at the patient. Do not be provocative.
Team leader establishes verbal contact with the patient.
Use clear, concise language.
Identify the patient's feelings and desires: "What are you hoping for?"
Listen, and restate what the patient said.
Set limits related to violent or disruptive behavior.
Offer choices and optimism.

Richmond JS, Berlin JS, Fishkind AB, et al. Verbal de-escalation of the agitated patient: consensus statement of the American Association for Emergency Psychiatry Project BETA de-escalation workgroup. *West J Emerg Med.* 2012;13(1):17–25.

Chemical Sedation

When verbal de-escalation is ineffective and a patient is identified as a risk to themselves or others, or if behaviors have quickly escalated to a dangerous level before verbal de-escalation can be used, patients and those around them must be kept safe. Medication administration will help calm the patient by decreasing their anxiety, treating their psychosis, or sometimes sedating them. The technician will often assist the nurses with persuading the patient to accept medications.

If a patient is willing to take oral medications, this is usually preferable. If not, intramuscular (IM) injections can be used. Multiple categories of antipsychotic medications can be given this way, (e.g., haloperidol) or benzodiazepines (e.g., lorazepam). There are often regional or institutional preferences for which medications to use. Although the onset of medications given by IM injection is slower than those administered intravenously, it is much easier to give an IM injection to an agitated patient than to start an IV. If the patient already has an IV placed, however, the IV administration route may be preferable.

Physical Restraints

Physical restraints are another tool that can be used to ensure safety if verbal de-escalation is insufficient. These are usually placed by a team of no fewer than five persons, often including the EDTs, nurse, and security personnel. A team leader coordinating the response assigns one person to each limb. A patient can often be safely restrained in the supine or side-lying position. Avoid restraining the patient in the prone position as this increases the risk for suffocation. The team leader is responsible for the patient's head to avoid cervical spine trauma and to maintain an open airway. Typically, if four-point restraints are used, one arm should be up while the other one is down. This is intended to reduce the possibility that the patient will be able to overturn the stretcher. With two-point restraints, the contralateral arm and leg should be used. A sheet or a lap belt may also be used alone or in addition to existing restraints if extra support is needed. Fig. 21.1 demonstrates a type of restraint that can be used to maintain a patient in a seated position, and Fig. 21.2 demonstrates a softer restraint that can be used for patients who need less constricting restraints. Every institution is required to have a detailed protocol for the use of restraints, including team activation, reasons for restraints, and which type of restraints may be used. All patients who are restrained should be reevaluated frequently and the restraints discontinued as soon as possible (https://www.acep.org/patient-care/policy-statements/use-of-patient-restraints).

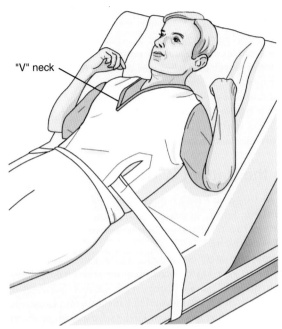

Fig. 21.1   Restraint vest. (From: Sorrentino SA and Remmert LN. Chapter 13:Restraint Alternatives and Restraints. In: Sorrentino SA and Remmert LN, eds. *Mosby's® Essentials for Nursing Assistants*, 7th edn. Elsevier;2023:144-158.)

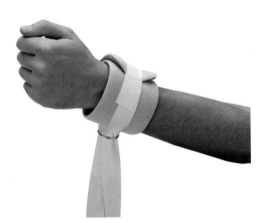

Fig. 21.2   Cotton extremity restraint. (From: Perry AG, Potter PA, Ostendorf WR, eds. *Clinical Nursing Skills and Techniques*, 9th ed. Elsevier;2018.)

Common Psychiatric Conditions

Knowledge of most common psychiatric conditions causing agitation is useful for ED staff.

Schizophrenia is a severe mental illness characterized by problems with cognition, emotion, and behavior. As many as 1% of the general population has schizophrenia, but this rises to 10% in people with a first-degree relative with schizophrenia. Schizophrenia is an illness in which the patient is disconnected from reality. Symptoms can include paranoia, hallucinations, delusions, disorganization, and negative symptoms. It is typical for symptoms to start in men from late adolescence to early adulthood; often, symptoms begin slighter later in women. Treatment is antipsychotic medication combined with psychosocial therapies. Although people with schizophrenia are more often victims of violence, they are at risk for agitation when they stop their medications or use intoxicants.

Bipolar disorder exists along a continuum and is characterized by the presence of hypomanic or manic episodes. At times the patient may be very depressed and potentially suicidal; other times the same patient may be euphoric and psychotic. Moods can be labile and irritable with impulsive behavior. Although it can start in childhood or adolescence, the typical age of onset for bipolar disorder is the mid-twenties and affects men and women equally.

Approach to the Patient With a Toxicologic Emergency

Often patients who are triaged as having a psychiatric complaint have also experienced an intentional or unintentional overdose or ingestion. In 2017 there were just under one million nonfatal drug overdose–related ED visits. Depending on the intoxicant, patients may present in an agitated, confused, or depressed state.

For agitated patients, the safety of the staff and the patient is of primary importance. For depressed patients, maintenance of oxygenation and breathing take priority. Restraint must be considered, but the physician will have to make a more detailed situational analysis when considering chemical sedation for an already intoxicated patient. In all patients with an overdose, it is important to make all possible attempts to identify the substance. A good resource for the providers is to call a regional Poison Control Center. Different centers cover different regions, but there is one national number (800-222-1222) in the United States, which will automatically direct the calls to your regional center.

Every attempt should be made to rapidly obtain a complete set of vital signs and blood glucose. If the patient is unstable (i.e., they have abnormal vital signs), resuscitation will focus on airway, breathing, and circulation. The technician is essential to rapidly placing the patient on a monitor, obtaining intravenous (IV) access, and administering supplemental oxygen. After quickly obtaining IV access, staff can provide the patient with medications and antidotes. IVs should be secured with gauze, and patients may require the use of restraints to minimize interference with ongoing medical resuscitation.

The technician may be asked to gather materials for decontamination that are unique to an overdose situation, such as an orogastric tube. Communication directly with the nurse and physician will aid in determining the most appropriate order of operations. Table 21.2 provides general guidelines for how the EDT should approach patients experiencing behavioral health emergencies.

Common Substances Associated With Toxicity In Overdose
ETHANOL (ALCOHOL)

Excessive ethanol use accounts for 95,000 deaths in the United States each year, including one in ten total deaths among working-age adults. Immediate health effects related to alcohol include increased risk of injury and increased risk of poisoning or overdose from other substances. Alcohol use is also associated with unintended pregnancy, poor pregnancy outcomes, and sexually transmitted infections. Long-term alcohol use is associated with high blood pressure, heart disease, stroke, liver disease, and cancer. Acute alcohol intoxication is often diagnosed based on clinical appearance and can be confirmed and quantitated using a breathalyzer or blood test. Exact levels of ethanol poorly correlate with a patient's observed level of intoxication, as patients who chronically consume ethanol become tolerant to some of its effects. Acutely intoxicated patients may be euphoric or combative. Severe intoxication results in slurred speech, nystagmus (rapid eye

TABLE 21.2 ■ Emergency Department Technician Flow for Patients Experiencing Psychiatric Emergencies

Step	Pearls	Pitfalls	Comments[a]
1. Safety	Safety of staff, patient, and others present in the emergency department is paramount	Failure to undress/properly expose a patient who is experiencing a psychiatric emergency	Policies and procedures vary by hospital
2. Patient placement	Appropriate room placement within the department Placing the patient in an environment where there is minimal stimulation Patients should be near nursing and physician staff areas	Having too much equipment in a room Placing the patient in a room without a sitter	Some departments will designate specific rooms for patients in this situation
3. Patient assessment	Gather vital signs, alert additional team members if anything appears abnormal Sepsis, meningitis, seizures, hypoxia, hypoglycemia, intoxication, and other conditions can mimic acute mental health disturbances	Failure to gather a complete set of vital signs (including temperature and oxygen saturation) Letting the patient leave the department after expressing suicidal or homicidal thoughts	Often patients will disclose important clinical information to the technician; it is important to convey this information to nursing staff and physicians
4. Patient restraint (chemical and physical) only if necessary	Identify a team of security, nursing staff, and other technicians who will be activated in the event that a patient acutely needs to be restrained Use simulated exercises to practice restraining patients	Not establishing a team to help restrain patients during the shift Failing to identify a patient who may require physical or chemical restraints	Occasionally, this will be the first step in your patient interaction, as the patient may be too agitated to be safely cared for
5. Communicate with team and gather additional materials	Discuss with the physician, nurse, and team leaders what additional materials and special equipment may be needed in the resuscitation of the patient	Failure to communicate as a team may result in delayed diagnosis, treatment, and deleterious consequences for the patient	A coordinated response ensures that all team members understand what the patient needs

[a]Always follow institutional protocols when available.

movements), and ataxia (difficulty walking) and can lead to coma. Alcohol use can also lead to hypothermia and hypoglycemia, particularly in children.

Alcohol withdrawal may begin as early as 2 to 6 hours after a reduction in alcohol consumption in habituated patients and may present as elevated blood pressure, elevated heart rate, and hand and foot tremors. If the patient has abnormal vital signs, it is important for the technician to alert additional staff, as alcohol withdrawal can precipitate extreme agitation or seizures and can result in death.

AMPHETAMINE AND METHAMPHETAMINE

Amphetamines are synthetic drugs that stimulate the central nervous system. They are commonly prescribed for treatment of attention-deficit/hyperactivity disorder (ADHD). Other amphetamines include a compound that is smoked, known as "ice" or "crystal meth." Some signs of amphetamine abuse that the technician may notice include hostility, insomnia, dilated pupils, fever, hyperventilation, and psychosis.

COCAINE

More than one in three drug use–related ED visits involve cocaine. Cocaine use is most often seen in individuals 35 to 44 years of age. Cocaine causes euphoria and increased alertness and energy levels. A cocaine overdose can lead to tachycardia, fever, respiratory failure, and seizures. High blood pressure secondary to cocaine use can lead to stroke, cerebral hemorrhage, and myocardial infarction.

PHENCYCLIDINE

Phencyclidine (PCP, or "angel dust") is a dissociative anesthetic that produces hallucinations and distorts reality. Commonly, a user smokes a marijuana cigarette that has been dipped into PCP. The most common sign of PCP intoxication is a blank stare. Other signs of PCP intoxication are hypertension; horizontal, vertical or rotatory eye movements (nystagmus); nausea/vomiting; drooling; agitation; violent behavior; tachycardia; odd affect; delusions; numb extremities; and myocardial infarction.

LYSERGIC ACID DIETHYLAMIDE

Lysergic acid diethylamide (LSD) is a substance that causes hallucinations. Most patients who present to the ED for an LSD-related problem are experiencing what is colloquially known as a "bad trip." Signs of a bad trip may include dilated pupils, anxiety, seizures, paranoia, mood swings, and thoughts of suicide.

OPIOIDS

Often called "narcotics," common examples of opioids include injectables such as heroin, fentanyl, morphine, and oral pain relievers such as oxycodone, hydrocodone, fentanyl, and methadone. The opioid epidemic in the United States is growing rapidly. In the last decade, 90% of opioid users were white adults aged 21 to 24, but persons of any age, gender, or ethnicity can have opioid use disorder.

The main cause of death from an opioid overdose is respiratory depression. Opioids are one of the intoxicants for which there is an excellent antidote (naloxone), which acts almost instantaneously when given intravenously; it can also be given intramuscularly or intranasally with slightly slower onset of action. Other signs of opioid intoxication include constricted pupils, decreased alertness, and changes in heart rate. Signs of opioid withdrawal include lacrimation, perspiration, piloerection, restlessness, irritability, fatigue, headache, nausea/vomiting, and fever.

The opioids fentanyl and carfentanyl are particularly dangerous. Carfentanyl is used for the sedation of large animals, and it is 10,000 times more potent than morphine. Fentanyl is also of concern, as it is 50 times more potent than heroin. These substances may be present on a patient as a white powder resembling cocaine and can cause dangerous exposures in first responders and hospital personnel through accidental inhalation or skin absorption.

SYNTHETIC CANNABINOIDS

Synthetic cannabinoids include "K2," "spice," and synthetic marijuana. K2 is a type of chemical commonly sprayed onto marijuana and smoked; it may also be mixed into a liquid and vaped, or added to tea or food and ingested. It is vital that these patients are kept on a monitor, as K2 use can be associated with a variety of neurologic, psychiatric, and physical side effects.

The physical side effects can range from nausea and vomiting to chest pain, kidney failure, and even death. Onset of symptoms and time to metabolize these substances vary depending on the route of exposure. Additionally, patients may also become addicted to synthetic cannabinoids. There is no antidote for intoxication with these substances, and most hospitals do not have toxicology screens to confirm their ingestion. The ED treatment is therefore observational and supportive, and most patients metabolize the intoxicant and are able to be discharged from the ED home.

References for Additional Reading

Akerele E, Olupona T. Drugs of abuse. *Psychiatr Clin North Am.* 2017;40(3):501–517. https://doi.org/10.1016/j.psc.2017.05.006.

Capp R, Hardy R, Lindrooth R, Wiler J. National trends in emergency department visits by adults with mental health disorders. *J Emerg Med.* 2016;51(2):131–135. E1. https://doi.org/10.1016/j.jemermed.2016.05.002.

Coburn VA, Mycyk MB. Physical and chemical restraints. *Emerg Med Clin North Am.* 2009;27(4):655–656. https://doi.org/10.1016/j.emc.2009.07.003.

DEA Issues carfentanil warning to police and public. Drug Enforcement Administration Web site. September 22, 2016. www.dea.gov/press-releases/2016/09/22/dea-issues-carfentanil-warning-police-and-public.

Downey LV, Zun LS, Burke T. Undiagnosed mental illness in the emergency department. *J Emerg Med.* 2012;43(5):876–882. https://doi.org/10.1016/j.jemermed.2011.06.055.

Excessive alcohol use. Centers for Disease Control and Prevention Web site. September 21, 2020. www.cdc.gov/chronicdisease/resources/publications/factsheets/alcohol.htm.

Figurasin R, Maguire NJ. 3,4-Methylenedioxy-Methamphetamine. In: StatPearls. Treasure Island, FL: StatPearls Publishing; January 2020. Updated May 24, 2020. Available from: https://www.ncbi.nlm.nih.gov/books/NBK538482/.

Greene S. General management of poisoned patients. In: Tintinalli JE, Stapczynski J, Ma O, Yealy DM, Meckler GD, Cline DM, eds. *Tintinalli's Emergency Medicine: A Comprehensive Study Guide.* McGraw-Hill; 2021. 8th ed.https://accessmedicine-mhmedical-com.proxygw.wrlc.org/content.aspx?bookid=1658&sectionid=109437481. [Accessed 03 January 2021].

Hsu CC, Chan HY. Factors associated with prolonged length of stay in the psychiatric emergency service. *PLoS One.* 2018;13(8):e0202569. https://doi.org/10.1371/journal.pone.0202569.

Isoardi K, Ayles S, Harris K, Finch C, Page C. Methamphetamine presentations to an emergency department: management and complications. *Emerg Med Australa.* 2018;31(4):593–599. https://doi.org/10.1111/1742-6723.13219.

Merck Manual Professional Version. https://www.merckmanuals.com/professional. Accessed February 2, 2021.

Moore G, Plaff JA. Assessment and emergency management of the acutely agitated or violent adult. UpToDate. https://sso.uptodate.com/contents/search. Published December 9, 2020. Accessed January 7, 2021.

Ng P, Long B, Davis W, Sessions D, Koyfman A. Toxic alcohol diagnosis and management: an emergency medicine review. *Intern Emerg Med.* 2018;13(3):375–383. https://doi.org/10.1007/s11739-018-1799-9.

What are the effects of MDMA? National Institute on Drug Abuse Web site. https://www.drugabuse.gov/publications/research-reports/mdma-ecstasy-abuse/what-are-effects-mdma. April 9, 2020. Accessed January 8, 2021.

Roberts J, Kowalski JM. Physical and chemical restraint. In: *Roberts and Hedges' Clinical Procedures in Emergency Medicine.* 7th ed. Philadelphia, PA: Elsevier; 2019.

Richmond JS, Berlin JS, Fishkind AB, et al. Verbal de-escalation of the agitated patient: consensus statement of the American Association for Emergency Psychiatry Project BETA De-escalation Workgroup. *West J Emerg Med.* 2012;13(1):17–25.

Tasman A, Kay J, Lieberman J, First M, Riba M. *Psychiatry*. 4th ed. John Wiley & Sons, Ltd; 2014.

Thomas KC, Owino H, Ansari S, et al. Patient-centered values and experiences with emergency department and mental health crisis care. *Adm Policy Ment Health*. 2018;45(4):611–622. https://doi.org/10.1007/s10488-018-0849-y.

Tucci V, Moukaddam N. Mental Health Disorders: ED evaluation and disposition. In: Tintinalli JE, Ma O, Yealy DM, eds, et al. *Tintinalli's Emergency Medicine: A Comprehensive Study Guide*. McGraw-Hill; 2020. 9th ed. https://accessmedicine-mhmedical-com.proxygw.wrlc.org/content.aspx?bookid=2353&sectionid=222326260. [Accessed 03 December 2020].

Vivolo-Kantor AM, Hoots BE, Scholl L, et al. Nonfatal drug overdoses treated in emergency departments — United States, 2016–2017. *MMWR Morb Mortal Wkly Rep*. 2020;69:371–376. https://doi.org/10.15585/mmwr.mm6913a3.

CHAPTER 22

Medical Ethics, the Law, and Cultural Competency

Yasmin Al-Atrache ■ Rita Manfredi ■ Kiara Brooks ■ Naja Wilson

Introduction

Medical ethics encompass the obligations health care professionals have to ensure patients' overall well-being and to respect their fundamental human rights. Medical ethics applies to every health-care provider and is a dynamic concept that varies among different societies, religious groups, and cultures. Implementing the basic principles of medical ethics is an essential component of patient care. There are four main pillars of medical ethics:

- *Autonomy:* Allow an individual freedom to make their own decisions.
- *Justice:* Treat all patients fairly and with equality.
- *Beneficence:* Do good on behalf of the patients and society as a whole.
- *Nonmaleficence:* Do no harm or protect from harm.

The four main pillars of medical ethics serve as a general guide in patient care and are adaptable to specific situations. There are inherent limitations to each of these principles. For example, autonomy may not be appropriate for a patient who lacks decision-making capacity due to severe dementia or intoxication.

These concepts not only dictate standards of care but also help us evaluate our own personal biases and behavior toward patients, their families, and our colleagues. Consider the concept of cultural sensitivity and how that fits into the pillars of medical ethics. In the ED, we often encounter patients of varied religious, cultural, and social backgrounds. Respect, professionalism, and consideration of such differences are imperative in implementing patient-oriented care in hopes of improving patient outcomes.

Everyone on the medical team should ensure that the patient's well-being is a priority during the ED visit and has an obligation to speak up with concerns or questions. Technicians are especially important in this process because they often have more frequent interactions with patients and their families and can provide an invaluable perspective.

Emergency Medical Treatment and Labor Act

Providing emergent, stabilizing care to all patients regardless of financial considerations is required by a Federal law called the Emergency Medical Treatment and Labor Act (EMTALA). EMTALA requires that all patients presenting to the ED receive a "medical screening exam" to ensure that the patient's complaints do not represent a life or limb threatening emergency. Patients then must receive whatever care the hospital can provide to treat and stabilize their condition.

Prior to the passing of EMTALA, patients were occasionaly turned away from hospitals unless the patient had a certain type of insurance or could pay for the treatment. This often resulted in patients being moved from private to public hospitals even if the private hospital could provide the needed treatments. A hospital may transfer a patient to another medical facility for higher level of care, such as trauma surgery or interventional radiology if those services are not provided at the original hospital. Additionally, EMTALA requires that larger, referral hospitals must accept transfer patients from less equipped hospitals if the referral hospital has the facilities required to treat the patient experiencing the emergency. The receiving facility cannot refuse such a transfer for financial reasons.

Health Insurance Portability and Accountability Act

Patient privacy is essential to fostering a safe and autonomous healthcare environment. Personal medical information and history is sensitive information that should be treated as such. The Health Insurance Portability and Accountability Act (HIPAA) protects the privacy of patients by describing with whom a patient's medical information can be shared. The purpose of HIPAA is to limit the distribution of protected health information (PHI) on a need-to-know basis. When providing care to patients, all members of the care team should be informed of the patient's condition and relevant medical history. Members of the care team are authorized "need-to-know" individuals.

PHI is any information that links a medical condition to an individual. Information such as a name, date of birth, address, and contact information are all considered PHI. HIPAA prohibits the sharing of PHI in written, spoken, and electronic formats. The majority of health information is stored electronically, so it is imperative that necessary practices are in place to protect patient privacy. Keeping computers locked when not in use, not sharing passwords, and employing encryption are the most common and effective methods to protect electronic patient information. Never share information about the patient outside of their treating healthcare team without patient consent. This includes not discussing specific patient issues with colleagues in public places such as hospital elevators or cafeterias and not sharing information with family members who are not the patient's designated guardian or surrogate.

Three Cs: Consent, Capacity, Competence

There are times when a patient's ability to consent to a procedure or specific care plan is unclear. For example, consider an elderly patient who has advanced Alzheimer dementia arriving at the ED for syncope and is later found to have advanced renal failure. The patient is in need of emergent hemodialysis and placement of a central line for access. How would a provider determine the patient's capacity to consent for the procedure while also respecting their autonomy?

A definition of the three c's includes: (Fig. 22.1):

Consent: A process in which an individual agrees to a particular procedure/treatment

Capacity: A measure of someone's ability to make a decision about a particular procedure/treatment, including an understanding of the risks, benefits, consequences, and alternative treatment options

Competency (legal term): An individual's ability to consent to a particular procedure/treatment being offered

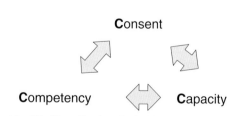

Fig. 22.1 The interrelationship of the Three Cs of medical ethics and law.

Consent, capacity, and competency are specific to a particular situation and can change from one moment to the next. Additionally, assessing a patient's capacity is needed to determine their competency. For example, a patient with dementia may be able to decide between chocolate and vanilla ice cream but might not have the capacity to make decisions regarding complex medical issues. Determining capacity can be complex and is often performed by an attending physician, advanced practitioner, and/or psychiatric team.

Against Medical Advice

Patients may choose to leave the ED against medical advice (AMA) for many reasons, such as prior obligations, family commitments, dissatisfaction with care, fear, frustration, and miscommunication. They may refuse further treatment or specific treatment plans, medications, evaluation, or other aspects of patient care. Although these situations can be frustrating and time-consuming, respecting patients' autonomy while balancing legal and ethical considerations is important.

Patients who leave AMA are at increased risk for readmission and mortality and thorough documentation on these patients is a must. The ED tech should ensure that any notes they make on the patient are consistent with those made by the RN's and providers.

If a patient chooses and has the *capacity* to decide to leave AMA, it is imperative that several steps be taken to protect the patient and providers.

1. Ensure that the patient is aware and *understands* the risks of leaving AMA. Most institutions have an AMA form for the patient and a witness to sign. In addition to completing the form, it is worthwhile for the provider to include a comprehensive narrative in the patient's chart that describes the provider's concerns, notes that they have the capacity to refuse treatment, and details the efforts they made to dissuade the patient from leaving.
2. Remove the patient's intravenous (IV) line, and allow them to dress in their own clothes.
3. Provide the patient with discharge instructions, including a statement that they are encouraged and welcome to return to the ED at any time.

When a patient decides to leave the ED prior to discharge and without going through the process of AMA counseling, it is called *elopement.*

Hospice and Palliative Care in the Emergency Department

The EDT will be treating many patients with serious illness in the ED, and these patients may benefit from palliative care. The word *palliate* means "make a disease or its symptoms less severe or unpleasant without removing the cause." The objective of palliative care is to aggressively treat disease symptoms in order to minimize the patient's suffering in the setting of serious or incurable illness (Table 22.1). Palliative medicine addresses the biological, psychological, social, and spiritual pain that patients experience. This type of care can be instituted in the ED and then continues in the inpatient setting or as an outpatient after being discharged.

The World Health Organization defines palliative care as "an approach that improves the quality of life of patients and their families faced with life-threatening illness by relieving physical, psychosocial, and spiritual suffering." Objectives of palliative care in the ED are outlined in Table 22.2.

Often when patients with serious chronic illness present to the ED, their medical status has changed and clinical the situation may have deteriorated. It is at this point emergency personnel may need to be aware of the patient's goals and desires for future care, especially if their condition

TABLE 22.1 ■ Diseases in Emergency Medicine that Qualify for Palliative Intervention

Congestive heart failure	Liver disease
Sickle cell anemia	Diabetes
COPD	AIDS
Cancer	Severe dementia
End-stage heart disease	Stroke
Failure to thrive, frailty	Degenerative neurologic diseases (e.g., ALS, MS)
End-stage kidney disease	COVID-19 infection with irreversable respiratory failure

AIDS, Acquired immunodeficiency syndrome; *ALS*, amyotrophic lateral sclerosis; *COPD*, chronic obstructive pulmonary disease; *MS*, multiple sclerosis.

TABLE 22.2 ■ Objectives of Palliative Care in the Emergency Department

Affirm life and regard dying as normal processes
Apply early in the course of illness, in conjunction with other therapies that are intended to prolong life, such as critical cardiac medications, chemotherapy, and radiation therapy
Enhance a patient's quality of life, which may positively influence the course of illness
  Use a team approach to help patients and their families cope with illness and bereavement
  Offer a support system to help patients live as actively as possible until death
  Do not intend to either hasten or postpone death
  Better understand and manage distressing clinical complications

requires artificial life support. These goals can be documented in advance directives, which are documents that provide instructions about a patient's healthcare wishes in the future when they may no longer be able to make their own independent healthcare decisions or speak for themselves. Living wills and durable powers of attorney for healthcare are both types of healthcare advance directives.

Often a healthcare proxy, agent, or surrogate has been chosen by the patient as the person who will speak on the patient's behalf when they are incapacitated and no longer able to make medical treatment decisions for themselves.

Patients may arrive in the ED with a medical order known as a MOLST or POLST (medical/physician order for life-sustaining treatment), which is signed by a physician. These standardized medical orders address key critical care decisions consistent with the patient's goals of care and are a result of shared informed decision-making between healthcare providers and patients with advanced progressive illness or frailty.

There are instances when a patient and family have decided that the patient does not desire artificial life support and does not want to be resuscitated. These decisions are converted into a DO NOT Resuscitate (DNR) order and indicate that the patient no longer desires cardiopulmonary resuscitation or ventilation by respirator in the event of cardiac arrest. If the patient desires full resuscitation, then a FULL CODE order is placed.

Frequently patients arrive at the final phase of their serious illness and find themselves at end of life. This is when hospice care is offered to patients and includes supportive care where the focus is on comfort and quality of life rather than cure (Fig. 22.2). The goal of hospice care is to ensure patients are comfortable and free of pain and other bothersome symptoms so they can live each

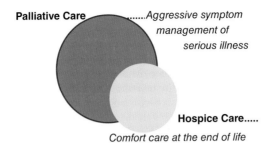

Palliative Care ......*Aggressive symptom management of serious illness*

Hospice Care.....
Comfort care at the end of life

Fig. 22.2   **The relationship between palliative care and hospice care.** Hospice care is a small subset of the larger, all-encompassing palliative care in seriously ill patients.

remaining day as fully as possible. Comfort care order sets may be instituted in these situations. Medicare Part A covers hospice care.

Hospice care is a small subset of the larger, all-encompassing palliative care in seriously ill patients.

Accountability

Accountability is the obligation or willingness to accept responsibility for one's actions. Accountability is an important aspect of practicing medicine, where there is both individual and organizational accountability. To be accountable, hospitals often have a set of policies and procedures to avoid such bad outcomes and protect patients. A culture of accountability is much more than an organization insisting their employees follow rules. In order to be accountable, a provider must be willing to engage in active introspection and pursue further education from reliable sources during their entire career.

Consider the following examples of accountability: individual and organizational.

EXAMPLE OF INDIVIDUAL ACCOUNTABILITY

An EDT was asked by staff to assist an elderly patient to the restroom. While the patient was in the restroom, the tech stepped away to help another colleague. During his brief absence, the patient fell, hit his head on the floor, and required additional imaging.

- How could the EDT practice self-accountability in this scenario?
  The EDT could address how this accident may have been prevented, speak to a supervisor about the error, and identify ways to avoid further incidents.

EXAMPLE OF ORGANIZATIONAL ACCOUNTABILITY

During an evening shift, an EDT was asked to assist with the placement of an ultrasound-guided peripheral IV line. While she was preparing to place the line, she noticed the patient's identifier wristband had the incorrect name and date of birth.

- What can the EDT do in this situation to maintain organizational accountability and correct the error?
  The tech should contact her supervisor immediately to correct the patient's wristband information and notify clinicians of the wristband error. The tech may become part of a multidisciplinary team examining patient identification issues in the ED.

Errors in the ED

Often, the technician is the first team member interacting with the patient and their family members. As such, the ED technician (EDT) is in prime position to recognize when errors may have occurred and to aid in their future prevention. Multiple types of medical errors can occur in the ED and lead to increased patient morbidity, mortality, litigation, and emotional turmoil for clinicians and patients involved. Most hospitals have a reporting system whereby staff can report both actual errors and "near misses." These systems are managed by the Risk Management Department whose main charge is to identify and help reduce medical errors.

Recognizing Implicit Biases: "Do Not Jump to Conclusions!"

Every person possesses implicit *biases*. Also known as implicit social cognition, implicit biases are attitudes or stereotypes that affect our understanding, actions, and decisions in an unconscious manner. Implicit biases are involuntary, residing deep in the subconscious, and are based on making certain assumptions about a person based on their race, ethnicity, age, or appearance.

Implicit biases have real-world consequences, and the ED is a pivotal location where medical providers engage with the full spectrum of humanity. A provider or EDT should consider using a "Self-Reflection Chart" (Table 22.3) to examine their own implicit biases by reflecting upon a situation or event in which they have felt uncomfortable, anxious, or angered.

Cultural Competence

We often encounter patients with diverse set of beliefs, practices, and values. Being able to adapt and understand these differences is vital in providing patient care and improving outcomes. To be culturally competent, one must be self-aware of their own culture and how it influences their views and practices. Self-awareness and openness to such differences is imperative in achieving cultural competency and sensitivity to cultural differences.

Lesbian, Gay, Bisexual, Transgender, Queer, +

There are significant healthcare disparities among the Lesbian, Gay, Bisexual, Transgender, Queer, + (LGBTQ+) community, especially in communities of color or lower socioeconomic status. Access to healthcare regardless of one's sexual orientation and gender identity is a fundamental human right and can often begin in the ED. In order to better address the needs of the LGBTQ+ community and provide supportive, sensitive care, it is important to know basic terms.

TABLE 22.3 ■ Example of a Self-Reflection Chart

Questions to Pose	Reflections on the Situation
What, where, and who? How did you feel before, during, and after? Why did it happen? What could have been done differently? What can be done in the future?	

L = Lesbian, women who are sexually or romantically attracted to other women

G = Gay, men who are sexually or romantically attracted to other men

B = Bisexual, a person who is sexually or romantically attracted to more than one gender

T = Transgender, someone who does not identify with the sex they were assigned at birth

Q = Queer, a reclaimed word that can encompass any identity that is not cisgender and/or heterosexual

The addition of "+" to the acronym is an acknowledgment that there are other noncisgender and nonstraight identities that are not included in the acronym. This is a shorthand or umbrella term for all people who have nonnormative gender identity or sexual orientation.

Using correct pronouns is also important in providing culturally sensitive healthcare. If the EDT is unsure of a patient's preferred pronouns, ask to clarify their preferences in a respectful way. For example, the EDT can start by identifying their own preferred pronouns before asking the patient to identify their pronoun. If an incorrect pronoun is used, it is appropriate to acknowledge the mistake and offer an apology.

Because a technician often encounters a patient before medical clinicians and other staff, use this opportunity to foster a respectful, safe environment for patients to express their concerns and receive care without judgment or ridicule.

References for Additional Reading

Acronyms Explained. Outrightinternational.org Web site. Published August 12, 2019. Accessed March 16, 2021. https://outrightinternational.org/content/acronyms-explained.

American College of Emergency Physicians. Cultural awareness and emergency care. *Ann Emerg Med.* 2008;52(2):189.

Buchanan A. Mental capacity, legal competence and consent to treatment. *J R Soc Med.* 2004;97(9):415–420. https://doi.org/10.1177/014107680409700902.

Creating a culture of accountability in healthcare. Powerdms.com Web site. Published March 1, 2018. Accessed March 16, 2021. https://www.powerdms.com/blog/creating-culture-accountability-healthcare/

Definition of ACCOUNTABILITY. Merriam-webster.com Web site. Accessed March 16, 2021. https://www.merriam-webster.com/dictionary/accountability

Donaldson LJ. Professional accountability in a changing world. *Postgrad Med J.* 2001;77(904):65–67.

Edemekong PF, Annamaraju P, Haydel MJ Health Insurance Portability and Accountability Act. In: StatPearls. StatPearls Publishing; 2021.

Emanuel LL. A professional response to demands for accountability: practical recommendations regarding ethical aspects of patient care. Working Group on Accountability. *Ann Intern Med.* 1996;124:240–249.

Iserson KV. *Ethical principles—emergency medicine. Emerg Med Clin North Am.* 2006;24(3):513–545. https://doi.org/10.1016/j.emc.2006.05.007.

Koshy K, Limb C, Gundogan B, Whitehurst K, Jafree DJ. Reflective practice in health care and how to reflect effectively. *Int J Surg Oncol (N Y).* 2017;2(6):e20.

Lee CA, Cho JP, Choi SC, Kim HH, Park JO. Patients who leave the emergency department against medical advice. *Clin Exp Emerg Med..* 2016;3(2):88–94. https://doi.org/10.15441/ceem.15.015.

Markose A, Krishnan R, Ramesh M. Medical ethics. *J Pharm Bioallied Sci.* 2016;8(Suppl 1):S1–S4. https://doi.org/10.4103/0975-7406.191934.

Palliative care. Who.int Web site. Accessed March 16, 2021. https://www.who.int/news-room/facts-in-pictures/detail/palliative-care

Understanding implicit bias. OSU.edu Web site. Accessed March 16, 2021. http://kirwaninstitute.osu.edu/research/understanding-implicit-bias/

Zibulewsky J. The Emergency Medical Treatment and Active Labor Act (EMTALA): what it is and what it means for physicians. *Proc (Bayl Univ Med Cent).* 2001;14(4):339–346.

CHAPTER 23

Patient Transport

Ayal Pierce ▪ Sarah Cronin ▪ Trent Nayve

Introduction

A significant amount of an emergency department (ED) technician's (EDT's) shift will be spent moving patients throughout the department and assisting them with various tasks outside the stretcher. Some patients in the department will be independent; some will be at risk to fall and hurt themselves; and some may be completely reliant on the tech's assistance to move or even go to the bathroom. It is a vital part of the EDT's job to know how to assess and assist patients in ways that are not only safe for the patient but also for the technician.

Initial Assessment

The EDT is often the first member of the ED team to assess a patient as they are transported throughout the department. Before transporting, moving, or allowing a patient to move throughout the hospital, it is important to perform an initial assessment. This assessment will include, but is not limited to, evaluating them as a fall risk, assessing any handicaps that require the tech's assistance, and knowing why they are in the ED in the first place, as this will affect their transport.

CLINICAL CONDITION

Before transporting a patient, the EDT must know why the patient is in the ED and how that might affect their transportation. If a patient is in critical condition, they should always be moved on a stretcher. The patient who presents to the ED for a twisted ankle will likely need a stretcher or wheelchair in order to be brought to their bed. Patients in critical condition often have multiple medications running through IVs as well as monitors that need to be transfered with them. Intubated patients must be transfered with their attached ventilator and may also have a respiratory therapist with them. Because each patient is unique, and before transporting them to a different location, assisting them in walking around the department, or even helping them use the restroom, it is the EDT's job to accomodate their specific needs. However, there will always be somebody the EDT can ask to help clarify the the patient's condition and needs. It is good practice for the EDT to review the patient's chart before transporting them.

FALL RISK

Falls in the hospital can cause anything from minor scrapes and bruises to severe disability and even death. It is important to assess a patient for how at-risk they are for a fall prior to leaving them alone, as patients can fall when standing on their own, when out of bed, or even when hospital staff are carrying them. It is often the EDT's job to identify patients who are at high risk for falls and to make sure they are given proper assistance to ensure a fall does not happen. Sometimes it is easy to identify people who are a low fall risk simply by clinical judgment (e.g., a 24-year-old male who walks into the ED for a finger laceration and does not seem to have any trouble walking). Sometimes it is easy to identify people who are a high fall risk just by judgment (e.g., the intoxicated patient who cannot stand up without swaying). Any patient in critical condition should be considered a high fall risk. However, for those more subtle but clinically relevant fall risk patients, there are decision tools that help, such as the Johns Hopkins Fall Risk Assessment Tool. Do not hesitate to ask a nurse, or other members of the care team for clarification of the patient's fall risk.

Once a patient at high fall risk is identified, it is important to provide a visual indicator on the patient so that all staff who interact with them know they are at risk for a fall. Different hospitals use different fall risk indicators. Some facilities will use a colorful wrist band while others may use color-coded gowns or socks (Fig. 23.1). Whatever the method, it is important to easily identify patients at high fall risk in order to prevent falls in the ED.

Special Populations

In addition to recognizing the specific needs of the critical patient, there are other special populations in the ED who require specific accomodations.

Different Languages

The ED staff may need translation assistance for patients who speak a diffrent language. It is a patient's legal right to receive care in the language they prefer. Hospitals will either have in-person interpreters for more common languages, or they will provide a phone or video conference for other languages. The EDT should never use a family member to translate, as this violates the patient's privacy, and they may not be willing to be forthcoming with you, except in emergent (life-threatening) situation. However, they are not to be relied upon for translation once a translator is obtained.

Obese Patients

Patients who are extremely obese and immobile may require extra assistance with transportation. One can simply ask the person if they need help getting up to walk or to use the bathroom in order to gauge what extra assistance is needed. Some may need special devices to move them from a chair to bed or from one bed to another, and some may need differently sized wheelchairs or hospital beds in order to accommodate their body habitus. Keep in mind that the patient may feel uncomfotable about the extra staff, equipment, or special needs that go into transporting them and it is the responsibility of the ED staff to ease that discomfort through compassion and respect.

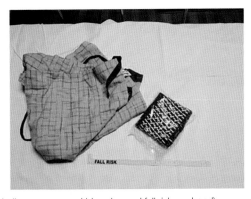

Fig. 23.1   Fall risk outfit (yellow gown, nonskid socks, and fall risk armband).

PHYSICAL DISABILITIES

Patients with various physical differences and disabilities will present to the ED. It is important to know that many patients live independently and may not require any assistance. Although patient safety is our top priority, patient autonomy is also important. One can simply ask a person with a physical disability what assistance they need, if any. Attempting to help patients with various tasks, without their permission or guidance may be percieved as disrespectful and may interfere with the patient's own abilities.

Preventing Provider Injury

In all aspects of patient care in the ED, the EDT must remain safe. This includes the EDT's physical safety during patient handling. To prevent musculoskeletal injury and to ensure patient safety, manual lifting of a patient should be avoided. Assistive devices should be used to replace manual lifting when possible. Some hospitals and institutions have "no lift" policies in which that require staff to use an assist device during patient movement. Be sure to talk to your supervisor and nursing staff for further clarification on when manually lifting a patient is permitted.

When handling patients, an EDT must consider the patient's size, strength, ability to follow and cooperate with instructions, physical abilities, and medical conditions. Determine the patient handling equipment that will be needed for the movement, such as a slide board, low friction draw sheet, or sling device. If you have any questions or concerns, follow your hospital's guidelines or ask someone around you for help and assistance.

Determine the support that you will need from other staff members. A patient should never be lifted by one individual. Prior to moving a patient, ensure that the bed is in locked position, all clutter is removed from the area, and that the bed is at hip level. Ensure that the bed is in an appropriate position, such as keeping the head of the bed flat or tilted downward when pulling a patient up in bed. Keep the patient close to you and directly in front of you when moving to eliminate awkward twisting motions. Legs should be kept at a wide stance to remain stable during the movement. Maintain a bend in the knees and use them to lift the patient. Avoid using the back to lift. Encourage patient participation when possible.

It is important to use assistive devices whenever possible to prevent staff member injury. Follow hospital and manufacturer guidelines on use for assistive devices. Eliminate lifting whenever possible.

Patient Positioning

A patient's position is not only important for their comfort but is also helpful for certain medical needs. Table 23.1 lists common names for patient positions.

TABLE 23.1 ■ Common Names for Patient Positions

Name	Description
Supine	Lying flat on the back
Prone	Lying flat, face down
Lateral recumbent	Lying on either side, often curled up
Fowler	Sitting, head of bed at 45 degrees, knees can be raised
Semi-Fowler	Sitting, head of bed at 30 degrees
Trendelenburg	Lying flat with entire bed angling the head down and feet up
Reverse Trendelenburg	Lying flat with entire bed angling head up and feet down

Special Considerations

INTUBATED PATIENT

Always make sure there is either a registered nurse (RN) or a respiratory therapist present before moving an intubated patient. This is critical because it is important to maintain their airway. A patient who is intubated should be positioned and transported with the head of the bed raised to approximately 30 degrees. This has been shown to decrease rates of pneumonia that are associated with the ventilator.

SPINAL PRECAUTIONS

In some situations, moving a patient's spine can cause or worsen an existing injury. Improperly moving a patient with a spinal fracture, or potential spinal fracture, can result in permanent paralysis. Patients with possible spinal fractures should have a cervical collar applied and be in the supine or semi-Fowlers position, depending on concern for thoracic or lumbar spinal injury. Ask the patient's nurse or medical provider if they should be on spinal precautions.

When a patient cannot move any part of the spine at all and it is necessary to turn the patient to look at their back, they must be "log-rolled." In this procedure, one person is at the head of the bed stabilizing the C-spine, and two people stand next to each other on one of the patient's sides. The two people cross their arms so one hand is on the patient's shoulder, above the hip, below the hip, and legs. Whoever is controlling the head needs to count, and then in one motion, the patient is turned to their side, so as not to twist the spine (Fig. 23.2A,B).

INTRACRANIAL HEMORRHAGE

When a patient has a brain bleed, it is important to keep pressure within the skull as low as possible to help prevent additional injury to the brain. Keep the head of the bed elevated to 30 degrees to help decrease intracranial pressure.

Preventing Falls

Preventing patient falls is a team effort that includes the EDT, nurses, medical providers, and the patient themselves. Ensuring that all precautions have been taken greatly increases patient safety and improves patient outcomes. This section will cover some of the practical considerations when facilitating patient movement throughout the department.

PATIENT AUTONOMY

Although it is important to keep the patient safe, it is equally as important to give the patient as much autonomy as possible given the circumstances. Patient autonomy affords the patient the opportunity to participate in their own care and increases their overall comfort.

ASSISTING THE PATIENT OUT OF BED

Patients who are able to stand with a steady gait may wish to walk around. If the EDT is concerned about the patient falling, they may elect to assist the patient in ambulating by placing an arm or hand under the patient's axilla and one hand on their back. Stand to the patient's side and try to walk as one would normally. With continuous assessment, the EDT may elect to reduce thir level of support or may choose to have the patient sit back down. Again, it is important to be transparent with the patient as to the decisions made about movement about the ED.

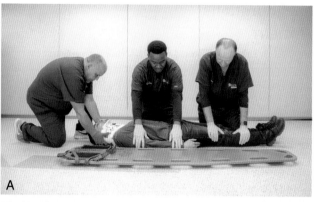

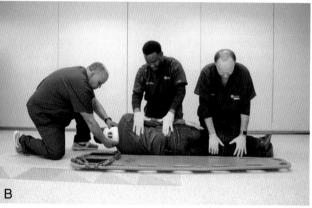

Fig. 23.2 (A, B) Log roll. (From Swartz MH, Phrampus PE. The acutely ill or injured patient. In: Swartz MH, ed. *Textbook of Physical Diagnosis: History and Examination*. 8th ed. Elsevier; 2021:612–623.e1.)

BATHROOM

One of the most common requests from patients is to use the restroom. Here, it is even more important to consider the patient's fall risk. If the patient is ambulatory, has normal vital signs, and has a stable clinical condition, they can be directed to the closest available bathroom. However, if the patient is a fall risk or if the risk is unknown, it is highly recommended that a provider either assist the patient to the closest bathroom or offer the patient alternatives such as a urinal, bedpan, or commode. Help the patient sit on the toilet, if necessary. To maintain the patient's comfortability and autonomy, you may leave the restroom and stand outside the door. If the bathroom is equipped with an emergency pull cord, educate the patient to pull the cord if they need help.

SELF-RELEASING ROLL BELT (POSEY)

Patients who are at risk of rolling out of bed or are inclined to slide out of bed may be braced to the hospital bed with a Posey self-releasing roll belt (Fig. 23.3). An altered patient is usually placed in a Posey belt so that they have freedom to change positions but not to the point of falling out of the hospital bed. It is important to note that the belt should not be covered, and

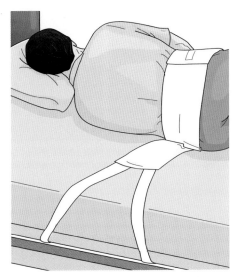

Fig. 23.3   Self-releasing roll belt (From: Sorrentino SA and Remmert LN. Chapter 13:Restraint Alternatives and Restraints. In: Sorrentino SA and Remmert LN, eds. *Mosby's® Essentials for Nursing Assistants*, 7th edn. Elsevier;2023:144-158.).

the patient should be able to release themselves from the belt if they so choose. Depending on the hospital's policy, a covered Posey belt may be considered a patient restraint and be documented as such. Be careful when applying the Posey. If it is placed too tight or misapplied to the body, it can cause injury such as skin damage or bruising or can even restrict their breathing.

SAFETY SITTERS

Safety sitters are an important part of the patient care team. Safety sitters are generally assigned to patients who endorse suicidal or homicidal ideation and/or who pose a risk to themselves if they get out of bed. These individuals are specifically assigned with a 1:1 sitter to patient ratio to best ensure patient safety. It is sometimes the job of the EDT to act as a safety sitter.

Assisting Patients With Alternative Waste Apparatuses
STANDARD BEDPAN

A bedpan is a basin that emulates the shape of a toilet and is used to catch bodily waste. It is particularly useful for patients who cannot get out of bed, including fall risk patients without cervical spine or fracture precautions.

If the patient can participate, lay the patient flat on the bed and ask for them to lift their hips toward the ceiling; insert the bedpan with absorbent underpad underneath. The patient can then be sat up to their comfort by raising the back of the bed. Do not forget that patients can slide or fall, so make sure they are stable. If the patient cannot fully participate, lay the patient flat on the bed. With the assistance of another provider, log-roll the patient one direction and

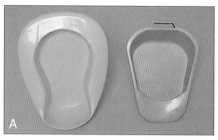 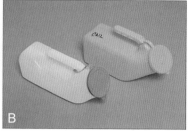

Fig. 23.4 (A) Regular and fracture bedpans. (B) Types of male urinals. (From Craig M. Essentials of patient care for the sonographer. In: Hagen-Ansert SL, ed. *Textbook of Diagnostic Sonography*. 8th ed. Elsevier; 2018:24–53.)

place the bedpan with underpad at an angle under the patient's buttocks. Then, with the assistance of the other provider, roll the patient back on their back while pushing the bedpan underneath the patient. Adjust the patient on the bedpan as necessary and then sit the patient up to their comfort (Fig. 23.4A). Place both side rails up, if not already, to ensure that the patient does not roll off the bed.

FRACTURE BEDPAN

A fracture bedpan is smaller wedge-shaped basin. It is best used on fall risk patients with cervical spine precautions or spinal fracture precautions; it is even useful for patients with back pain. It can also be used for female patients who only need to urinate.

If cervical spine precautions are taken, have one provider hold the patient's C-spine. The rest of the process is similar to that of a standard bedpan, but the wedge design allows for easier positioning. The handle should be positioned toward the patient's feet. It is important to note that when rolling a patient with a fracture, roll the patient onto their noninjured side. If the patient is unable to be log-rolled, stand at the foot of the bed or to the side of the bed so that your dominant hand is at the foot of the bed. With underpad underneath, place the wedge bedpan in between the patient's legs. Slowly wedge the bedpan underneath the patient with the handle toward the foot of the bed.

MALE PORTABLE URINAL

A male urinal is a bottle with an angled and wide opening with a lid. It can be used for male patients who cannot leave their room or stretcher to use the restroom. Educate the patient to urinate into the urinal and to secure the lid of the urinal and attach to the side rail when finished (Fig. 23.4B).

COMMODE

A commode is a portable device with a toilet seat over a bedpan that allows a patient to relieve themselves as they would sitting on a toilet without having to leave the room or ambulate very far. It is best used on patients at moderate fall risk who can ambulate independently or with minimal assistance for short periods of time or for patients who are in isolation rooms.

Set up the commode as recommended by the manufacturer. Set up the commode so that it is perpendicular to the bed and has enough distance in between the bed and commode to turn the patient 90 degrees. Assist the patient into a sitting position on the bed. (Hint: Use the bed to sit the patient up fully.) Have the patient swing their legs off the bed. (Important: If the patient is unable to stay in a seated position without assistance, elect to use a standard or wedge bedpan.) With one hand under the patient's armpit and one supporting their back, assist the patient into a standing position. Assist the patient in turning 90 degrees and sitting on the commode.

URINARY CATHETER

There are three common types of urinary catheters: condom catheters, which are attached to the outside of the penis like a condom; wick catheters, which are attached on the outside of the vagina; and indwelling catheters, which are inserted sterilely into the urethra, and an inflatable balloon is filled inside the bladder to keep it in place.

In some hospitals, the placement of some types of urinary catheters may be an assigned EDT procedure. More commonly, it is the nurse's or medical provider's responsibility to place urinary catheters. However, it is important to be familiar with how they are used, as the EDT may be called to assist in placing them, as well as educating patients on their use. For non-indwelling catheters, patients may have to be encouraged to urinate despite not being on a toilet.

Use the hospital's standard protocols and product's instruction manual for the placement and care of indwelling urinary catheters.

Passport to Leave/Ticket to Ride

Before transporting a patient anywhere, be sure to get permission from the patient's nurse or the charge nurse. It is vital to know where patients are at all times.

Transporting Patients

INTRODUCTION

Whenever possible, patients should be assisted throughout the department and hospital on an ED stretcher, hospital bed, or a wheelchair, thereby limiting the chances of falling. Choosing which provider should transport the patient is also of utmost importance to ensure optimal patient safety. This section will cover the considerations of patient transport.

TRANSFER FORMS

For patient safety, many hospitals have created transfer forms (sometimes called a *ticket to ride*) for patient transfer to other units. These forms can include items such as the transferring and receiving nurses' names and phone numbers, special considerations for the patient (e.g., isolation or fall risk), a recent set of vital signs, and an admitting diagnosis. The transfer form can assist the transporting EDT in evaluating patient needs prior to and during transport. It is also helpful to have contact information for the transferring and receiving nurses in case there is an issue during transport. An EDT should always carry a phone with the capability of calling either the sending or receiving unit, as well as calling codes or rapid responses during transport. If a patient is in critical condition, there must always have an RN with you when transporting.

Patient Ticket to Ride
Sending Location: <u>Emergency Department</u> Sending Nurse: <u>Liz</u> Extension: <u>4857</u>
Receiving Location: <u>4 South</u> Receiving Nurse: <u>Bradley</u> Extension: <u>5253</u>
Admitting Diagnosis: <u>Pyelonephritis</u>

Vital signs
Time: <u>1558</u>
BP: <u>118/74</u>
HR: <u>97</u>
RR: <u>16</u>
Spo$_2$: <u>98</u>
Temp: <u>37.5</u>

Special Considerations
☐ Isolation: _____
☐ Fall Risk
☐ Hard of Hearing
☐ Blind
☐ Police Custody
☐ Other _____

PATIENT BELONGINGS

A patient's belongings typically should stay with the patient at all times. The EDT can preserve patient belongings in special bags throughout the duration of their stay. Special considerations can be made so their belongings can stay in their ED space while they go to radiology, or that their belongings can be checked into security for safekeeping. It is recommended that large items (e.g., standard wheelchair, electric wheelchair) are checked into security throughout the duration of the patient's stay. It is very important to keep the patient involved in the decision-making process to prevent loss of belongings. Thorough documentation can also help track patient items.

TRANSPORT TO MEDICAL/SURGICAL FLOORS

Attached equipment (e.g., intravenous [IV] infusion, supplemental oxygen, telemetry box with predetermined cords, catheter with urine bag, IV infusion warmer) may require nurse transport for proper handoff and maintenance. The patient's nurse or medical provider should be asked about IV infusion before transport to determine whether the infusion can be discontinued to avoid entanglement during transport. Supplemental oxygen should be transferred to the stretcher tank and set to the same flow rate. The patient should be informed of the momentary discontinuation of supplemental oxygen. The nurse or medical provider may determine that supplemental oxygen can be discontinued fully during transport, if indicated. If the patient requires continuous cardiac and/or pulse oximetry, the telemetry box should be attached to the patient's cardiac leads and pulse oximeter turned on. The patient should be informed of this attachment and educated that it must remain in place until removed by a nurse. Patients attached to an IV infusion warmer must be transported with a nurse.

The patient is brought to their predetermined room and assisted to the hospital bed. The patient should be oriented to their room, if possible, and the bed brought to the lowest position with guardrails raised. Their belongings, if present, should be placed at the bedside to eliminate the risk of the patient reaching for their belongings and falling. The call button should be given to the patient. The patient's folder is given to the secretary to bring the patient onto their respective patient-tracking board. If the patient is on supplemental oxygen, transfer tubing from the mobile oxygen tank to the wall oxygen at the same flow rate. If the patient is on IV infusion pump, keep the patient attached and transfer the pump and fluids to the IV pole in the room. If unable to safely transfer a patient to a bed with IV infusion attached, ask the receiving nurse or ED nurse if IV infusion can be discontinued during transfer.

TRANSPORT TO INTENSIVE CARE UNIT

When transporting a patient to the intensive care unit (ICU), the EDT will be assisting the nurse during transport. An EDT should never transport a patient to the ICU independently. The patient will likely have multiple pieces of equipment that will accompany them during transport. IV infusion pumps, Foley catheters, ventilators, monitors, and defibrillators are just some of the equipment that can be transported with a patient to the ICU. It is important that the EDT remain aware of the locations of all lines, tubes, drains, and cables. The EDT must ensure that the equipment is an appropriate distance from the patient so as not to inadvertently remove any equipment from the patient or pull out lines, tubes, or drains.

TRANSPORT TO OPERATING ROOM

Emergent surgery is often required for ED patients. When transporting a patient emergently to the operating room (OR), the EDT will be accompanying a nurse. Follow all the same guidelines as for transporting the patient to the ICU, with some additional considerations.

Prior to transport to the OR, the patient must be completely undressed. This can be a function of either the nurse or the EDT. All belongings should be given to the patient's family member(s) or sent to a secure location, following hospital protocols.

Often when transporting a patient to the OR, there will be a handoff location. It is important that the EDT remain outside the OR and not enter any prohibited areas in the unit. This is to keep a sterile environment in the OR.

TRANSPORT TO RADIOLOGY

Patients should be prepared for radiology according to the imaging ordered. To ensure optimal image quality, patients should be undressed and gowned according to the images that will be taken (e.g., everything above the beltline for a chest x-ray or below the beltline as comfortable for leg or pelvic injuries). Depending on the image needed, the patient may be able to keep articles of clothing on to their comfort. To avoid interference, all metallic items (e.g., earrings, rings, necklaces, hair clips and pins) should be removed.

Magnetic resonance imaging (MRI) involves the use of very strong magnets. Patients are preemptively screened to identify any metal in their body (such as shrapnel or pacemaker) that may react with the magnets and cause serious injury or death. Patients must be provided a specific gown with no metal and the EDT must ensure that no metal is brought into and left in the room.

TRANSPORT TO LABOR AND DELIVERY

Depending on hospital policy, patients approximately 28 weeks or more into their pregnancy experiencing an emergency relating to the pregnancy (e.g., signs of labor, bleeding) should be brought straight to the labor and delivery department. If there is uncertainty if the patient's chief complaint relates to the pregnancy, ED staff should consult with labor and delivery staff.

Morgue Prep

When a patient dies in the ED, it is often the responsibility of the EDT to ensure that the patient's body is prepared for and transported to the morgue appropriately. It is vital that all hospital policies and state and local regulations are followed during this process.

After a death in the ED, there will be paperwork to complete. Specific paperwork details will vary among different hospitals and jurisdictions. Some items that may be included are the time of death, the name and signature of the provider declaring the time of death, the time and date of medical examiner (ME) notification, and the time and date of local organ donation agency notification.

It is important to facilitate family viewing of the body prior to preparation for transport to the morgue. If the patient was a victim of violence (VOV) or if there is a possibility that the case will be referred to the ME, check with law enforcement and hospital policies prior to allowing family to view the body. Law enforcement may prohibit visitors or may require a chaperone for viewing. For patients who were not VOV or are not ME cases, the body may need to be cleaned prior to family viewing. Any patient that was a VOV or is an ME case should remain uncleaned so as not to disturb any evidence that may be on the body.

The body may need to remain in the department or in a designated area while waiting for family to arrive to view the body. Be sure to follow state and local department of health laws and guidelines, as well as hospital policies and protocols, for limiting the time between patient time of death and transport to the morgue.

When all appropriate agencies are notified about the time of death, the patient's body should be prepared for the morgue. If the patient was a VOV or if there is a possibility that the body will be taken by the ME, all lines, tubes, and drains must remain in place. Do not extubate the patient's body or discontinue any IV or intraarterial lines. A tag with the patient's name, date of birth, and medical record number (preferably typed) should be tied to the patient's great toe or other designated location per hospital protocol. Proper tagging of the patient's body is essential to identify the body once in the morgue, either for transport to the ME or the funeral home.

Once the body is tagged, place the body in an appropriately sized body bag. The bag should completely enclose the body. Depending on the quality of the bag and the size of the patient, a second bag may be required. After the body is secured in the bag, a second identification tag should be tied to the zipper of the bag. Ensure that the identification tag on the zipper matches the one on the toe.

After the patient's body is enclosed in the body bag, it must be transported to the morgue. Your facility may have a special cart to transfer the body to the morgue, or it may be transferred using a regular stretcher. Two hospital personnel should transport the body. Upon entering the morgue, complete the paperwork or log as required by your institution. Once in the morgue, use the morgue lift to maneuver the body to the morgue slot. The morgue lift may be crank-operated or electric. Follow facility protocol and manufacturer recommendations for use.

The process of preparing and transferring a patient's body to the morgue is often an essential function of the EDT. It is important that all hospital policies and procedures, as well as regulations from state and local regulatory bodies, are followed in the process.

Conclusion

An EDT should be thoughtful about ensuring that their patients are safely and efficiently transported throughout the hospital. From the initial assessment, to assist devices, to proper body mechanics, it is vital that the EDT can transport patients of all levels of need to anywhere in the department or hospital.

CHAPTER 24

Pediatrics

Rita Manfredi ▪ Ayal Pierce ▪ Lexington Lemmon

General Approach

Children are not just small adults. Pediatric patients include a spectrum of children up to 18 years of age: newborns, neonates, infants, toddlers, preschoolers, school-age children, preteens, and adolescents. Their anatomy and physiology constantly change as they grow, as well as their emotional disposition and comfort with the healthcare system. Children account for about 20% of all emergency department (ED) visits with a large proportion of children 4 years or younger, so it is vital that the ED environment be child friendly and child safe. Children are almost always accompanied by an adult when presenting to the ED and family should be allowed to stay with the child whenever possible. Be sure to inquire what name to call the child, and then address the child by name. As the ED technician (EDT), you may be the first provider in the ED who interacts with the patient and family, so displaying competence and compassion is critical to set the stage for a successful visit.

Privacy is important regardless of the age of the child. Always use nonmedical terminology when speaking with the child and parents or caregivers so that all involved will comprehend results, interventions, and treatment. Be sure to acknowledge and compliment the child's good behavior by encouragement and praise. Stickers or books can be used as rewards for good behavior. Allowing the child to make simple age-appropriate choices, such as which arm to use for measuring blood pressure, allows the child a sense of control in a medical situation that most likely will provoke anxiety. Encouraging the child to play during the examination and any procedures may have a calming effect. Diversion techniques, such as blowing bubbles to blow the hurt away or singing a favorite song with parents and caregivers are methods that provide distraction. As the EDT, you might ask older children to visualize a favorite place and describe it in detail with all five senses. Remember to give the child permission to express any feelings, reminding them it is "OK to cry." Be mindful of what you might say aloud in the presence of an awake or presumed unconscious child, just as you would with an adult. Empathy is essential when caring for children.

When providing treatment for a child, interactions with the family play a fundamental role in the ED experience. Effective communication with family members facilitates obtaining an accurate history so optimal care can be delivered. Often family members will exhibit significant anxiety and emotional stress, especially if the child is injured or ill. The reaction of the parent or caregiver will directly affect how the pediatric patient behaves and how the ED team approaches the patient. In situations such as these, providing a supportive environment is critical for cooperation from the family and the patient. The presence of the family during procedures has been shown to decrease patient stress, and evidence indicates that family members do not interfere with the duties of healthcare providers. It is important to assess first whether the family member will be able to cope with the events that might occur during the procedure.

Initial Assessment of the Pediatric Patient

Children who are ill and potentially critical present differently than adults, so it is essential to recognize when a child requires urgent attention. The Pediatric Assessment Triangle (PAT) is an assessment tool that should be performed prior to the physical examination (see Fig. 24.1). The PAT is a 15- to 20-second evaluation that assesses general appearance, work of breathing, and circulation to the skin. This efficient method determines whether a patient is critically ill. If one of the three components of the PAT is abnormal, then the EDT should alert a nurse or physician immediately.

Physiologic Differences

In neonates, presenting symptoms are vague, nonspecific, and subtle. Many visits are due to parental concerns related to feeding, weight gain, stooling, breathing patterns, and sustained crying. Physiologic differences compared with adults that are important to recognize in neonates and infants include the following:

    Larger head-to-body ratio
    Faster relative heart rate
    Lower relative blood pressure
    Larger tongue
    Hyperextension of neck easily obstructs airway
    Chubby arms and legs so difficult to place intravenous (IV) line
    Body heat lost more easily

Normal Vital Signs

Vital signs are the purview of the EDT. You may be expected to obtain vital signs and report abnormal findings to the nurse or medical provider. Abnormal findings may indicate critical

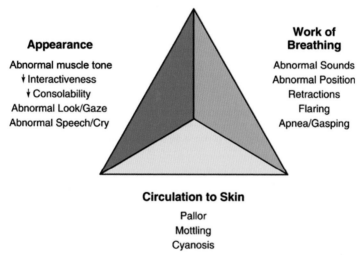

Fig. 24.1 Pediatric Assessment Triangle. (From Horeczko T, Enriquez B, McGrath NE, et al. The pediatric assessment triangle: accuracy of its application by nurses in the triage of children. *J Emerg Nurs.* 2013;39(2):182–189.)

TABLE 24.1 ■ **Age-Dependent Normal Vital Signs**

Age	Respiratory Rate	Heart Rate	Systolic Blood Pressure
Newborn	30–60	120–160	50–70
Infant (1–12 months)	25–30	100–150	70–100
Toddler (1–3 years)	20–40	90–130	80–110
Preschool (3–5 years)	20–30	80–120	80–110
School age (6–12 years)	18–30	70–110	80–120
Adolescent (13+ years)	12–16	60–105	100–120

illness in the patient, so it is important to recognize both normal and abnormal vital signs in the pediatric patient. As children grow and develop, their vital signs change. Table 24.1 summarizes normal vital signs.

The Pediatric Advanced Life Support formula for the 50th percentile of blood pressure is 90 + (2 × age in years). A normal newborn blood pressure is 60 mm Hg.

The rare event of pediatric cardiac arrest is most often the result of respiratory failure, so respiratory rate and oxygen saturation are crucial measurements in every child.

Intravenous Access

IV access in pediatric patients can be extremely difficult and will depend on the skill level of the EDT. Placing an IV in children is frequently made challenging by anatomic factors such as vein size and mobility and limited patient cooperation where the child may move, cry, or pull away from the technician.

Before attempting IV access on a pediatric patient, an EDT must be proficient with obtaining IV access in adult patients. Placing an IV should not constitute an episode that might cause psychological trauma to the pediatric patient. Using a child life specialist to ease discomfort during ED visits and educate children on health issues and topics is extremely helpful. Child life specialists are pediatric healthcare professionals who work closely with children and their families to help everyone cope with medical procedures, pain, and other challenges in the hospital setting. Their job is to provide children with age-appropriate preparation for painful medical procedures and coping strategies.

To cultivate trust, an EDT must be honest with the patient. If the child is old enough to understand why the procedure must be done, then the following language can be used in the explanation: "After the needle comes out, there is just a plastic straw that stays in your body and the needle does not stay in your skin." Always ensure there is a parent or guardian present for the procedure with a nurse or other helper to safely keep the patient still while you attempt IV access. Many EDs use topical anesthetics (e.g., EMLA) applied to the skin site 20 minutes prior to insertion of the IV to reduce pain. Unlike the usual IV antecubital fossa access in adults, optimal access in children may be found in the forearms, wrists, and hands. When attempting to locate venous access, the use of an LED-based transillumination vein finder may be a useful solution (Fig. 24.2).

Another important factor in successful IV insertion is careful selection of catheter size. The typical sizes used in children are 26 G or 24 G in neonates, 22 G in infants, and 20 G in children. Once the IV is successfully obtained, place a stiff board at the site under the extremity and wrap with gauze. This will ensure integrity of the IV with a gauze covering that will decrease emotional distress.

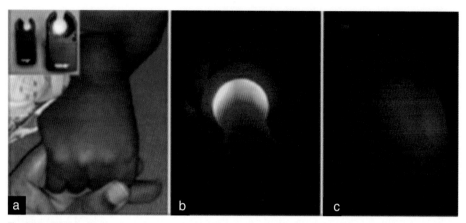

Fig. 24.2 (A) Transillumination of vein in hand. (B) transillumination vein finder device (C) transilluminated vein on hand. (From Naik VM, Mantha SSP, Rayani BK. Vascular access in children. *Indian J Anaesth.* 2019;63(9):737–745. doi:10.4103/ija.IJA_489_19.)

Restraining Techniques for Procedures

Pediatric patients may require restraints for procedures such as IV placement, laceration repair, or lumbar puncture. Patients will require evaluation by a medical provider or nurse to assess if they can independently tolerate a procedure or need restraint. Patients may be restrained manually or with specific assistive devices.

A lumbar puncture, especially in an infant, is one common procedure where restraint by an EDT is required. Any infant under 30 days of age who presents with a fever will need a lumbar puncture as part of the workup. The restraint techniques used by the EDT for the procedure often determines the success of the procedure itself. Therefore it is important for the EDT to be trained in holding the child securely and safely without compromising the patient's airway or disrupting the sterile field. Nurses or physicians may ask an EDT to provide sucrose (sugar water) on a pacifier to help soothe the patient.

Another common procedure that may require restraint is a laceration repair. Depending on laceration size and cooperation of the patient, the EDT may be able to simply hold the patient gently but firmly while the provider is repairing the laceration. Frequently an assistive device is needed, such as a papoose (Fig. 24.3). This can sometimes be scary for children, so it is important to explain the entire process and have a child life specialist and parent present.

Musculoskeletal and Wound Care

Pediatric patients often visit the ED for fractures (broken bones) and skin lacerations. In some EDs, the EDT will be trained to apply splints to extremities where there may be a fracture. Your exact role will be determined by your departmental supervisor, so it is important to discuss this beforehand as different departments may have different protocols.

As with any procedure, it is important to explain the entire process to the patient to alleviate some of the emotional stress. A parent or guardian present at the bedside is beneficial in calming the patient. Sometimes you may need to involve your team of nurses, medical providers, and other EDTs when extra providers are required.

The EDT role in laceration repairs may consist of two functions: restraining the patient and preparing for wound closure. If the wound is extremely painful, the medical provider will anesthetize (numb) the wound with topical anesthetic prior to irrigating. As the medical provider

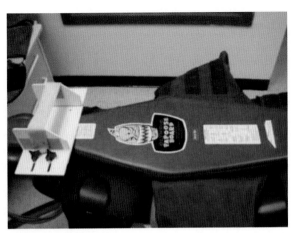

Fig. 24.3 **Pediatric papoose board.** (From: Malamed SF. The pediatric patient. In: Malamed SF. *Sedation: A Guide to Patient Management.* 6th ed. Elsevier; 2018: 497–520.)

is repairing the laceration, it is important to make sure the patient remains still to provide the best cosmetic results. The presence of the child life specialist and the patient's parents may calm the patient. If an assistive restraint device is required, remember to discuss this with the medical provider and nursing staff and describe what will happen during the procedure to the patient and their parents. Be aware that sometimes parents may opt to remain outside the room during the procedure. Reassurance is a key aspect if that occurs.

Nonaccidental Trauma

Children may present to the ED with nonaccidental trauma (previously known as *child abuse*). The EDT may first recognize some of the signs and symptoms and must notify the nurse or medical provider immediately. Presentations may include signs of head trauma, such as ecchymoses (bruising), lacerations, scalp contusions, bruises behind the ear, bruises around the eyes; extremity tenderness, edema, bruising; or deformity that suggests a fracture. There may also be multiple bruises at different stages of healing encountered on a patient at an age where they should be crawling or walking but have not yet achieved those milestones. To safeguard the child, reporting suspected nonaccidental trauma is a mandatory process with, protections from any retaliation in place.

Respiratory Distress: Cough and Wheezing

Respiratory distress is one of the most common pediatric emergencies, and prompt recognition is vital. Whereas older children may be able to identify and communicate their symptoms (including difficulty breathing, wheezing, and cough), infants and toddlers must be observed for signs of respiratory distress: nasal flaring, noisy respirations, grunting, skin mottling, pallor or cyanosis, altered mental status, and bradycardia or tachycardia.

Use the previously discussed PAT: appearance, work of breathing, and circulation. To assess appearance, look for alertness, the ability to make eye contact, muscle tone, interactiveness, presence of sweating, and changes in phonation. To assess breathing, listen for breath sounds and observe patient positioning, presence of retractions, nasal flaring, apnea/gasping, presence of coughing, and wheezing. To assess circulation, examine skin for changes in color, such as pallor, mottling, or cyanosis; abnormal temperature; capillary refill; and pulse quality. The following is a list of respiratory distress signs and symptoms in a pediatric patient:

- *Grunting:* A grunting noise may be heard each time the patient exhales as a means of maintaining air in the lungs.
- *Retractions:* The chest will appear to sink in below the Adam's apple (thyroid cartilage) or below the rib cage with each breath to inhale more air.
- *Wheezing:* A tight, whistling, or musical sound heard with each breath, indicating that the airway is narrowed.
- *Stridor:* A high-pitched, wheezing sound heard in the upper airway when the child inhales. This can be a sign of imminent respiratory arrest.
- *Accessory muscle use:* The patient uses the muscles of the neck and between the ribs during inspiration in an attempt to inhale more air.

The signs of respiratory distress may masquerade as other medical conditions, so it is important to recognize and address these with the medical team immediately to avoid respiratory arrest.

Fever

Fever in children younger than 3 years of age is the most common chief complaint in the ED. Fever is a physiologic response to an invading microorganism characterized by a core body temperature of 38°C (100.4°F) or greater. The most common causes of fever in children are infections, but some noninfectious causes include immune-mediated and inflammatory conditions.

Body temperature can be measured in the axilla, rectum, mouth, and ear and over the skin. There are substantial differences among measurement sites, and as an EDT you should be comfortable with each of these methods of measurement. *Rectal temperature* measurement is the most accurate for estimating core body temperature, and its use is dictated by illness severity, clinical safety guidelines, and physical discomfort. *Oral temperature* measurement is one of the most accurate methods to assess for fever but is not suitable for younger or nonverbal children. *Axillary temperature* measurement is practical and only fairly accurate, with accuracy decreasing as age increases. *Tympanic infrared thermometers* represent a possible alternative, but they are not accurate in children under 3 months of age. *Temporal artery thermometers and forehead noncontact infrared thermometers* represent emerging techniques. With all of this in mind, be sure to ask the nurse or medical provider which method is preferred when obtaining temperature measurements.

Techniques for obtaining a temperature in the pediatric patient:
1. Rectal temperature
   a. The child or infant should lie prone (on their belly).
   b. Cover the thermometer tip with the plastic disposable probe cover.
   c. Apply a small amount of lubricant gel to the thermometer.
   d. Gently spread the buttocks and carefully insert the thermometer approximately 2 cm (no more than 1 inch) into the child's rectum.
   e. Hold the thermometer in place until the thermometer produces a final number or beeps.
2. Oral temperature
   a. Cover the thermometer tip with the plastic disposable probe cover.
   b. Place the tip of the thermometer under the child's tongue in the mouth. Ask the child to hold the thermometer with their lips.
   c. Keep the lips sealed around the thermometer until the thermometer produces a final number or beeps.
3. Axillary temperature
   a. Cover the thermometer tip with the plastic disposable probe cover.
   b. Place the tip of the thermometer in the child's dry axilla (armpit).

   c. Hold the thermometer in place by holding the child's elbow against the chest until the thermometer produces a final number or beeps.

4. Ear temperature
   a. Cover the thermometer with the plastic disposable probe cover.
   b. Hold the ear probe in the child's ear for approximately 2 seconds.

5. Temporal artery temperature
   a. Cover the thermometer with the plastic disposable probe cover.
   b. Run the thermometer across the forehead and in front of the ear.
   c. The thermometer will produce a number after the movement is completed.

Neurologic Complaints: Seizures

Although neurologic complaints are not as common in the pediatric population compared with adults, children may present with seizures, and it is important to treat them quickly. Seizures are bursts of abnormal and uncontrolled electrical activity in the brain and are sorted into two categories. A *generalized seizure* occurs when the patient loses consciousness in the setting of rhythmic shaking (convulsions) of the entire body. *Focal seizures* occur when a localized part of the body may rhythmically shake while the patient often remains alert and is able to talk to you. Both are medical emergencies, and as an EDT, it is important that you recognize the presence of a seizure as you may be the first to identify it and must alert other team members for intervention.

Common causes of seizures in children are rapidly rising fevers, hypoglycemia, and epilepsy. When a seizing child presents to the ED, start with the ABCs (airway, breathing, circulation). Do not put anything into the child's mouth. (There is a prevailing myth that you must hold the tongue so the child won't swallow it. This is blatantly untrue and may cause injury to the child.) Protect the child by removing objects that may hurt them and, if they are not on a stretcher, place a pillow under their head so they do not strike their head on the hard floor. Be prepared to set up the wall suction unit so the medical team can suction secretions from the airway. EDTs will be expected to connect the patient to the vital signs monitor to include telemetry, blood pressure measurement, and pulse oximetry. Careful attention must be given to a low oxygen saturation (Sao_2) reading (<90%) on the pulse oximeter, as the most common cause of pediatric cardiac arrest is respiratory arrest and may be heralded with a decreased Sao_2. IV access in seizure patients is critical and often requires the placement of two IVs. A point-of-care blood glucose should be obtained to rule out hypoglycemia (low blood sugar) as the etiology or cause of the seizure. Children may also experience a postictal confused state seen in adults.

Gastrointestinal Complaints: Vomiting and Abdominal Pain

Up to 14% of children will visit a physician for abdominal pain, yet most will have no identifiable organic cause. Common sources of abdominal pain range from constipation, viral illness, gastroesophageal reflux, urinary tract infection, and milk protein allergy, to more serious illnesses like appendicitis, intestinal obstruction, and congenital conditions. Because infants cannot verbalize if they are experiencing pain, they may present with vomiting, poor feeding, or fussiness. The role of the ED is to identify and rule out emergencies, diagnose the cause of the pain, and provide relief to the child. The EDT is vital in expediting these diagnostic tests. As with every patient, start with the ABCs and PAT. If the child is in critical condition, immediate IV access and continuous monitoring will be required.

For the noncritical patient, an IV or radiologic imaging (x-rays or computed tomography [CT] scans) may or may not be indicated. Be sure to ask about the expected course from the physician or nurse. Because most adult patients with abdominal pain will require an IV and CT scan imaging, in pediatrics this may not be the case unless there is significant abdominal trauma or high suspicion of a condition that might require surgery. The use of ultrasound for abdominal diagnoses has recently increased.

It is important to monitor the patient for any change in status, such as vomiting or variation in vital signs. Before a patient can be allowed to eat or take anything by mouth, check with the nurse or medical provider, as patients often need to remain with nothing by mouth should a surgical problem be discovered.

Cardiopulmonary Resuscitation

EDTs are expected to participate in cardiopulmonary resuscitation (CPR), most likely performing cardiac compressions according to Basic Life Support guidelines and EDT scope of practice. The American Heart Association (AHA) recommends "push hard and push fast" during compressions.

Pediatric cardiac arrest is rare and most commonly the result of respiratory failure from pneumonia, asthma, bronchiolitis, or aspiration. According to the AHA guidelines, CPR should be performed when the heart rate of newborns and neonates is less than 60 beats per minute, unlike adults where CPR is started when the heart rate is zero. Typically, pediatric defibrillation/cardioversion pads should be available to fit the patient's smaller torso. If these smaller pads are not available, adult pads may be used. One adult-size pad should be applied to the front of the chest and the other to the child's back if pediatric pads are unavailable.

The chest compression rate is 100 to 120 beats per minute, at a depth of at least one-third of the patient's chest diameter. As you learned in your CPR class, the compression-to-breath ratio is 30:2 in one-rescuer CPR but changes to 15:2 if there are two or more rescuers present.

References for Additional Reading

Adams J, et al. Emergency Medicine Clinical Essentials. 2013;2(14-25):113–208.

Clark B. PALS Algorithms 2020 (Pediatric Advanced Life Support). United Medical Education. https://www.acls-pals-bls.com/algorithms/pals. Accessed March 02, 2021.

Dionne JM, Bremner SA, Baygani SK, et al. Method of blood pressure measurement in neonates and infants: a systematic review and analysis. *J Pediatr*. 2020;221:23–31. e5. https://doi.org/10.1016/j.jpeds.2020.02.072.

McDermott KW, Stocks C, Freeman WJ. Overview of Pediatric Emergency Department Visits, 2015: Statistical Brief #242. In: *Healthcare Cost and Utilization Project (HCUP) Statistical Briefs*. Rockville (MD): Agency for Healthcare Research and Quality (US); 2018.

Naik VM, Mantha SSP, Rayani BK. Vascular access in children. *Indian J Anaesth*. 2019;63(9):737–745. https://doi.org/10.4103/ija.IJA_489_19.

New Jersey Department of Health and Senior Services. Pediatric Assessment. https://www.nj.gov/health/ems/documents/reg-enforcement/peds_assess.pdf. Accessed November 29, 2020.

Scott-Warren VL, Morley RB. Paediatric vascular access. *BJA Education*. 2015;15(4):199–206. https://doi.org/10.1093/bjaceaccp/mku050.

Tintinalli JE, Ma OJ, Yealy DM, et al. Sedation: a guide to patient management. In: *Tintinalli's Emergency Medicine: a Comprehensive Study Guide*. New York: McGraw Hill Education; 2020:497–520 Figure 35.1.

CHAPTER 25

Documentation

Sarah Cronin ■ Ksenya Badashova ■ Emmanuel Chukwuma

Documentation in the healthcare setting should be clear, concise, objective, timely, and accurate. The medical record documents a patient's trajectory through the healthcare system. It is used as a communication tool among all participants in the patient's care team to coordinate patient care, and much of the record is now shared directly with the patient through online portals. The patient's medical record is also a legal document and will be a very important part of any medico-legal proceedings. It is important that the emergency department (ED) technician develops good documentation skills.

Use of Documentation

The ED technician (EDT) is part of a provider team caring for the patient, all of whom contribute to the patient's record. In most EDs, the EDT is responsible for documenting all procedures they perform, including patient transport, so the range of documentation will parallel their scope of practice. Examples of EDT documentation are intravenous catheter insertion, patient transport, collection of patient belongings, point-of-care testing, electrocardiograms (ECGs), vital signs, and splint application (Table 25.1).

Table 25.2 describes the specific elements of common note types. Some documented information, such as vital signs and point-of-care test results, can communicate aspects of the patient's current health status that determine the patient's plan of care. All members of the healthcare team are responsible for clear, concise, and timely documentation.

Electronic Medical Record

In 2014, Federal legislation required that all hospitals implement an electronic medical record (EMR) system in order to participate in Medicare and Medicaid. Although there are a variety of hospital EMRs, the three largest are Epic (29% of US market), Cerner (26%), and Meditech (17%). EMRs can have hospital-specific modifications, resulting in slight variations of the charting system among different hospitals using the same platform. The EDT should follow guidelines for documentation based on their hospital's policies and procedures.

In the ED, the tracking board is the central display in all EMRs. The tracking board attempts to present large amounts of data in a concise way and allows healthcare providers to pinpoint the patient's physical location within the ED and the status of their evaluation. Standard information displayed on the tracking board includes the patient's age, gender, vital signs, Emergency Severity Index triage level, patient-specific attributes (such as allergies), and the status of certain tasks. There may also be a staff comments section used for short notes for intradepartmental communication that often does not become part of the permanent medical record. Tasks to be completed and patient-specific attributes are often represented by tracking board icons. See Fig. 25.1 for an example of a tracking board.

Associated with each patient in the unit is an extensive collection of individual entries which, when aggregated, constitute the chart. Analogous to sections of a paper record, the patient's EMR is divided into sections, with different types of information residing in each section. There may

TABLE 25.1 ■ Example of ED Technician Documentation Notes

Vital signs	Postmortem care
Patient safety checks	Blood draw
Patient ambulation	Swab/culture specimen
Suspected abuse	Suctioning
Maintenance of seizure precautions	Placing patient on oxygen
Immobilization/restraints	Assisting physician in orthopedic reduction
Cardiopulmonary resuscitation	Assisting physician with cast
Electrocardiogram	Splint application
Orthostatic vital signs	Orthopedic devices application
Intravenous access	Providing crutch training
Wound care	Waste disposal
Type of device, location of device, distal pulse, Patient transport	Facilitating environmental services

TABLE 25.2 ■ Specific Elements of Different Types of Notes

Procedure	Essential Documentation Components
Intravenous access	Catheter size, insertion site, number of attempts, skin prep used, patency, dressing type, special equipment used (such as ultrasound)
Wound care	Wound site, site condition, dressing type
Orthopedic devices	Type of device, location of device, distal pulse, motor and sensation pre- and postdevice application, instructions given
Patient ambulation	Steadiness of gait, amount of assistance needed, safety precautions in place
Electrocardiogram	Time and date of completion, time and date shown to provider, name of provider shown
Patient transport	Method of transport (e.g., wheelchair, stretcher, ambulatory), destination, specialty equipment or monitoring devices used in transport

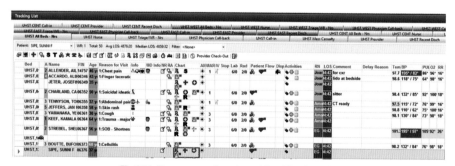

Fig. 25.1 Emergency department tracking board.

also be summary pages that pull information from different sections of the record. Figs. 25.2–25.5 provide examples of how the data entry screens appear for several different types of notes that might be completed by the EDT.

Barcode Scanning

When collecting patient specimens, EDTs will be required to scan laboratory labels. When a physician orders a lab test on an individual patient, a label is created to be affixed to the sample.

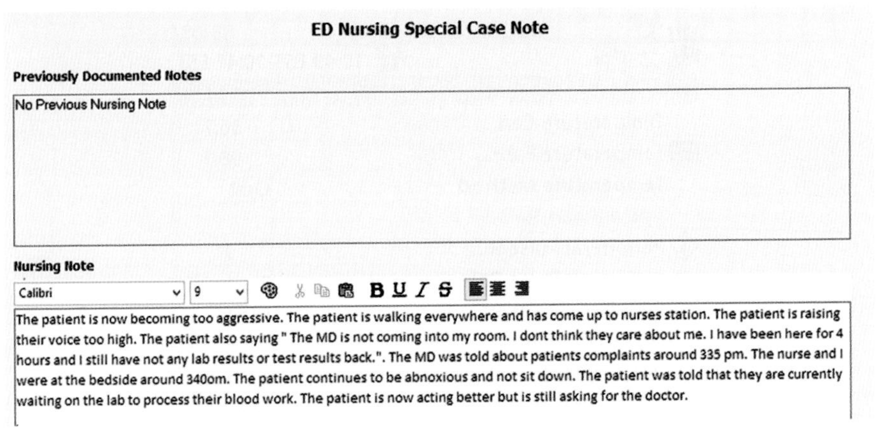

ED Nursing Special Case Note

Previously Documented Notes

No Previous Nursing Note

Nursing Note

| Calibri ⌄ | 9 ⌄ | 🌐 | ✂ 📋 📷 | **B** U *I* S | ▦ ▦ ▦ |

The patient is now becoming too aggressive. The patient is walking everywhere and has come up to nurses station. The patient is raising their voice too high. The patient also saying " The MD is not coming into my room. I dont think they care about me. I have been here for 4 hours and I still have not any lab results or test results back.". The MD was told about patients complaints around 335 pm. The nurse and I were at the bedside around 340om. The patient continues to be abnoxious and not sit down. The patient was told that they are currently waiting on the lab to process their blood work. The patient is now acting better but is still asking for the doctor.

Fig. 25.2 Emergency department nursing special case note.

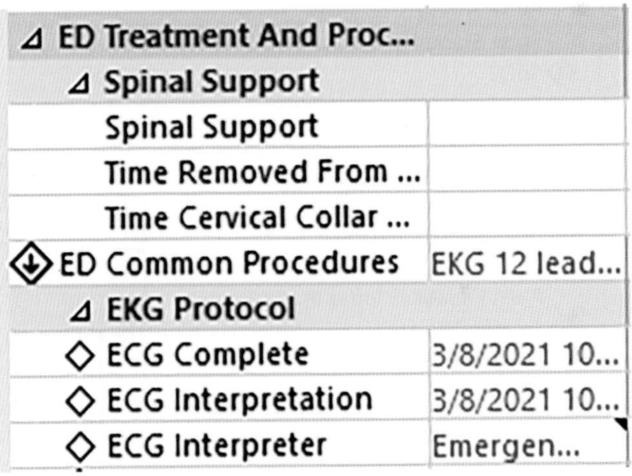

Fig. 25.3 Electrocardiogram documentation.

Each patient is given a wristband identifier upon initial arrival in the ED. By using a barcode scanner connected to the device used for documentation (i.e., phone, tablet, computer), the EDT can scan both the barcode on the patient's wristband and the barcode on the laboratory label, ensuring that the specimen label matches the patient on whom the specimen was ordered. An additional benefit of barcode scanning is that the EMR will create a time stamp to specify the time of collection.

Equipment Association

Some EMR platforms can receive information such as ECGs and vital signs transmitted into the chart from various devices used in the department. For instance, vital signs can be transmitted directly from the monitor or vital sign machine into the patient's chart without the EDT entering each vital sign individually into the EMR. EDTs should learn the process for associating the machines with the patient's EMR for ease and accuracy of documentation.

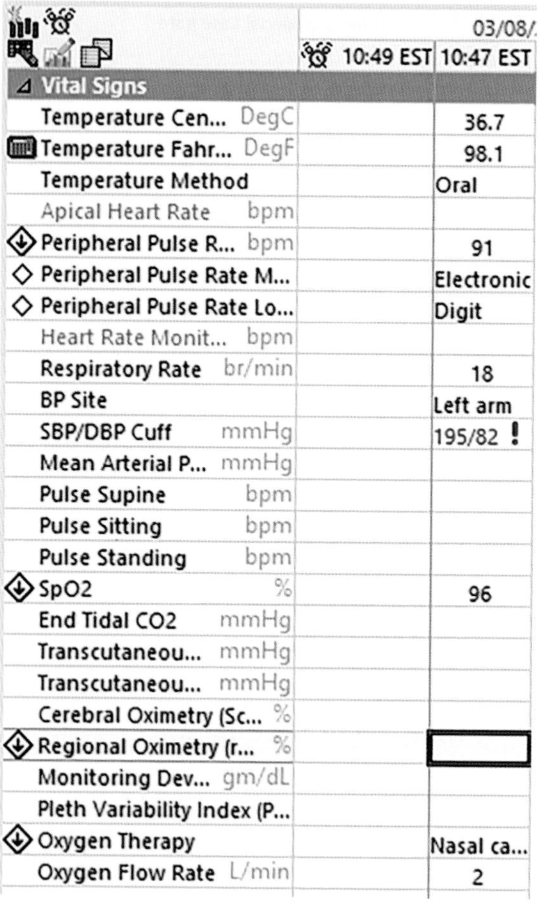

	03/08/
	10:49 EST	10:47 EST

△ Vital Signs	
Temperature Cen... DegC	36.7
Temperature Fahr... DegF	98.1
Temperature Method	Oral
Apical Heart Rate bpm	
Peripheral Pulse R... bpm	91
Peripheral Pulse Rate M...	Electronic
Peripheral Pulse Rate Lo...	Digit
Heart Rate Monit... bpm	
Respiratory Rate br/min	18
BP Site	Left arm
SBP/DBP Cuff mmHg	195/82 !
Mean Arterial P... mmHg	
Pulse Supine bpm	
Pulse Sitting bpm	
Pulse Standing bpm	
SpO2 %	96
End Tidal CO2 mmHg	
Transcutaneou... mmHg	
Transcutaneou... mmHg	
Cerebral Oximetry (Sc... %	
Regional Oximetry (r... %	
Monitoring Dev... gm/dL	
Pleth Variability Index (P...	
Oxygen Therapy	Nasal ca...
Oxygen Flow Rate L/min	2

Fig. 25.4 Vital sign documentation.

Registration

It may be in the scope of the EDT's practice to register patients in the EMR. This may be within the same system used for documentation or a separate registration system that communicates with the EMR. Regardless of the system's configuration, it is important that the EDT be accurate when entering patients into the EMR. Once entered into the EMR, the patient's previous visits will populate into the patient's history in the chart. If the wrong information is entered, previous visits will not populate for the medical team to review. It is also possible to misidentify a current patient as a similarly named patient, thereby associating the current patient with the wrong historical record. The EDT should confirm information with the patient, such as name, date of birth, and possibly Social Security number, to ensure the accuracy of the entered information.

Best Practices

1. Documentation should be timely. Documentation should occur as close to the actual time of activity as possible. An EDT should never "predocument," which is the documentation of an activity before the activity actually occurs. It is possible that unforeseen circumstances

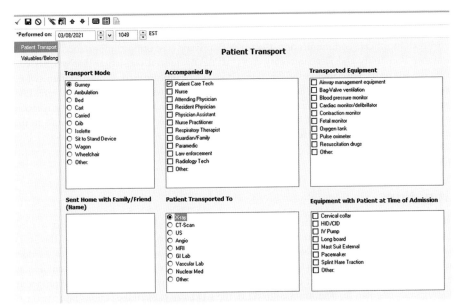

Fig. 25.5 Patient transport.

could arise when the EDT attempts to complete an activity. Only after a task has been completed can it be documented accurately. Excessively late charting must also be avoided, as accuracy may deteriorate with time. EMR platforms allow the provider to document the time an activity took place as well as the time the documentation occurred. As documentation is a communication tool among the care team, it is important that the team has access to the information as close to real time as possible.

2. Documentation should be objective and accurate. The EDT should avoid subjective documentation and opinions when charting. Entries should provide objective information without bias. Direct quotations can be used to express what the patient has stated. It is also important when the EDT is documenting that they do not document by "autopilot" and that they consider each part of their documentation. Hasty documentation can lead to errors and contradictory information in the chart. When a patient decides to leave against medical advice (AMA), it is important to document the situation in an unbiased and factual way. Simply stating that the patient has decided to leave AMA and their reason is a good approach. Direct quotations from the patient's explanation can be included. The key is to remain nonjudgmental and to refrain from blaming or berating the patient.

3. Documentation should use only hospital-approved abbreviations. Medical terminology consists of many words that can be abbreviated or included in an acronym. It is important to use only hospital-approved abbreviations when documenting. Consult with your supervisors to determine what is acceptable in your workplace.

4. Ensure you are documenting on the correct chart. It is important to double-check that you are documenting on the correct patient. In a hectic environment such as the ED, it is easy to document in error. It is therefore important for the EDT to double-check the patient's name and date of birth on the chart when documenting. If the EDT finds that they have documented on the incorrect patient, the record with incorrect information can be amended, identifying the documentation that was inaccurate. Even when documentation is labeled as in error, the errant documentation will still be visible and will not completely delete from the chart.

Patient Privacy

As with all healthcare communication, the patient's privacy is of utmost importance. The Health Insurance Portability and Accountability Act (HIPAA) is federal legislation that was passed in 1996. The law protects a patient's information within the healthcare setting, making it unlawful to disclose any protected health information to individuals not involved in the patient's care. EMR systems are protected by username and password. The EDT should never share their username or password. It is also important for the EDT to only access the charts of those patients in their direct care. EMR systems can track and record all staff who access a given patient's record. It is a violation of HIPAA for an EDT to access a patient's chart without being part of the direct patient care team.

Litigation

Clear and precise documentation is also important for legal reasons. A patient's chart is a legal document, and there may be times when it is reviewed as part of a legal proceeding. The goal of documentation is to create an accurate record of findings and actions. Courts can review documentation and use their findings to determine the quality of care provided to the patient. It could be years from the time of patient care to the time a case is reviewed in court. Through proper and thorough documentation, if summoned to court, the EDT can explain the actions taken while the patient was in their care.

Downtime

Although an EMR is generally reliable, there are times in which the EMR is not functioning properly or the staff are unable to access the EMR. The EMR may go into downtime for routine maintenance or for unplanned issues such as natural disasters or cyber attacks. Each hospital has paper forms in the event of downtime. EDTs should be familiar with downtime procedures and forms. Follow individual hospital policies and protocols for downtime procedures.

Whether documenting in the EMR or on paper downtime forms, the EDT has the responsibility to objectively document the patient's care in a timely manner. In a busy ED, it is imperative that the entire care team uses documentation as a communication tool for the current ED visit and beyond.

References for Additional Reading

American Nurses Association. ANA's principles for nursing documentation: guidance for registered nurses. 2010. Accessed June 11, 2022. www.nursingworld.org/~4af4f2/globalassets/docs/ana/ethics/principles-of-nursing-documentation.pdf.

Emergency Nurses Association. Handbook for implementing an emergency department electronic medical record system. 2014. https://www.ena.org/shop/catalog/learn/toolkits-resources/handbook-for-implementing-an-emergency-department-electronic-medical-record-system/c-23/c-94/p-203.

Goodwin D. Documentation skills for nursing students. *Nursing Made Incredibly Easy!* 2019;17(2):16–21.

Prideaux A. Issues in nursing documentation and record-keeping practice. *Br J Nurs.* 2011;20(22):1450–1454.

Selvi S. Documentation in nursing practice. *Intl J Nurs Educ.* 2017;9(4):122–123.

CHAPTER 26

Disasters and Mass Casualty Events

Jordan Selzer ▦ Elise Milani ▦ Cody Johnson ▦ Maggie McEnery

Introduction

From the horrors of the terrorist attacks on September 11, 2001, to the chaos in the aftermath of the Joplin, Missouri, category EF5 tornado in 2011, disasters are a scary but very real aspect of working in the emergency department (ED). Before understanding how to prepare for and respond to a disaster, it is first important to understand the term *disaster*. The World Health Organization defines a disaster as a "serious disruption of the functioning of a community or a society causing widespread human, material, economic or environmental losses that exceed the ability of the affected community or society to cope using its own resources." Key to this definition is the concept that the event overwhelms the available resources. In fact, a disaster does not have to be a large-scale event, and it is context and location dependent. A three-car accident may be a disaster to one hospital while barely impacting another. It is the disruption of normal functioning that requires additional consideration and training.

Disasters can be broken up into a variety of categories including natural versus man-made, internal or external, and even acute versus prolonged (Table 26.1). Understanding the nature of a disaster is essential in creating an effective plan to mitigate and respond. Disaster science has advanced significantly in recent decades, and the Federal Emergency Management Agency (FEMA) has become the lead agency in the US government's federal response. According to FEMA, an all-hazards approach (one that accounts for the full spectrum of emergencies and disasters) is key to adequately preparing for a disaster.

Disaster Cycle

Although a disaster may be a singular event or series of events, the disaster cycle is a continuous spectrum of activities (Fig. 26.1). This cycle can be broken down into four phases: response, recovery, mitigation, preparation (Table 26.2).

Although a deep dive into hospital emergency management is beyond the scope of this text, many resources are available on this topic, including https://www.FEMA.gov.

Disaster Declarations

A common saying in disaster management is that "all disasters are local." Although this saying is true, the response to a disaster can vary widely depending on the severity of the event and resources available. At each level of response, there are different organizations and groups that are responsible. To initiate the appropriate response, a disaster must first be declared. This can be done at the institutional, local, state, regional, national, or international level.

Institutional: At the hospital level, this declaration will typically be made by a predesignated set of senior staff, such as the nursing house supervisor, ED attending physician, or chief medical officer. A hospital disaster declaration will initiate a number of processes and resources available to

TABLE 26.1 ■ Disaster Types and Terms

Type of Disaster	Example
Natural disaster	Tornado, hurricane, flood, tsunami, earthquake, volcanic eruption, pandemic
Technical/man-made disaster	Mass shooting, bombing, vehicle ramming, cyber attack, plane crash, chemical or biological attack
Internal disaster	Power outage, IT failure, flooded hospital unit
External disaster	Terrorist attack, plane crash, chemical plant explosion
Acute disaster	Tornado, mass shooting, bombing
Prolonged disaster	Pandemic, drought, prolonged civil unrest
No-notice event	Terrorist attack, volcanic eruption, cyber attack
Common Terms	**Definition**
CBRNE	Chemical, biological, radiologic, nuclear, explosive
Weapon of mass destruction (WMD)	A device typically using a chemical, biological, radiologic, nuclear, or explosive source to cause harm to a large number of people

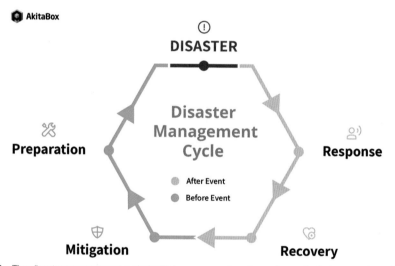

Fig. 26.1 The disaster management cycle facilitates a comprehensive and coordinated approach to disaster management.

TABLE 26.2 ■ The Phases of the Disaster Management Cycle

Phase of Disaster Cycle	Definition
Mitigation	Actions to minimize probability of a disaster occurring or its negative impacts, such as morbidity and mortality, through structural and nonstructural means
Preparation	Ongoing planning, training, evaluating, and corrective action, ensuring the highest level of readiness
Response	Actions taken after a disaster occurs to prevent further morbidity or mortality
Recovery	Actions taken to restore, resume, and ideally improve normal operations

the institution in order to minimize damage to life and property and restore normal functioning as quickly as possible.

Municipal/State: If an event impacts more than one institution, a disaster may be declared at the municipal or state level. These designations are made by a mayor or governor, respectively. This designation makes additional resources available and allows public officials to exercise emergency powers to preserve life, property, and public health.

National: A national disaster declaration can only be made by the US president; this is referred to as invoking the Stafford Act. This allows federal organizations such as FEMA to provide assistance to disaster victims. Additional federal resources available include teams of medical professionals including physicians, nurses, paramedics, pharmacists, and respiratory therapists, as well as logisticians known as disaster medical assistance teams. There are also material supplies, known as the Strategic National Stockpile (SNS), which include large quantities of mechanical equipment such as ventilators and cardiac monitors, personal protective equipment (PPE), and medications, such as antibiotics and antidotes for chemical attacks. These stockpiles are distributed throughout the US in secured locations.

Disaster Planning and Operations

Planning and preparing for a disaster is fundamental to success. To standardize and assist in these planning efforts, FEMA has developed the National Response Framework, which describes best practices including the Incident Command System (ICS). The ICS describes planning and management functions for responding partners to work in a coordinated and systematic approach by defining common terminology, coordinating resource management, and defining job titles and roles. This resource has been adapted to better fit the hospital environment and is known as the Hospital Incident Command System (HICS).

Beyond identification of roles and responsibilities, a key to successful disaster preparedness is the development of an emergency operations plan. This is an institution-specific document that details the plan and procedures using an all-hazards approach, as well as disaster-specific guidelines. These plans are developed and maintained by a hospital emergency manager or emergency management committee. Once developed, the plan must be tested with drills, which can range from virtual, tabletop exercises to full-scale scenarios using real equipment to treat simulated victims. These drills and the subsequent knowledge gained from them are essential to an institution's success in preparing for and responding to a disaster.

ED Operations

The environment during a disaster can be vastly different from normal operations. Patients and healthcare workers will likely be under significant stress, and standard operations can be critically disrupted. One way operations may differ is the need to rezone or restructure patient flow in order to streamline appropriate care. An example is creating red, yellow, and green zones in which patients with similar levels of injury or medical need can be grouped together. Additionally, it is common that patient documentation and tracking will be completed on paper charts and using whiteboards, as using computer systems may be too slow or burdensome.

It may also be necessary to work beyond the normal ED technician (EDT) scope of practice for your hospital (e.g., giving basic medications or starting intravenous lines). It is essential that under these circumstances, explicit permission has been designated by the hospital administration or appropriate authority and that the requisite skills and proficiencies are already established. Conversely, ED staff may find themselves asked to perform seemingly unskilled tasks, such as patient movement or equipment stocking. It is necessary to remain flexible under these stressful circumstances.

Disaster Triage

During a disaster incident, hospital resources are overwhelmed, and the approach to patient triage is different. The goal of triage during a disaster is to "do the most good for the greatest number of people." This means that resources should be directed to saving the most patients, not necessarily the sickest patients. It is for this reason that during a disaster, patients that exhibit no signs of life or injuries with very little chance of survival are not triaged at the highest priority. Instead, resources are directed toward the many sick patients that have a better chance of survival. If and when the hospital system is no longer overwhelmed, then triage should resume back to prioritizing the sickest patients.

During a disaster, patients are triaged into one of four categories that corresponds to a colored tag:

Immediate (red tag): these patients are critically ill and have a chance of survival with immediate treatment.

Delayed (yellow tag): these patients have serious and often life-threatening injuries that need urgent care; however, they are likely to survive with delayed treatment.

Minor (green tag): these patients have minor injuries and are likely to survive if care is delayed several days.

Deceased/expectant (black tag): these patients are either already dead or very unlikely to survive given the severity of injury and/or the availability of resources.

This simplified system helps quickly sort patients based on acuity of illness and chance of survival with immediate, delayed, or prolonged treatment. Red tag patients are treated first, followed by yellow tag patients, and finally green tag patients. Black tag patients that exhibit signs of life should be given palliative care such as pain medication, supplemental oxygen, and other comfort measures.

There are two widely accepted disaster triage algorithms: the START (Simple Triage and Rapid Transport) system (Fig. 26.2) and the SALT (Sort, Assess, Lifesaving interventions, Treatment/Transport) system (Fig. 26.3).

Staffing/Shift Change

A critical aspect of disaster management is appropriate staffing. Hospitals should have a paging system in place, typically through a phone tree or automated messaging system, which is activated by hospital incident command and/or hospital administration. This paging system not only informs healthcare workers of the mass casualty event but also calls in additional staff to assist with the increased patient burden. These additional staff can be referred to as the "activation team." Which staff are called in as part of the activation team is determined by the department chairs and the nature of the disaster event. Additionally, some healthcare workers may be pulled from other departments that are less impacted by the disaster to assist in highly burdened areas—typically the ED, critical care units, operating rooms, and hospital floors. It is also critical for departments to activate a "relief team." In the ED, the relief team is the group of healthcare workers that are assigned to come in for the subsequent shift and relieve the current team from duty. It is just as important to have a relief team as it is to have an activation team, as healthcare workers can become overextended and burned out.

ED Flow in a Surge

If many patients suddenly arrive simultaneously, it can overwhelm the department's ability to evaluate and treat them all in a timely manner. A small amount of forewarning might allow first receivers to prepare for this. One of the first steps of responding to an expected surge, which

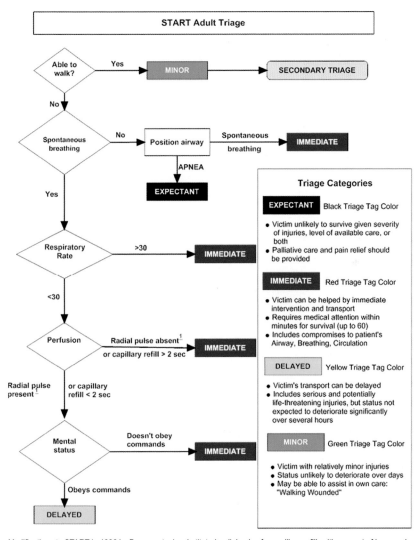

START Adult Triage

Modifications to START in 1996 by Benson et. al. substituted radial pulse for capillary refill, with a report of improved accuracy, especially in cold temperature.[1]

1.Benson M, Koenig KL, Schultz CH. Disaster triage: START, then SAVE-a new method of dynamic triage for victims of a catastrophic earthquake. Prehospital Disaster Med. 1996; Apr-Jun; 11(2): 117-24

Fig. 26.2   START triage. (From https://chemm.hhs.gov/startadult.htm.)

should occur simultaneously with securing the ED and establishing a triage point, is the decompression of the department.

Senior physicians should rapidly round in the department and determine which patients can be safely discharged and who needs to be admitted to complete as an inpatient what would normally be an ED evaluation. With the department newly emptied, the typical structure might change. Be aware that typical room staffing assignments may change, and the ED may

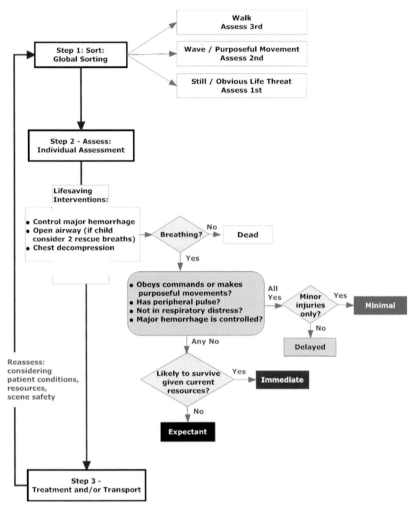

Fig. 26.3 SALT triage. (From https://remm.hhs.gov/salttriage.htm. Adapted from Lerner EB, Cone DC, Weinstein ES, et al. Mass casualty triage: an evaluation of the science and refinement of a national guideline. *Disaster Med Public Health Prep*. 2011;5(2):129-137.)

be blocked into abnormal sections and staff redistributed accordingly. You may be asked to staff an unusual pattern of rooms and should listen to senior physicians or hospital command center (HCC) staff.

Pandemics and instances of highly infectious diseases provide unique challenges, as limiting healthcare personnel and patient interactions is necessary to limit risk to staff and limit spread. As it is still necessary for in-person interactions to occur for direct patient care, the largest difference that will be seen is the donning of less commonly used PPE. If the use of this PPE is unfamiliar to you, you should request just-in-time training on its use and proper donning and doffing. The flow of patients through the department will likely change, and patients will be asked screening questions before being allowed into a typical room. If you are responsible for moving patients from their rooms to different sites within the hospital for testing, you should be educated on what PPE you will need and any different patterns for trafficking patients.

The HCC is a structure that will direct the hospital's response to a large surge and is formed as part of the HICS. The HICS is required to be used and tested regularly by the Joint Commission, the body that regulates hospitals. It is staffed by upper administration who can make decisions for the institution with subject matter experts built into its modular organization as consultants. There are several guiding themes of the HICS, some of which include modular organization that can expand/contract as needed for the size of the incident, universal command staff so all facets of the response go through one decision-making body, and a manageable span of control so that each individual providing oversight is not overwhelmed by people reporting to them. More information and at-home certifications are available through FEMA online (https://www.FEMA.gov) and can be done at your leisure to further your knowledge of hospital emergency management.

Role and Challenges of the ED in a Disaster

The ED is the hospital's front line for disaster response and management. Although the entire hospital is impacted by disaster incidents, it is the ED that will be the initial point of contact for mass casualty events, and an organized, deliberate ED response is critical to maintain functional operations within the hospital. As the first point of contact, the ED is responsible for triaging patients, stabilizing those patients, and adapting patient treatment to the means of injury (e.g., chemical exposure, blunt trauma). During a disaster, the primary objective of the ED is to provide patient care. This becomes difficult when resources are depleted by the large influx of patients presenting with similar injury patterns. ED providers need to be resourceful. During the 2017 Las Vegas mass shooting at the Route 21 Harvest Festival, ED physicians at Sunrise Hospital ran out of chest tubes, so they improvised by using endotracheal tubes as alternatives. When they ran out of ventilators, they used a single ventilator to ventilate two patients. This ability to quickly develop creative solutions is critical.

Personal Protective Equipment

In the ED, the EDT must be prepared to see various types of infectious diseases. The ED staff must first protect themselves when coming into contact with these patients in order to prevent further spread of the infection. Understanding modes of transmission will help the EDT protect themselves. The EDT should don (apply) the appropriate PPE before interacting with patients with an infectious disease. Doffing (removal) of PPE must occur when leaving a space with a possible infected patient and before interacting with any other patient. Used PPE should be removed and placed in the appropriate discard location when exiting the patient's room. PPE will be covered more in depth in Chapter 27.

Hospital Security in a Mass Casualty Incident

During a mass casualty incident (MCI), the chaos caused by the event needs to be mitigated by the preparedness of the responding hospital. The first group of patients to arrive at the hospital may not be the most injured, as many people who are able to self-refer to the hospital will come of their own accord. This is in comparison to people significantly affected by an event who are too injured to get themselves to the hospital and must be brought in by emergency medical services (EMS). Additionally, there may be an overcrowding of family or friends in search of loved ones who may have been brought to the hospital. To keep finite resources available for severely injured patients, hospital security is an essential part of disaster response and must be deployed early and deftly to secure key areas of the hospital.

A point should be predesignated as the triage point where the severity of patients' illness or injury is determined and where they can be sorted to the appropriate area to receive care. To maintain an orderly influx of patients and control foot traffic in crowded hospital spaces, additional security is essential. External sources of security may also be available but cannot be relied upon, as they will likely need to be deployed in their primary job capacities in response to the incident.

With familiarity of the hospital and specifically the ED layout, EDTs hold valuable knowledge of ED structure and ingresses and egresses. In the early phases of response to an MCI, technicians may be called upon by hospital security to assist in securing the ED. All external points of ingress to the ED (i.e., all doors that do not lead further into the hospital) should be secured, except for one agreed-upon entrance through which only triaged patients can enter. In some cases, doors between the ED and the rest of the hospital may need to be limited as well. In-house security may ask technicians to assist in this process, or if external law enforcement or security is present, they may require technician knowledge of ED and hospital layout. Early control of these access points is essential, but technicians should not take it upon themselves to assist in securing them, as it may hinder security and law enforcement in their duties. Others who may have access to additional information in the HICS chain of command may give other instructions regarding lockdown, and these should be followed.

If the safety of staff and patients in the ED is compromised by the incident, senior hospital staff and/or law enforcement may ask that you evacuate the department. You should comply with these orders. If you are unsure why you are being evacuated or if you believe there is a compromise of safety in the department, you should seek advice from your immediate supervisor. If your immediate safety is compromised, you should follow your facility's protocol for an active threat in the department.

Hospital Decontamination

If there is a release of chemical, biological, radiologic, nuclear, or explosive material that has the potential to cause ongoing harm to those affected, or to contaminate and cause harm to others, patients will need to be decontaminated before entering the hospital except the most critically ill. EDTs may be called upon before an event to participate in hazardous materials training, which should include different levels of PPE, how to don and doff this equipment, and how to evaluate patients for possible contamination. This training should be voluntary. If trained to do so, you may be requested to participate in decontamination; no individual who is not specifically trained in the use of these special equipment and procedures should be involved, as they may cause harm to themselves or others.

Those not directly involved in the decontamination procedures should ask clinical supervisors what, if any, additional PPE they should be using while in the ED and request just-in-time training on its use, if needed.

Infectious Disease Outbreaks

Recently, the world was forever changed by the emergence of the SARS-CoV-2 virus, which caused the COVID-19 pandemic. Nearly every institution and healthcare worker has been heavily impacted by this deadly disease. Profound as the impact has been, this is far from the first global pandemic, or even the worst. It is worth briefly describing the difference between an *epidemic* and a *pandemic*. According to the CDC, an epidemic is defined as "an increase, often sudden, in the number of cases of a disease above what is normally expected in that population in that area." In contrast, a pandemic is defined as "an epidemic that has spread over several countries or continents, usually affecting a large number of people."

Pandemics have been written about as far back as 430 BCE with what is suspected to have been typhoid, spreading through Libya, Ethiopia, Egypt, and Greece. One of the most well-known pandemics occurred in Europe during the Middle Ages. In 1347, plague hit the continent, and in 4 short years it killed almost one-third of the population, claiming nearly 200 million lives. It was during this pandemic that the concept of quarantine was invented. First attempted in the Venetian ports, a 30-day period of isolation was mandated for all new merchants arriving. More recently, the 1918 influenza pandemic claimed an estimated 50 million lives worldwide, making it the most deadly in recent times. In the last 20 years, we have seen numerous pandemics emerge including 2003 SARS, 2009 swine flu (H1N1), and 2012 MERS. Unfortunately, with continuous urbanization and climate change, human-animal contact is increasingly frequent, setting up the conditions for novel diseases to develop. Further, global travel has never been easier, making rapid global transmission nearly inevitable.

Role and Challenges of the ED in an Outbreak

An infectious outbreak is a unique type of disaster incident that is of particular importance in the ED. Similar to its role in mass casualty events, the ED acts as the first point of contact for many infected patients. It falls to the emergency medicine provider to diagnose these infections, making timely identification, isolation, and treatment of the illness of critical importance. All attempts should be made to reduce patient crowding to prevent disease propagation through the waiting room and patient care areas. In the case of respiratory transmission, masks should be made available to all patients. Handwashing stations should be readily available. Given available resources and weather conditions, the ED waiting room may be moved to an outdoor staging area to reduce the risk of indoor transmission. Additionally, there is the added challenge of protecting ED staff from becoming infected themselves. Important measures to keep ED staff safe include appropriate PPE, patient screening tools, coordination with prehospital staff, and patient education.

References for Additional Reading

Bahrami P, Ardalan A, Nejati A, Ostadtaghizadeh A, Yari A. Factors affecting the effectiveness of hospital incident command system: findings from a systematic review. *Bull Emerg Trauma*. 2020;8(2):62–76.

Brouqui P, Puro V, Fusco FM, et al. Infection control in the management of highly pathogenic infectious diseases: consensus of the European Network of Infectious Disease. *Lancet Infect Dis*. 2009;9(5):301–311.

Burgher S, Klein J. The night Dallas seemed more like Afghanistan. *ED Manag*. 2016;28(9):97–100.

Chinn RYW, Sehulster L. Guidelines for environmental infection control in health-care facilities; recommendations of CDC and Healthcare Infection Control Practices Advisory Committee (HICPAC). 2003. Accessed June 11, 2022. https://stacks.cdc.gov/view/cdc/7190.

Ciottone GR. *Ciottone's Disaster Medicine*. 2nd ed. Elsevier; 2016.

Dalton J. Coronavirus: timeline of pandemics and other viruses that humans caught by interacting with animals. *The Independent*. April 27, 2020. Accessed February 14, 2021. https://www.independent.co.uk/news/uk/home-news/coronavirus-pandemic-viruses-animals-bird-swine-flu-sars-mers-ebola-zika-a9483211.html.

de Jongh FHC, de Vries HJ, Warnaar RSP, et al. Ventilating two patients with one ventilator: technical setup and laboratory testing. *ERJ Open Res*. 2020;6(2).

Disaster medical services. *Ann Emerg Med*. 2018;72(4):e39.

Disaster Medical Assistance Teams. Public health emergency. September 9, 2017. Accessed June 11, 2022. https://www.phe.gov/Preparedness/responders/ndms/ndms-teams/Pages/dmat.aspx.

Emergency management plan for mass casualty incidents. Kings County Hospital Center. Accessed June 11, 2022. https://www.downstate.edu/emergency_medicine/pdf/KCHCSection03.pdf.

Esmailian M, Salehnia M-H, Shirani M, Heydari F. Reverse triage to increase the hospital surge capacity in disaster response. *Adv J Emerg Med*. 2018;2(2):e17.

Freund Y. The challenge of emergency medicine facing the COVID-19 outbreak. *Eur J Emerg Med*. 2020;27 (3):155.

Golabek-Goldman M. Adequacy of US hospital security preparedness for mass casualty incidents. *J Public Health Manag Pract*. 2016;22(1):68–80.

Hick JL, Penn P, Hanfling D, Lappe MA, O'Laughlin D, Burstein JL. Establishing and training health care facility decontamination teams. *Ann Emerg Med.* 2003;42(3):381–390.

Hojman H, Rattan R, Osgood R, Yao M, Bugaev N. Securing the emergency department during terrorism incidents: lessons learned from the Boston marathon bombings. *Disaster Med Public Health Prep.* 2019;13 (4):791–798.

Hospital Incident Command System. California Emergency Medical Services Authority. 2014. Accessed June 11, 2022. https://emsa.ca.gov/disaster-medical-services-division-hospital-incident-command-system-resources/.

Hospital medical surge planning for mass casualty incidents. Florida Department of Health. Accessed June 11, 2022. https://www.urmc.rochester.edu/MediaLibraries/URMCMedia/flrtc/documents/WNY-Hospital-Medical-Surge-Planning-For-Mass-Casualty-Incidents.pdf.

Lee CH. Disaster and mass casualty triage. *Virtual Mentor.* 2010;12(6):466–470.

Lerner EB, Brooke Lerner E, Cone DC, et al. Mass casualty triage: an evaluation of the science and refinement of a national guideline. *Disaster Med Public Health Prep.* 2011;5(2):129–137.

Menes K, Tintinalli J, Plaster L. How one Las Vegas ED saved hundreds of lives after the worst mass shooting in U.S. history. Emergency Physicians Monthly. November 3, 2017. Accessed June 11, 2022. https://epmonthly.com/article/not-heroes-wear-capes-one-las-vegas-ed-saved-hundreds-lives-worst-mass-shooting-u-s-history/.

National Response Framework. FEMA. 2019. Accessed June 11, 2022. https://www.fema.gov/sites/default/files/2020-04/NRF_FINALApproved_2011028.pdf.

O'Mara E, Cole P, Wynn A, Collison R. A fit for purpose training programme for the decontamination of personnel. *J Radiol Prot.* 2015;35(2):249–256.

Onion A, Sullivan M, and Mullen M. Pandemics that changed history. History. January 30, 2020. Accessed June 11, 2022. https://www.history.com/topics/middle-ages/pandemics-timeline.

Park J-H, Lee S-G, Ahn S, et al. Strategies to prevent COVID-19 transmission in the emergency department of a regional base hospital in Korea: from index patient until pandemic declaration. *Am J Emerg Med.* 2021;46:247–253.

Phelps S, Russell R, Doering G. Model "code silver" internal lockdown policy in response to active shooters. *Am J Disaster Med.* 2007;2(3):143–150.

Principles of epidemiology. Centers for Disease Control and Prevention. May 11, 2020. Accessed March 7, 2021. https://www.cdc.gov/csels/dsepd/ss1978/lesson1/section11.html.

Qureshi MN, AlRajhi A. Challenge of COVID-19 crisis managed by emergency department of a big tertiary centre in Saudi Arabia. *Int J Pediatr Adolesc Med.* 2020;7(3):147–152.

Roos D. How 5 of history's worst pandemics finally ended. History. March 17, 2020. Accessed June 11, 2022. https://www.history.com/news/pandemics-end-plague-cholera-black-death-smallpox.

Silvestri S, Field A, Mangalat N, et al. Comparison of START and SALT triage methodologies to reference standard definitions and to a field mass casualty simulation. *Am J Disaster Med.* 2017;12(1):27–33.

START adult triage algorithm. Accessed March 7, 2021. https://chemm.hhs.gov/startadult.htm.

Strategic National Stockpile. Public Health Emergencies. February 26, 2021. Accessed June 11, 2022. https://www.phe.gov/about/sns/Pages/default.aspx.

CHAPTER 27

Infection Control in the Emergency Department

Alexa Tovsen ▪ Lareb Altaf

Introduction

Infection control is a crucial component of maintaining a safe, clean, and healthy environment for both patients and staff in the emergency department (ED). The ED presents unique challenges in infection control due to the high turnover of patients, varying levels of patient acuity, frequent interaction between healthcare staff and patients, and the simultaneous care of multiple patients. EDs are busy, multifaceted environments where overcrowding is common and infections can easily spread. It is of the utmost importance that all ED staff members follow strict protocols to protect themselves and their patients from the unnecessary spread of infection.

Hand Hygiene

The most effective way to prevent the spread of infection is by strict adherence to good hand hygiene practices. Hand hygiene in the ED consists of both handwashing and the use of alcohol-based hand rubs. The Healthcare Infection Control Practices Advisory Committee at the Centers for Disease Control and Prevention strongly recommends performing hand hygiene in a variety of clinical scenarios (Table 27.1).

When hands are visibly soiled, they must be washed thoroughly with soap and water for at least 20 seconds. When hands are not visibly soiled, an alcohol-based hand rub is an acceptable alternative and is often preferred over handwashing due to evidence of better compliance. There is usually a dispenser of alcohol-based hand rub outside of every patient room in the ED, but there is not always a sink nearby. Whichever method is chosen, the key is to develop good habits of routine hand hygiene throughout any period of time in the ED.

Personal Protective Equipment

Use of personal protective equipment (PPE) is a critical component in infection control in the ED. When deciding when to wear certain PPE, healthcare workers must consider the established or potential risks in the immediate area. Healthcare workers wear PPE in order to protect themselves, the patients, and others from chemical, biological, and radiologic elements. Common PPE worn by ED staff includes, but is not limited to, gloves, gowns, face masks (surgical masks and N95 respirators), shoe and hair coverings, and eye protection (face shield or goggles). It is not only important to choose the correct PPE, but also to don (put on) and doff (take off) the PPE in the correct manner and order (Fig. 27.1).

A surgical mask (Fig. 27.2) creates a physical barrier between the mouth and nose of the wearer and potential contaminants in the immediate environment. It is loose-fitting, disposable, and is intended to be used only once. Surgical masks are effective at blocking large-particle droplets, splashes, or sprays that may contain infectious particles. However, a surgical mask does not

TABLE 27.1 ■ Common Indications for Hand Hygiene in the Emergency Department

Indications for Hand Hygiene

Immediately before and after touching a patient or the patient's immediate environment
Before performing an invasive procedure or handling invasive medical devices
Before moving from work on a soiled body site to a clean body site on the same patient
After contact with blood, body fluids, or contaminated surfaces
Immediately after glove removal

From Hand hygiene guidance. Centers for Disease Control and Prevention. Accessed June 11, 2022. https://www.cdc.gov/handhygiene/providers/guideline.html.

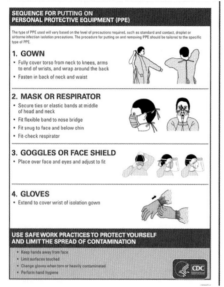
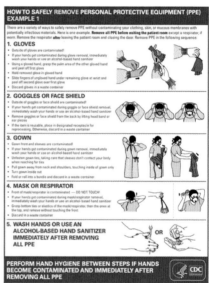

Fig. 27.1   The Centers for Disease Control and Prevention describes proper donning and doffing techniques. (From PPE sequence. Centers for Disease Control and Prevention. Accessed June 11, 2022. https://www.cdc.gov/hai/pdfs/ppe/ppe-sequence.pdf.)

filter or block small aerosolized particles in the air that may be transmitted by coughing, sneezing, or certain medical procedures. Historically, surgical masks were only worn during sterile medical procedures (e.g., lumbar puncture or central line placement), when caring for patients with high likelihood of respiratory droplet spread (e.g., active influenza infection) or body fluid exposure (e.g., during incision and drainage of an abscess). However, surgical masks are now commonly used to decrease the spread of disease, such as COVID-19, from the wearer to others in public as well as healthcare settings.

An N95 respirator (Fig. 27.3) is a protective mask designed for efficient filtration of airborne particles. The name "N95" is based on a US standard that requires these masks to be able to filter out at least 95% of very small particles. N95 masks are intended to cover the nose and mouth completely and fit tightly on the wearer's face. There are multiple manufacturers and styles of N95 respirators. Every healthcare worker must undergo yearly fit testing to ensure that they are matched with a brand, size and fit that provides full protection. Wearing a respirator that has not been fit-tested to the wearer may not protect them. Similar to surgical masks, N95 masks are intended to be single-use devices and are discarded after each patient encounter.

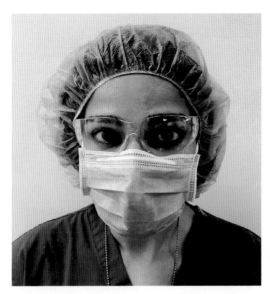

Fig. 27.2 **Safety goggles with surgical mask.** (From Lauer JK, Acker KP, Saiman L, et al. PPE during a pandemic: the experience of obtaining PPE and lessons learned from a department of obstetrics and gynecology in New York city. Semin Perinatol. 2020;44(6):151293.)

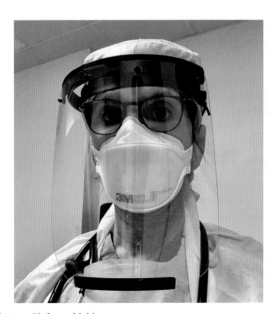

Fig. 27.3 N95 Respirator with face shield

A powered air purifying respirator (PAPR) (Fig. 27.4) provides battery-powered positive airflow through a filter to a hood or face mask and provides a higher level of protection from aerosolized particles. PAPRs can be worn on multiple occasions but must be cleaned and sanitized according to the manufacturer's recommendations between each use. A PAPR is a good alternative to an N95 mask if the N95 mask does not fit properly due to an individual's face shape or facial hair.

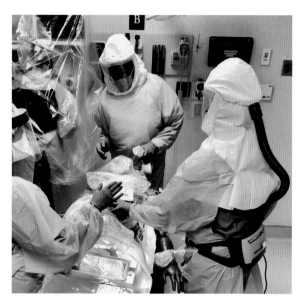

Fig. 27.4   A powered air purifying respirator covers the entire face and is used to prevent the wearer from inhaling aerosolized particles.

Infection Control Precautions

The first tier of infection prevention measures that are used on every patient in the ED are called standard precautions. These comprise the minimum protection required for the care of all patients, regardless of infection status. They are also referred to as universal precautions, because they should be applied at all times when administering patient care. These precautions include hand hygiene, use of PPE, safe disposal of sharps, cough etiquette (coughing into your arm or a tissue), safe injection of medications, use of sterile instruments and devices, and maintenance of a clean and disinfected environment.

When standard precautions are not enough to prevent transmission of infection, they are supplemented with transmission-based precautions. This second tier of infection prevention is used when patients have known or suspected infections that can spread through contact, droplet, or airborne routes. In the ED, patients requiring transmission-based precautions will have a sign on their door indicating the level of necessary precaution, as well as a cart outside of their room containing the necessary PPE. This PPE must be worn every time a staff member enters the patient's room and is discarded immediately after leaving the room. This serves to protect the health of the staff member and to decrease the risk of transmission to other patients and staff in the department.

Contact precautions (Fig. 27.5A) are used for patients with known or suspected illness that spreads through physical touch (direct or indirect). ED staff must wear the appropriate PPE, including gloves and a gown, when taking care of patients placed on contact precautions. This PPE must be properly donned each time before entering a room and then doffed and disposed of upon exiting the room. Common skin infections that require contact precautions include methicillin-resistant *Staphylococcus aureus* (MRSA), herpes zoster (shingles), and monkeypox (Table 27.2). ED staff also adhere to contact precautions when patients have an insect infestation such as bed-bugs, lice, and scabies. The rooms of patients on contact precautions must be properly cleaned every day and after patient discharge. In cases of insect infestation, the patient room will require additional cleaning (a terminal clean), which is performed by environmental services.

Enteric precautions (see Fig. 27.5B) are contact precautions used when caring for patients with known or suspected infectious diarrhea. These precautions are necessary to prevent infections that are transmitted primarily by direct or indirect contact with fecal material. Common intestinal infections that are transmitted by contact via the stool are *Clostridioides difficile*, vancomycin-resistant *Enterococcus* (VRE), and norovirus (common cause of the "stomach flu") (see Table 27.2).

Droplet precautions (see Fig. 27.5C) are used for patients with a known or suspected infection that is transmitted by respiratory droplets when coughing, sneezing, or talking. Proximity is required for spread, as droplets do not remain suspended in the air. Patients and healthcare workers should

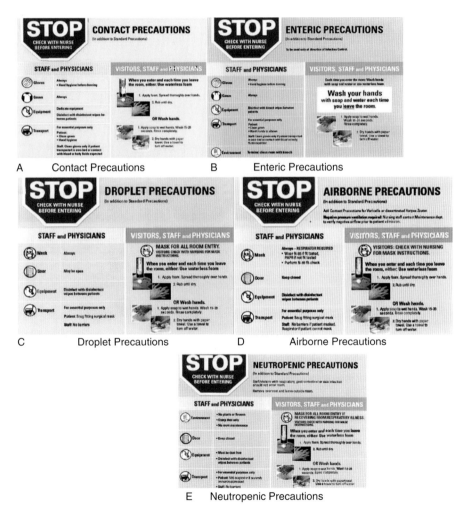

Fig. 27.5 Commonly-used signs that are displayed outside a patient's room to indicate the need for (A) contact precautions, (B) enteric precautions, (C) droplet precautions, (D) airborne precautions, and (E) neutropenic precautions. (From Environmental Services Cleaning Guidebook. Minnesota Hospital Association. Accessed June 11, 2022. https://www.mnhospitals.org/Portals/0/Documents/ptsafety/CDICleaning/4.%20Environmental%20Services%20Cleaning%20Guidebook.pdf.)

TABLE 27.2 ■ Infectious Organisms That Require Contact and Enteric Precautions, Along With Their Characteristics, Treatment, and Prevention

Organ	Disease	Pathogen	Characteristics	Treatment	Prevention
Dermatologic	Chicken pox		Typically a vesicular childhood rash starting on the face and trunk	Analgesics, antiviral, antihistamines	Vaccine
	Shingles	Varicella zoster virus	Usually in adults, limited to a single dermatome, does not cross midline		
	Infection	Methicillin-resistant Staphylococcus aureus (MRSA)	Organism with acquired resistance to common methicillin antibiotics . Particularly worrisome in setting of declining antibiotic treatment options	Antibiotic	Good hand and body hygiene Good antibiotic stewardship
Gastrointestinal	Colitis	Clostridioides difficile	Causes severe watery diarrhea Associated with antibiotic use Commonly a nosocomial (hospital-acquired) infection	Discontinue prior antibiotic and start an antibiotic targeted to C. difficile	Good hand and body hygiene Good antibiotic stewardship
	Infection	Vancomycin-resistant Enterococcus (VRE)	Organism with acquired resistance to the antibiotic vancomycin Particularly worrisome in setting of declining antibiotic treatment options	Antibiotic	Good hand hygiene Good antibiotic stewardship
	Gastroenteritis	Escherichia coli	Little or no fever, severe abdominal cramps, watery diarrhea followed by bloody diarrhea	Fluid repletion	Food and water safety Good hand hygiene
		Campylobacter jejuni	Watery diarrhea followed by foul smelling bloody diarrhea (10 or more stools/d), intense abdominal pain, fever, vomiting	Antibiotic	Food and water safety
		Salmonella	Inflammatory diarrhea with/without visible blood, nausea, vomiting, fever, abdominal cramps, myalgia, and headache Lasts 2–7 d	Usually resolves spontaneously	Food and water safety

From Nepal H, Tewodros W. (2020) Microbiology lectures at Trinity School of Medicine, St. Vincent and the Grenadines.

wear a surgical mask, gown, gloves, and eye protection at all times to prevent the spread of droplets. Common infections that are spread via droplets include influenza, parainfluenza, respiratory syncytial virus, meningococcal meningitis, mumps, pertussis, and rubella (Table 27.3).

Airborne precautions (see Fig. 27.5D) are used for patients with a known or suspected infection that is transmitted by airborne particles. This differs from droplet precautions because airborne droplet nuclei remain suspended in the air for long periods of time. These patients need to be placed in a designated negative-pressure isolation room that is equipped with a filtered ventilation system that continuously pulls contaminated air out of the room. This creates a pressure gradient so that air pressure in the patient's room remains lower than the air pressure outside the room. As a result, when the door is opened, contaminated air from inside the room does not flow outside the room and contaminate the ED. Staff must wear N95 respirators or a PAPR when taking care of patients with airborne precautions, and patients should wear surgical masks at all times. Common infections that are spread via airborne particles include COVID-19, tuberculosis (TB), disseminated varicella zoster (chicken pox), and measles (Table 27.4).

A patient with respiratory symptoms may require an aerosol generating procedure (AGP), or a procedure that is likely to cause the patient to cough and produce droplets or aerosols that contain respiratory pathogens. AGPs that are commonly performed in the ED include positive pressure ventilation, endotracheal intubation, airway suction, and nebulizer treatments. AGPs should be avoided in patients with airborne precautions, if possible. AGPs are made safer by the use of PPE such as PAPRs. During the COVID-19 pandemic, barrier devices such as the Airway Procedure Tent (Fig. 27.6), were used during AGPs to help protect healthcare providers from exposure to aerosols.

When patients are suspected of having an infection that requires transmission-based precautions, they will be tested for the particular infection in question, if available. If the test results reveal that the patient does *not* have the suspected infection, the transmission-based precautions can be discontinued, and staff should continue using standard precautions only.

Neutropenic precautions (see Fig. 27.5E) are necessary when caring for patients with neutropenia, or a low neutrophil count. Neutrophils are white blood cells that aid in the body's immune response and are most commonly depleted during chemotherapy treatments used to treat cancer. A neutropenic patient has a weakened immune system and is susceptible to unique pathogens and infections. Therefore ED staff must comply with standard precautions and avoid unnecessary visits to neutropenic patients' rooms. Invasive procedures such as catheter insertions, rectal temperatures, and insertion of nasogastric tubes should also be avoided when possible. If patients are markedly immunosuppressed, staff may be required to use additional PPE, such as a surgical mask and gown. Neutropenic patients must wear a surgical mask when leaving their room at all times and cannot have fresh flowers or raw foods due to the high risk of bacterial colonization.

Cleaning and Disinfecting

All areas of the ED are routinely cleaned by both healthcare workers and environmental services to maintain a sufficient level of cleanliness. All high contact surfaces, including the stretcher mattress and bed rails as well as equipment used, must be sanitized with a hospital grade disinfectant after the patient is discharged or transfered. It is often the responsibility of the ED technician to perform this important procedure. Environments and equipment used during the care of patients on transmission-based precautions require terminal cleaning (Table 27.5). During terminal cleaning, all contact surfaces are cleaned with hospital grade disinfectants, such as quartenary ammonium compounds (quat or QAC) and EPA List N cleaning agents, specifcally designated as effective against the suspected or confirmed infectious organism in order to prevent transmission of infectious particles to the next patient in the room. Terminal cleaning is typically performed by trained environmental service providers and may

TABLE 27.3 ■ Infectious Organisms That Require Droplet Precautions, Along With Their Characteristics, Treatment, and Prevention

Disease	Pathogen	Characteristics	Treatment	Prevention
Influenza	Influenza virus	Dominant influenza strain varies year-to-year Presents as fever, cough, sore throat, fatigue, body aches	Antivirals can shorten duration of infection	Vaccine
RSV	Respiratory syncytial virus	Viral respiratory illness, more common in infants and young children Can progress to life-threatening pneumonia	Bronchodilators; Oxygen therapy	Monoclonal antibodies for high-risk patients
Meningococcal meningitis	*Neisseria meningitidis*	Meningitis: abrupt onset of fever, intense headache, chills, vomiting, stiff neck Meningococcemia: sepsis-disseminated infection	Antibiotics	Prophylactic antibiotics if exposed Vaccine
Whooping cough	*Bordetella pertussis*	Major cause of childhood fatality before vaccination Uncontrollable, violent coughing, rhinorrhea	Antibiotics	Prophylactic antibiotics if exposed Vaccine
Rubella/ measles/ mumps	Rubella virus/rubeola virus/ rubulavirus	**Measles** Children: low-grade fever, rash starts on face, moves to trunk/extremities and usually fades after 3 d Adults: mild illness, but some may have more severe presentations including arthralgia, arthritis, and postinfectious encephalopathy **Congenital rubella syndrome** Maternal infection during first trimester results in growth retardation and congenital birth defects **Mumps** Fever, fatigue, body aches, classic swelling of the parotid glands	Antipyretics; supportive care	Vaccine

From Nepal H, Tewodros W. (2020) Microbiology lectures at Trinity School of Medicine, St. Vincent and the Grenadines.

TABLE 27.4 ■ Infectious Organisms That Require Airborne Precautions, Along With Their Characteristics, Treatment, and Prevention

Disease	Pathogen	Properties	Treatment	Prevention
COVID-19	Coronavirus SARS-CoV-2	Cough, short of breath/difficulty breathing, fever, chills, muscle pain, sore throat, new loss of taste or smell, congestion or runny nose, nausea or vomiting, diarrhea	Antivirals; monoclonal antibodies	Vaccine
Tuberculosis (TB)	*Mycobacterium tuberculosis*	Coughing for ≥ 3 wk, bloody or mucous sputum, unintentional weight loss, more common in underdeveloped/developing countries	Antibiotics	Early detection of latent TB with PPD testing and treatment

From Nepal H, Tewodros W. (2020) Microbiology lectures at Trinity School of Medicine, St. Vincent and the Grenadines.

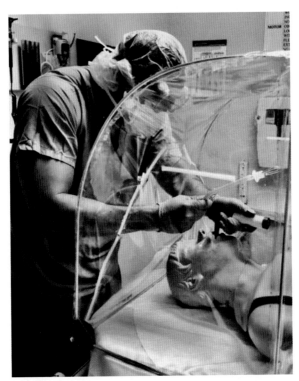

Fig. 27.6 An Airway Procedure Tent (APT) is used during a mock endotracheal intubation. APTs add an extra layer of protection between healthcare providers and the aerosols produced by the patient during the procedure.

TABLE 27.5 ■ Infectious Organisms and Infection Control Methods

Precaution	Indication	PPE in Area When Occupied by Patient	PPE in Area When Unoccupied by Patient	Cleaning Procedure After Discharge
Contact	MRSA, impetigo, bedbugs, lice, scabies	1. Gloves 2. Isolation gown	1. Gloves 2. Isolation gown	Routine cleaning/disinfecting
Droplet	Influenza, parainfluenza, RSV, meningococcal meningitis, mumps, pertussis, rubella	1. Surgical mask	None required	1. Routine cleaning/disinfecting 2. Quat detergent for floor cleaning
Enteric	*Clostridioides difficile*, VRE, norovirus	1. Gloves 2. Isolation gown	1. Gloves 2. Isolation gown	1. Bleach cleaning/disinfecting (especially around toilet) 2. Quat detergent for floor cleaning
Airborne	Tuberculosis, measles, chicken pox, COVID-19	1. N95 mask or PAPR 2. Add isolation gown and gloves for contact precautions	1. N95 mask or PAPR within 1 h of discharge 2. Add isolation gown and gloves for contact precautions	Routine cleaning/disinfecting
Neutropenic	Immunocompromised patients who are at high risk for hospital-acquired infections	Surgical mask if healthcare worker has symptoms of respiratory infection	None required	Routine cleaning/disinfecting

MRSA, Methicillin-resistant *Staphylococcus aureus*; *PAPR*, powered air purifying respirator; *PPE*, personal protective equipment; *RSV*, respiratory syncytial virus; *VRE*, vancomycin-resistant *Enterococcus*.
From Nepal H, Tewodros W. (2020) Microbiology lectures at Trinity School of Medicine, St. Vincent and the Grenadines.

also involve the use of UV lights. Once the patient has been discharged or transfered, the ED technician should block off the room on the tracking board in order to prevent it's use until terminal cleaning is complete. Additionaly, the ED technician should immediately contact environmental services to request a terminal clean and inform them as to which transmision precaution was in place as well as the suspected or confirmed organism.

Drug Resistance

Drug resistance is a growing public health problem worldwide and is caused in large part by unnecessary prescription and overuse of certain medications.

When exposed to the same antibiotics, antivirals, antifungals, and antiparasitics time and time again, bacteria, viruses, fungi, and parasites learn ways to adapt and survive in these environments. They can share this knowledge with other organisms, leading to multiple infectious microbes that are resistant to the effects of the medication. If a patient only takes a portion of their prescribed course of medications, some microorganisms may survive and will not be affected by the antimicrobial agent the next time they are used. These resistant organisms become "superbugs" that are very difficult to treat and can cause serious and life-threatening illnesses. MRSA, TB, malaria, and VRE are common drug-resistant organisms. Human immunodeficiency virus (HIV) can mutate and reproduce, rendering many HIV medications inefective thereby limiting treatment options and forcing prescribers to turn to more expensive, harmful, or less accessible antiviral medications.

In the United States alone, at least 2.8 million people are infected with drug resistant bacteria or fungi every year, and more than 35,000 people die as a result. Although new antimicrobial drugs are being developed to combat the rise in resistant organisms, these drugs are few and far between, enormously costly, and will likely meet the same fate if prescribing practices do not improve. Healthcare providers must be judicious when deciding if and when patients definitively require an antimicrobial medication, and patients must be sure to take the full course of medication as instructed.

Conclusion

Infection can easily spread in the ED due to the high volume of people, many of whom are actively and present in close proximity to one another. Fortunately, there are simple steps that healthcare workers can take to protect themselves and others from spreading infectious particles throughout the department. Best practices including wearing proper PPE, routine hand hygiene, and the appropriate cleaning and disinfecting of shared spaces. Strict adherence to infection control practices must be one of the top priorities for every healthcare worker.

References for Additional Reading

About antibiotic resistance. Centers for Disease Control and Prevention. Accessed June 11, 2022. https://www.cdc.gov/drugresistance/about.html.

Environmental Services Cleaning Guidebook. Minnesota Hospital Association. Accessed June 11, 2022. https://www.mnhospitals.org/Portals/0/Documents/ptsafety/CDICleaning/4.%20Environmental%20Services%20Cleaning%20Guidebook.pdf.

Hand hygiene guidance. Centers for Disease Control and Prevention. Accessed June 11, 2022. https://www.cdc.gov/handhygiene/providers/guideline.html.

Healthwise Staff. Hospital isolation rooms. University of Michigan Health. Accessed June 11, 2022. https://www.uofmhealth.org/health-library/abo4381.

Liang S, Reithman M, Fox J. Infection prevention for the emergency department. *Emerg Med Clin N Am*. 2018;36(4):874.

Nepal H, Tewodros W. (2020) Microbiology lectures at Trinity School of Medicine.

Nirenberg A, Bush A, Davis A, Friese C, Gillespie T, Rice R. Neutropenia: state of the knowledge part II. *Oncol Nurs Forum*. 2006;33(6):1202–1208.

N95 respirators, surgical masks, and face masks. US Food and Drug Administration. Accessed June 11, 2022. https://www.fda.gov/medical-devices/personal-protective-equipment-infection-control/n95-respirators-surgical-masks-and-face-masks.

Powered air purifying respirator (PAPR). Minnesota Department of Health. Accessed June 11, 2022. https://www.health.state.mn.us/facilities/patientsafety/infectioncontrol/ppe/comp/papr.html.

PPE sequence. Centers for Disease Control and Prevention. Accessed June 11, 2022. https://www.cdc.gov/hai/pdfs/ppe/ppe-sequence.pdf.

Standard precautions. Centers for Disease Control and Prevention. Accessed June 11, 2022. https://www.cdc.gov/oralhealth/infectioncontrol/summary-infection-prevention-practices/standard-precautions.html.

Tran K, Cimon K, Severn M, Pessoa-Silva C, Conly J. Aerosol generating procedures and risk of transmission of acute respiratory infections to healthcare workers: a systematic review. *PLoS One*. 2012;7(4):e35797.

Transmission-based precautions. Centers for Disease Control and Prevention. Accessed June 11, 2022. https://www.cdc.gov/infectioncontrol/basics/transmission-based-precautions.html.

CHAPTER 28

Case Studies in Emergency Triage

Eleanor Rubin ▪ Megan Hoffer ▪ Aaran Drake

Patients present to the emergency department (ED) with a variety of complaints of varying severity. The process by which ED providers prioritize patient complaints is called "triage." Triage originates from the French word *trier*, which means "to sort." In this setting, the "sorting" is completed through assignment of an Emergency Severity Index (ESI) Score from 1 to 5 to each patient, where an ESI of 1 is reserved for patients requiring immediate, life-saving interventions. This system prioritizes the treatment of sicker patients (lower ESIs) ahead of the less acute patients (higher ESIs). Although triage is generally a nursing responsibility in the United States, the ED technician (EDT) should be able to recognize patients who require immediate attention to assist nursing with this important function. This chapter highlights common ED presentations, outlines actions that should be taken on the patient's arrival, and describes "red flag" signs to recognize in order to more efficiently identify time-sensitive emergencies.

There are several core triage principles that should be applied to every patient to ensure rapid identification of emergent presentations.

- All patients should receive a *complete set of vital signs* on their arrival to the ED (heart rate, blood pressure [BP], respiratory rate, oxygen saturation, temperature). Abnormal vital signs suggest a patient should be seen quickly and assigned a more acute triage score (lower ESI). Marked abnormality of any vital sign or a combination of abnormal vital signs should prompt immediate notification of a provider.
- *Red flags* are those signs and symptoms that suggest the patient is suffering from a more severe illness. Red flags are disease specific and would justify placing the patient in a higher priority category.
- Time is of the essence in many patient presentations so the assignment of an accurate triage category is very important. All efforts should be made to expedite placing the patient into a treatment room ("rooming") for provider assessment.
- Intravenous (IV) access, cardiac monitoring, and oxygen administration are the EDTs priorities in rooming a patient with abnormal vital signs or red flag symptoms.
- Patients who present with abnormal vital signs or with red flag symptoms that suggest a serious illness should not be allowed to eat or drink (i.e., made NPO, from the Latin *non per os*, meaning "nothing by mouth"), as there is a higher likelihood that they will require an invasive procedure or intervention.

Chest Pain

A 65-year-old man presents ambulatory to triage with a chief complaint of chest pain. He states that his pain began about 1 hour ago, and that it feels like a crushing substernal pressure that radiates to his left shoulder. You notice that he is sweating, short of breath, and appears uncomfortable.

Chest pain is the second most frequent nontraumatic complaint evaluated in the ED and can represent a wide range of pathologies, from benign to life-threatening. A primary function of the ED visit is to consider and rule out life-threatening illness and identify and treat the cause of the patient's symptoms. Chest pain may be the first sign of acute coronary syndrome (blood clot in the coronary arteries that can lead to heart attack), heart rhythm disturbances (either slow or fast), pulmonary embolism (PE; a blood clot in the pulmonary arteries), aortic dissection (a tear in the aorta that can cause low blood flow to critical organs), pericarditis (inflammation of the membrane surrounding the heart), or pneumothorax (lung collapse). Chest pain may also have a noncardiac etiology that should be considered once more serious pathology has been ruled out. Costochondritis, an inflammation of the costal cartilage, is a common benign cause of chest pain that is reproducible on palpation of the chest wall. Gastroesophageal reflux and esophageal complaints may also present as chest pain often associated with eating and with nausea (Table 28.1).

CRITICAL ACTIONS FOR THE ED TECHNICIAN

- Take vital signs.
- Electrocardiogram (ECG) should be taken within 10 minutes of arrival.
- Place the patient on the cardiac monitor. Continuous rhythm, rate, and saturation monitoring are key. Periodic BP cycling frequency should be discussed with the registered nurse or treating provider.
- Apply oxygen to any patient with oxygen saturation less than 92% or who is on home oxygen.

RED FLAGS

- Abnormal vital signs
- Altered mental status or neurologic signs
- Diaphoresis (sweating)
- Pallor (pale, cool skin)
- Increased work of breathing: tachypnea, accessory muscle use, tripod position, short sentences when speaking
- New or escalating oxygen requirement

Any patient with a complaint of chest pain should have an ECG within 10 minutes of arrival. Note that the computerized interpretation found on the ECG may not be accurate, so most EDs require a provider to review the ECG shortly after it is obtained.

It is important to anticipate what the providers may order given the complaint and to prepare accordingly when starting your care. In addition to an ECG, lab work (complete blood cell count, comprehensive metabolic panel, troponin, pro–brain natriuretic peptide) and a chest x-ray (CXR) are often ordered. Other lab studies, such as coagulation tests (how well the blood clots) or D-dimer test (a measure of excess clotting in the blood), may be ordered depending on the

TABLE 28.1 ■ Characteristics of Chest Pain

Coronary artery disease/ myocardial infarction	Midsternal, left-sided, worse with exertion, radiating to arm or jaw
Pneumothorax	Unilateral, pain with inspiration, often traumatic but may be spontaneous in tall individuals or those with chronic lung disease such as chronic obstructive pulmonary disease
Pulmonary embolism	Pain with inspiration occasionally accompanied by unilateral leg swelling, history of long travel, recent surgery, or estrogen use
Aortic dissection	Severe, sudden onset, radiating to back, hypertensive, asymmetric blood pressures
Pericarditis	Pain with inspiration, improves with leaning forward
Abdominal aortic aneurysm	Chest and abdominal pain, pulsating abdominal mass
Gastroesophageal reflux	Epigastric pain, worst after eating, nausea
Costochondritis (musculoskeletal)	Reproducible chest wall tenderness

clinical suspicions of the provider. If in doubt of which tubes to draw, collect all tubes and follow the hospital's process for labeling and storing extra samples.

Reliable IV access is key for these patients, particularly for patients requiring computed tomography (CT) with IV contrast (to evaluate for PE or aortic dissection), as IV contrast needs to be placed through a larger-bore catheter (20 gauge or larger in most hospitals) and located preferably in the antecubital fossa. Even if not going for a contrast study, many of these patients may receive IV fluids or medications requiring free-flowing, stable access.

Shortness of Breath in a Younger Person

A 25-year-old woman presents to the ED via emergency medical services (EMS) with a chief complaint of shortness of breath (SOB). EMS reports that she has a history of asthma and that she has had increasing wheezing during the past few days. They report that she has been using her albuterol inhaler more frequently until this morning when it was empty. On initial assessment, she has increased work of breathing and has audible wheezes. Her oxygen saturation is 89%.

Patients frequently present to the ED with SOB, and this complaint frequently indicates a significant illness. It most frequently indicates either a problem with the heart, a problem with the lungs, or both. Less frequently, SOB can be due to severe metabolic disturbance or as the result of an overdose (e.g., aspirin). A complaint of SOB can represent serious illness in both the young and old. In a younger population, SOB is often seen in asthma or pneumonia. In an older population, SOB may be a presenting complaint in chronic obstructive pulmonary disease (COPD), congestive heart failure (CHF), or pneumonia. Anxiety as a cause of SOB is a diagnosis of exclusion, meaning that other more dangerous etiologies must be considered and evaluated first, and deemed less likely, before ascribing a patient's SOB to anxiety.

CRITICAL ACTIONS FOR THE ED TECHNICIAN

- Take vital signs.
  - Initiate supplemental oxygen if Spo_2 is less than 92%.
  - Assess general work of breathing. This can be done through observation of the patient's effort to breathe or talking to the patient if applicable to evaluate.
- Apply a pulse oximeter for continuous pulse oximetry measurement.
- Alert a provider if the patient appears to be in respiratory distress or requires supplemental oxygen.
- Use caution, as these patients may look well initially but may rapidly decompensate while in the ED.

RED FLAGS

- Previous history of intubation or intensive care unit (ICU) admission for asthma
- Increased work of breathing: intercostal retractions, accessory muscle use, tripod positioning
- Patient requires an increasing amount of supplemental oxygen to maintain the pulse ox above 92%
- Altered mental status
- Pallor
- Diaphoresis
- Cyanosis (bluish coloring of the skin)

The patient described above is most likely experiencing an acute asthma exacerbation. Providers may initiate some combination of bronchodilators (nebulized albuterol), ipratropium, steroids,

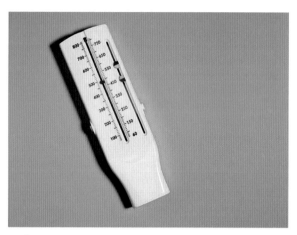

Fig. 28.1 Peak flow meter.

magnesium, and epinephrine depending on the severity of the exacerbation. IV access is important in moderate to severe exacerbations. Ideally, a peak expiratory flow measurement (requires the patient to forcefully exhale into a device that measures airflow) would be completed before the treatments and then at regular intervals to monitor the patient's improvement (Fig. 28.1). It is sometimes difficult to obtain this measurement on patient arrival until their breathing improves with treatment.

Expect that all patients with a severe lung problem will have an increased heart rate, and some asthma treatments may increase this further. You may also see a transient, mild decrease in the patient's oxygen saturation after initiation of bronchodilators. You can anticipate the providers may order an ECG or cardiac monitoring due to the patient's tachycardia or to rule out a cardiac cause for their acute SOB.

These patients may be at risk for developing complications like pneumothorax and pneumo-mediastinum (air in the tissues between the lung and heart) and often will need a CXR early in their ED stay.

Shortness of Breath in an Older Person

A 70-year-old woman presents to the ED with a chief complaint of SOB that has been worsening over the past 3 days. She reports a history of COPD and a 50 pack-year history of smoking. She uses 2 L of oxygen at home at night, but this week she has been needing to use her oxygen continuously. On arrival, she has increased work of breathing on her home oxygen and has "pursed-lip" breathing.

CRITICAL ACTIONS FOR THE ED TECHNICIAN

- Take vital signs.
  - Initiate supplemental oxygen if needed, with goal of 92%.
  - Assess general work of breathing.
- Initiate continuous pulse oximetry and cardiac monitoring.
- ECG is a priority in these patients, as they are more likely to have cardiac comorbidities.
- Alert provider if patient appears to be in respiratory distress or requires supplemental oxygen.

RED FLAGS

- Previous history of intubation or ICU admission for COPD
- Increased work of breathing: retractions, accessory muscle use, tripod positioning
- Requiring supplemental oxygen or more than baseline
- Altered mental status
- Pallor (pale skin)
- Diaphoresis (sweating)
- Cyanosis (bluish coloring of the skin)
- History of CHF or other cardiac comorbidities
- Concurrent chest pain

This presentation suggests that the patient is experiencing a COPD exacerbation. In general, the pathophysiology and treatment is similar to the young asthmatic, but COPD patients are typically older, have less ability to compensate for the increased work of breathing, and may decompensate quickly. Additionally, they are more likely to have concurrent heart problems. Cardiac comorbidities like CHF or coronary artery disease may complicate the picture.

Both asthma and COPD result from obstruction of the bronchi and destruction of alveoli where the blood is oxygenated. Patients cannot fully expel inspired air, and their lung volume expands. The oxygen saturation goal in both COPD and asthmatic patients is at least 92%. When in extremis, these patients will breathe faster to try to increase blood oxygenation and will often exhale more carbon dioxide than usual. As they tire, they may actually retain carbon dioxide which, when combined with low oxygen levels, is a deadly combination. Providers can monitor where the patient is on this continuum by analyzing the patient's blood gas. EDTs can also help monitor the patient's CO_2 levels by placing the patient on end-tidal CO_2 monitoring according to their hospital protocols.

IV access is even more important in the suspected COPD exacerbation than in an asthma patient due to the wider differential diagnosis and the higher likelihood of decompensation. You can also anticipate a wide array of labs to be drawn, including a venous blood gas. Pre- and post-treatment peak flow measurements are ideal for helping track response to treatment. As with asthmatics, these patients can develop a sudden pneumothorax and pneumomediastinum. Although a mild asthmatic may not require CXR, it is routine in an older COPD patient.

Abdominal Pain

A 72-year-old woman presents to the ED complaining of generalized abdominal pain for 2 days. She is resting with her eyes closed and appears to be uncomfortable. She is unable to localize the pain but points to the center of her abdomen as the site of worst pain.

Abdominal pain is the most common nontraumatic chief complaint in the ED. The differential for these patients is broad and includes problems arising from structures within the abdominal cavity (e.g., intestines, liver, or spleen), structures behind or below the abdominal cavity (e.g., kidney, aorta, uterus, ovaries, bladder), or even structures in the chest. Pain can be caused by inflammation with or without infection or lack of blood flow to key organs.

CRITICAL ACTIONS FOR THE ED TECHNICIAN

- Vital signs
- IV access
- ECG
- NPO

RED FLAGS

- Abnormal vital signs
- Tachycardia, hypotension
- Diaphoresis
- Intractable nausea and vomiting
- Severe pain

Evaluation of undifferentiated abdominal pain in the elderly patient includes ECG and a broad range of blood and urine tests. The patient may require IV fluids and antiemetics if they are experiencing significant vomiting or diarrhea. After evaluation, they often require abdominal imaging, including ultrasound or CT. Elderly patients have significant morbidity and mortality associated with abdominal pain, and good IV access is imperative for administering medications and providing IV contrast for CT imaging.

Syncope

A 26-year-old woman presents to the ED with abdominal pain and syncopal episode before arrival. She states that she has had about 2 days of vaginal bleeding and her last period was about 6 weeks ago. She reports lower pelvic pain and dizziness.

CRITICAL ACTIONS FOR THE ED TECHNICIAN

- Vital signs
- IV access (two large-bore IVs)
- Type and screen
- Point-of-care (POC) pregnancy test for every female with abdominal pain
- NPO

RED FLAGS

- Any history of syncope with abdominal pain
- Missed period
- Vaginal bleeding
- History of previous ectopic pregnancy

In addition to the general abdominal pain etiologies discussed above, in young female patients, we must also consider pregnancy-related causes of pain. This vignette is a characteristic presentation of a patient with a ruptured ectopic pregnancy (Fig. 28.2). Ectopic pregnancy is a developing pregnancy outside of its normal location in the uterus, most frequently in a fallopian tube. Generally, patients with this condition will present in their mid to late first trimester (4–13 weeks gestation) with abdominal pain, vaginal bleeding, or both. As the tubal pregnancy enlarges, there is slow but continuous venous bleeding into the abdominal cavity. Sometimes the blood itself causes pain, but if this internal blood loss occurs surreptitiously, a patient can present in severe hypovolemic shock that requires rapid transfusions. Determining the pregnancy status of a woman in her childbearing years with abdominal pain or vaginal bleeding is crucial to making this diagnosis. Pregnancy is most rapidly determined by a urine POC human choriogonadotropin test, so encouraging the patient to provide a urine sample or collecting a blood sample for a lab pregnancy test is critical to their management.

The hemodynamic stability of the patient will determine if the patient is sent to radiology for a formal transvaginal ultrasound. ED providers will often use a bedside ultrasound to determine if there is free fluid (in this context, blood) in the abdomen. Patients with ruptured ectopic pregnancies often proceed directly to the operating room after an obstetrics/gynecology

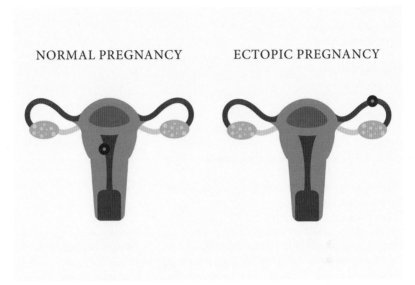

NORMAL PREGNANCY   ECTOPIC PREGNANCY

Fig. 28.2 Normal versus ectopic pregnancy.

consultation. To prepare your patient for the operating room (OR), ensure you have collected a type and screen and inserted two large-bore IVs. Remember, all OR-bound patients should remain NPO.

Trauma

A 28-year-old man is driven to the ED by a friend after being struck and falling from a motorized scooter while not wearing a helmet. He presents to triage reporting a headache and abdominal pain following the incident. He is ambulatory and has obvious signs of trauma and dried blood on his face. In triage, he shows you bruising on his abdomen. His initial vital signs show a temperature of 36.7°C, heart rate of 108, BP of 98/60, and respiratory rate of 16.

Trauma is a common reason for ED visits, regardless of whether the hospital carries a formal trauma designation, as patients with traumatic injuries often present to their nearest health facility. It is important for patients with the potential for severe traumatic injuries to be identified quickly, as they can decompensate rapidly. Any abnormal vital signs, severe mechanism of injury, or concerning examination findings in these patients should be escalated promptly to a senior provider.

CRITICAL ACTIONS FOR THE ED TECHNICIAN
- Take vital signs.
- Assess for red flags, including severe mechanisms of injury or head trauma.
- If abnormal vital signs or red flags are present, notify provider for immediate evaluation and activation of the trauma team if available at your facility.
- Place blunt trauma patients into cervical collar, as indicated below.
- Establish IV access (two large-bore IVs).
- Ask about use of blood thinners, tetanus status, and any medication allergies.

RED FLAGS

- Abnormal vital signs
- Signs of head trauma
- Altered mental status, seizure, or other neurologic symptoms
- Abdominal bruising
- Unequal pupils
- Significant mechanism
  - High-speed motor vehicle collision
  - Significant intrusion on the passenger compartment of a vehicle
  - Ejection from a vehicle
  - Death of another person in their vehicle
  - Fall from higher than 10 feet
- Penetrating trauma, like a stab or a gunshot wound
- Anticoagulant use
- Trauma in an elderly patient

In patients with head and neck trauma, such as in this case, evaluation is geared toward identifying any vertebral column, spinal cord, or intracranial injuries. Until the extent of head and neck injuries has been assessed, patients with neck pain after any trauma should be placed in a cervical collar (c-collar). Cervical immobilization is also indicated for patients with significant mechanisms of injury, altered mental status (including intoxication), midline spinal tenderness, new neurologic complaints (tingling, numbness, weakness), or in those who have other severe injuries that could distract from a neck injury. When in doubt, place the c-collar until the patient can be assessed more thoroughly by a provider.

Please note that patients with suspected intracranial or cervical spine injuries should be kept supine on a stretcher until they have been fully evaluated. Rolling of these patients from side to side ("log-roll") should only be completed with a provider at bedside and a qualified individual stabilizing the cervical spine during the maneuver.

Even in cases in which most of the complaint seems localized to the head and neck, care should be taken to exclude injuries of the chest or abdomen that may not be obvious at first. Most trauma patients receive an immediate FAST (focused abdominal sonography in trauma) examination by a provider with a bedside ultrasound to screen for any intraabdominal free fluid, which may indicate injury. Large-bore IV access and labs should be a priority in these patients. If the FAST examination is positive, the patient will proceed immediately to CT or to the operating room at the discretion of the attending trauma surgeon or ED physician. Bruising on the abdomen (often called the "seatbelt sign" after a motor vehicle accident), as in the vignette above, is concerning for intraabdominal bleeding. For these patients it is especially important to closely monitor vital signs and their level of consciousness.

Most hospitals will have specific protocols for the personnel who will manage patients with traumatic injuries. Become familiar with your local institution's protocols to be able to function most effectively on the treatment team.

Unilateral Weakness and Slurred Speech

A 62-year-old man presents to triage with his wife, who states that he had slurred speech, a left-sided facial droop, and left arm weakness. She states that he was previously healthy and that these symptoms started abruptly 1 hour ago.

CRITICAL ACTIONS FOR THE ED TECHNICIAN

- Recognize the presentation of common stroke symptoms.
- Alert a provider for immediate evaluation, preparation of the patient for a noncontrast head CT, and activation of the hospital's stroke protocol.

- POC glucose should be taken.
- Establish IV access.
- Determine time of onset.

RED FLAGS

- Presence of unilateral symptoms (facial droop, weakness on one side compared with the other)
- Altered mental status
- Unequal pupils
- Anticoagulant use

A stroke occurs either when a blood clot interrupts the blood supply to a portion of the brain (ischemic stroke) or when a hemorrhage within the brain itself disrupts and destroys brain cells (hemorrhagic stroke). The acronym FAST (not to be confused with the posttraumatic bedside sonogram) has been developed by the National Stroke Association as a first-line tool for detection of stroke:

*F*acial droop

*A*rm weakness

*S*peech difficulties

*T*ime to call 911

Although there are many other presenting symptoms that could suggest stroke, these are among the most common.

As with suspected heart attacks and high-risk traumas, most institutions have a protocol for alerting a team to expedite suspected stroke care because minutes matter. Patients with symptoms concerning for stroke should proceed quickly for a noncontrast head CT to exclude hemorrhagic stroke. The rapid administration of a clot-busting medication (thrombolytic) is indicated for many acute ischemic strokes. The decision to administer thrombolytics is complex and time sensitive. It often involves a neurologist who may be evaluating the patient in person or via telemedicine and is typically limited to patients who present within 4 to 6 hours of symptom onset. The American Heart Association's guidelines for acute stroke management recommend a door-to-CT time of less than 25 minutes and a door-to-needle time for the thrombolytic medication of less than 60 minutes.

Quickly acquiring a blood glucose level through a POC glucose test is also important because low blood sugar can mimic an acute stroke. Next, IV access for these patients is important for obtaining labs (anticipate specific coagulation tests ordered), providing IV contrast for additional brain imaging and administering medications.

Conclusion

ED triage prioritizes the care of patients with more serious complaints. The EDT is often instrumental in helping to identify these patients and bringing them to the attention of a provider. Of course, patient care experience will improve one's ability to make these determinations, but begin with a strict adherence to obtaining a complete set of vital signs for every patient while maintaining a watchful eye for red flags.

CHAPTER 29

Obstetrics and Gynecology in the Emergency Department

Margaret Klein ▪ Mary Taylor Winsten ▪ Samuel Winsten

Introduction

Women frequently present to the emergency department (ED) with obstetric (pregnancy-related) or gynecologic (non–pregnancy-related) symptoms that originate from issues of the female genital tract. As genital tract organs are colocated within the abdominal cavity with organs of the gastrointestinal and urologic systems, the evaluation of symptomatic patients often requires a careful evaluation to pinpoint which of these three systems is involved.

Anatomy

The female genital tract consists of:
1. The external genitalia
    a. Labia majora
    b. Labia minora
2. The vagina
3. The uterus
4. Two fallopian tubes
5. Two ovaries (Fig. 29.1)

Physiology

The menstrual cycle is governed by relationships between the pituitary gland and the organs of the female genital tract. The cycle is designed to give the woman a chance to become pregnant approximately once every month. The ovaries are active "endocrine-type" organs providing a source of ova (eggs) that become available for fertilization, as well as source of estrogen and progesterone, the major female hormones. Estrogen and progesterone target multiple genital tract tissues, but they primarily regulate a cycle at the beginning of which their levels rise, leading to uterine wall thickening to prepare for a potential pregnancy. If a pregnancy does not occur, the levels of estrogen and progesterone fall, leading to sloughing of the uterine wall each month, which causes vaginal (menstrual) bleeding.

A patient becomes pregnant when an egg cell is extruded from the ovaries and comes into contact with sperm cells in the fallopian tube. One sperm cell fertilizes the ovum (i.e., adds its genetic material to the cell), and cell division follows. The fertilized egg or zygote now exits the fallopian tubes and implants in the lining of the uterus (endometrium) where cell division and tissue differentiation continue. The developing fetus produces a hormone (human chorionic gonadotropin [HCG]) that stimulates the ovary to continue secreting high levels of estrogen and progesterone to maintain the developing pregnancy. A portion of this hormone (the β subunit) is virtually unique to a developing pregnancy, although several types of cancers can produce HCG. HCG's

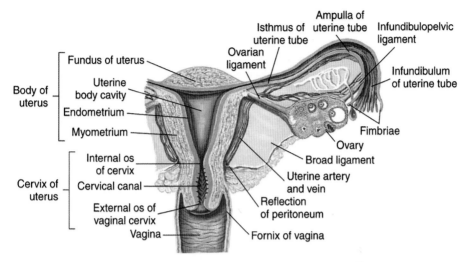

Fig. 29.1   Structures of the female reproductive system. (From Ball JW, Dains JE, Flynn JA, Solomon BS, Stewart RW. Female genitalia. In: Ball JW, Dains JE, Flynn JA, Solomon BS, Stewart RW, eds. *Seidel's Guide to Physical Examination*. 10th ed. Elsevier; 2023:448–498.)

β subunit is the substance that is measured by all types of pregnancy tests. The unit of measurement of HCG is international units per liter.

General Approach to the Patient With Abdominal Pain or Vaginal Bleeding, Unknown Pregnancy Status

In addition to the vital signs, determining whether the patient is pregnant is the key step in evaluating all women of childbearing age with abdominal or vagina complaints. The ED technician (EDT) can play a key role in speeding up the evaluation of these patients, almost all of whom require a pregnancy test by collecting urine for this test even before it is formally ordered.

There are two types of pregnancy tests. A qualitative test (generally done in the ED) determines whether a woman is pregnant, but it does not provide the exact level of HCG in the bloodstream. In order to determine a quantitative HCG level, blood must be sent to the lab and the results may take an hour. For some clinical situations, the ED qualitative test suffices, but in other situations, both the qualitative test (for speed of diagnosis) and the quantitative test (which contextualizes the findings on exam and sonogram) are both required.

There are generally three ways to perform a point-of care (POC) pregnancy test in the ED:

1. *Urine card test:* This is the simplest test and is also the basis for all home pregnancy tests. Most card tests use a technique called enzyme-linked immunosorbent assay. The test's sensitivity using a randomly collected urine sample corresponds to a serum level of about 20 international units per liter. This means that the test can be positive even before the missed period. The test performs quite well if done on a urine sample collected anytime during the day, and it is not necessary to get a first morning sample.

2. *Whole blood on a urine card:* If a woman is unable to produce urine, the EDT can perform a finger stick, place three drops of whole blood on a urine pregnancy test card, and read the result in about 10 minutes. For more accurate testing, tape a red-top tube of the patient's blood to a wall and allow to clot for about 10 minutes, leaving clear serum at the top of the

tube. Carefully draw the serum from the tube using a needle and syringe, then place the same number of drops on the card as instructed by the testing kit.

3. *Commercial POC cartridge machine:* A variety of commercial cartridge-based POC systems are available that can do bedside qualitative and quantitative HCG testing on heparinized whole blood. These systems are available in most EDs for a variety of tests. They take about 10 minutes to run the assay and are considered very accurate.

Once a patient's pregnancy status has been established, it is important to determine what other information is needed. Dating the pregnancy and determining the patient's obstetric history can help provide clinical context. Other information that may be helpful to gather during the initial patient triage includes any history of ectopic pregnancy, sexually transmitted diseases, or preeclampsia. A thorough understanding of patients' history of gynecologic or obstetric complications provides the care team with an idea of their risk factors for the disease processes that will be described below.

Pelvic Exam Setup

When a patient presents with vaginal bleeding, abnormal discharge, or other complaints of potential OBGYN pathology, the provider may need to perform a pelvic exam in the ED. The EDT (particularly if female) may be asked to assist with the exam. Having all the materials prepared for a pelvic exam is very important, as sometimes the provider is not sure of what they will need before they begin the examination. Most EDs have a "pelvic cart" with multiple drawers containing a variety of devices and diagnostic tests that could be needed for the exam.

The exam should be performed in the most private and quietest space available, and the EDT should thoroughly explain the procedure and facilitate the provider's answering any more complex questions.

Materials needed for a pelvic exam are a disposable speculum (see Fig. 29.2), a light source to illuminate the vagina (may either be built into the speculum or be an external light source), wall suction with appropriately sized catheters, sterile lubricant, sterile gloves, and disposable pads

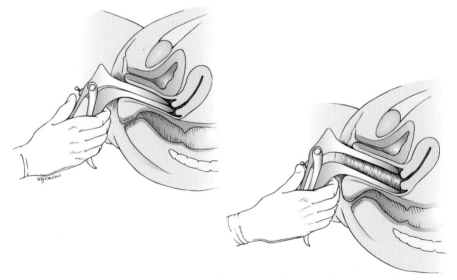

Fig. 29.2 **Pelvic examination using a speculum.** (From Swartz MH, Nentin FG. Female genitalia. In: Swartz MH, ed. *Textbook of Physical Diagnosis: History and Examination.* 8th ed. Elsevier; 2021:404–428.e2.)

(Table 29.1). Ensuring correct speculum size and understanding that there are options for different speculum sizes is important for patient comfort.

In patients with significant bleeding or copious vaginal discharge, gauze and large-tip cotton swabs to clear the clinician's visual field should be available at bedside. Positioning is also essential for proper exam and visualization of the cervix. As an EDT, helping a patient to the foot of the bed, with rolls of blankets or a bedpan underneath the patient's lower back and sacrum to allow for adequate pelvic positioning, can be very helpful to complete the exam quickly and with minimal discomfort if stirrups are not available on the types of ED stretchers used.

General Approach to the Known Pregnant Patient

The duration of a pregnancy is measured in weeks beginning on the date that the last menstrual period (LMP) began. A pregnancy is divided into three 12-week "trimesters." Table 29.2 outlines key developmental milestones in each trimester.

In addition to measuring and classifying pregnancy by trimester, the number of weeks a fetus spends in development designates the "term" classification for the pregnancy's duration as outlined in Table 29.3.

Patients in their second and third trimesters who appear to be having pregnancy-related symptoms often bypass the ED and go directly to the hospital's labor and delivery (L&D) unit, whereas in smaller hospitals any obstetric patient will be evaluated in the ED.

TABLE 29.1 ■ Material That May Be Needed for a Pelvic Exam

Equipment	Test
Red-top tube, saline flush, sterile swabs	Vaginal "wet prep" for bacterial vaginosis and *Trichomonas*
Cervical swabs	Gonorrhea and chlamydia
Potassium hydroxide solution	Vaginal yeast infection

TABLE 29.2 ■ Milestone Development in Different Semesters

Trimester	Weeks			
First	0–12	Heartbeat 6–8 wks		
Second	13–25	Can determine sex on sonography	Growth of hair	Baby moves for first time
Third	26–39	Baby moves frequently	Definitive viable baby	

TABLE 29.3 ■ Term Classification in Pregnancy

Gestational Age	Completed Postmenstrual Weeks
Postterm	>42 wks
Term	Completed >37 wks
Preterm	Born before 37 completed wks
Late Preterm	Born between 34 wks 0/7 d and 36 wks 6/7 d

Initial Assessment and Triage Information

The initial evaluation of a woman with a potential genital tract issue is as follows:
1. Is she pregnant?
   a. If so, is the pregnancy responsible for the symptoms?
   b. If not, what other processes could be causing them?
2. 2. If she is not pregnant, are her symptoms caused by genital tract or nongenital tract organs?

A gynecologic history on a menstruating woman should include the following elements at a minimum:
1. Date of LMP.
2. An accounting of the gravida number (total numbers of past pregnancies) and parity number that describes the outcomes of all of her pregnancies. Parity is often expressed as a four-part number:
   a. Full-term pregnancies
   b. Premature pregnancies
   c. Number of abortions (spontaneous and medically induced)
   d. Number of living children
3. Whether the woman is sexually active with a male and if so, the type of contraception (if any) is she using.

Vital signs are an important step, as they are for any patient, and intravenous (IV) access should be established.

For known pregnant patients, it is important to determine what other information is needed. Dating the pregnancy and determining the patient's past obstetric history can help provide clinical context. Other information that may be helpful to gather during the initial patient triage includes any previous history of ectopic pregnancy, sexually transmitted disease, or preeclampsia. A thorough understanding of patients' history of gynecologic or obstetric complications provides the care team with an idea of their risk factors for the disease processes that are covered next.

Vaginal Bleeding, Known Pregnancy

SPONTANEOUS ABORTION

Twenty percent of pregnant women experience some bleeding in the first trimester of pregnancy, and about half of the women who bleed will go on to have a normal pregnancy. Table 29.4 describes the risk factors for miscarriage. The ED evaluation of these patients is oriented toward identifying the location and viability of the pregnancy. The pace of the evaluation

---

TABLE 29.4 ■ Risk Factors for Spontaneous Miscarriage

Vaginal bleeding, especially >3 d, carries with it a 15%–20% chance of miscarriage
Advancing maternal age
Two or more prior miscarriages
Significant underlying maternal health issues, such as uncontrolled diabetes, thyroid disease, or other endocrine disturbances
Illicit substance use
Obesity
Alcohol, smoking, and excessive caffeine intake
Use of fluconazole in pregnancy is associated with a statistically significant increased risk of spontaneous miscarriage

TABLE 29.5 ■ Different Types of Abortion

Abortion	Description
Threatened	Slight vaginal bleeding and mild uterine cramping with a closed cervical os
Inevitable	Moderate vaginal bleeding and moderate uterine cramping with an open cervical os, gross rupture of membranes
Incomplete	Heavy vaginal bleeding and severe uterine cramping with an open cervical os and tissue in the cervix, incomplete expulsion of the products of conception
Complete	Slight vaginal bleeding with mild uterine cramping with a closed cervical os, complete expulsion of the products of conception
Missed	Slight vaginal bleeding and absent uterine contractions with a closed cervical os, prolonged retention of dead products of conception
Septic	Malodorous vaginal bleeding/discharge and absent uterine contractions with a closed cervical os, fever, intrauterine infection

Adapted from Kippenhan M. Disorders of early pregnancy. In: Adams JG, Barton ED, Collings JL, DeBlieux PMC, Gisondi MA, Nadel ES, eds. *Emergency Medicine*. 2nd ed. Elsevier; 2013:1023–1033.e1, table 119.1.

should be dictated by the rapidity of bleeding and the patient's vital signs. Of note, complications of medically induced abortion may present similarly to a spontaneous abortion, and depending on the jurisdiction, patients may not be forthcoming about admitting to having taken the medication that induces an abortion (mifepristone and misoprostol). Table 29.5 outlines the different types of abortions (miscarriages) experienced by patients.

It is important to understand the nomenclature of spontaneous pregnancy loss. Once a diagnosis of spontaneous abortion is made, either by pelvic examination, ultrasound, or laboratory workup, the patient's management will be based upon their level of stability, which is related to the amount and rapidity of bleeding. A pelvic exam may be performed to allow for manual removal of clots and passed tissue, during which the EDT may be asked to help with positioning and sample collection.

Spontaneous abortion is a sensitive subject, and it is important to respect the privacy of patients who are going through such an event, regardless of whether the patient was aware they were pregnant at the time. It can be a very emotionally charged diagnosis, and patients can react in any number of ways to the news. It is important for every member of the ED team to be cognizant of patients' feelings and to allow patients and their families privacy and support as needed during their visit. As an EDT, it is appropriate to advocate for closed-door rooms for bleeding patients and to minimize unnecessary intrusion depending on a patient's level of stability and mood.

Many ED protocols for treating patients with spontaneous abortions require sending a type and Rh test to the lab. Women whose Rh type is negative can become sensitized to Rh⁺ fetal red blood cells of the current pregnancies and will then produce antibodies against fetal tissues on subsequent pregnancies. Future problems can be avoided by administering preformed anti-Rh antibodies (RhoGAM) to Rh⁻ women having a miscarriage, thus minimizing the chances of Rh sensitization.

ECTOPIC PREGNANCY

All pregnant women who present with abdominal pain, with or without vaginal bleeding, should be suspected of having an ectopic pregnancy. An ectopic pregnancy occurs when a zygote implants outside of the uterus. This can occur anywhere along the route taken by the fertilized egg in moving toward the uterus, but the vast majority of ectopic pregnancies implant in the fallopian tubes. There are several reasons that abnormal implantation can occur, including history of previous sexually transmitted disease, tubal surgery, or previous ectopic pregnancy, as these processes result in scarring or narrowing of the fallopian tubes. Live birth is not a viable outcome because the fallopian tube can neither expand nor supply the developing pregnancy with sufficient nutritional support. As the ectopic pregnancy enlarges, there is occult venous bleeding into the peritoneal cavity that can lead to life-threatening hypovolemia. Fig. 29.3 demonstrates the different locations for an ectopic pregnancy in the female genital tract.

Ectopic pregnancy should be suspected in a female patient of reproductive age presenting with vaginal bleeding, abdominal pain, syncope, altered mental status, dizziness, hypotension, or any combination thereof. When ectopic is suspected in a woman with a positive pregnancy test, the next step is for the provider to either perform a bedside ultrasound or order a pelvic sonogram done in the radiology suite. These studies allow the provider to determine where the developing embryo is within the genitourinary system.

Once the diagnosis of ectopic pregnancy is established, consultants will be contacted to determine the treatment and follow-up. Depending on the patient's stability and the size and location of the ectopic, either medical or surgical management will be recommended. Medical treatment involves the administration of methotrexate, a chemotherapy-type agent that interferes with the rapidly dividing cells of the embryo. Surgical management is done laparoscopically and is generally performed on patients who are hemodynamically unstable, have a larger ectopic pregnancy, or have failed medical management. While awaiting the consultant's decision, the EDT may be asked to draw a blue-top tube for coagulation studies, blood for a type and screen, and Rh factor, and to obtain COVID-19 testing.

There are clinical situations in which a patient is known to be pregnant, but the sonogram is not definitive as to the location of the pregnancy. This is known as a pregnancy of unknown location (PUL). In this situation, patients are monitored with serial β HCG testing within 48 hours, and if they are unable to obtain this testing at an outpatient OBGYN office, they will often return

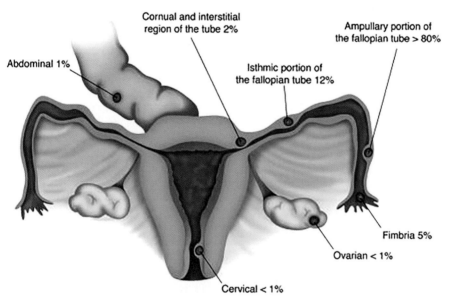

Fig. 29.3 Potential locations and frequency of ectopic pregnancy. (From Promes SB, Nobay F. Pitfalls in first-trimester bleeding. *Emerg Med Clin North Am*. 2010;28(1):219–234. [Adapted from: Breen JL. A 21-year survey of 654 ectopic pregnancies. *Am J Obstet Gynecol*. 1970;106(7):1004–1019.])

to the ED for repeat testing. Triage for these patients is much the same and should involve assessment for worsening of their symptoms, repeat serum pregnancy testing, and a repeat ultrasound.

OTHER OBSTETRIC CONDITIONS

Hypertension in Pregnancy

Vital signs are a critical part of the evaluation of pregnant patients, and it is important to remember that blood pressure elevations that are easily tolerated in nonpregnant patients can be harbingers of serious pregnancy-related conditions, such as preeclampsia.

Gestational hypertension is defined as a systolic blood pressure measurement of ≥140 mm Hg or a diastolic measurement of ≥90 mm Hg after week 20 of the pregnancy. Pressures this high are not necessarily an emergency but are definitely a pertinent finding requiring the EDT to notify someone on the provider team. Elevated blood pressure, especially in patients without a history of hypertension, can be a sign of more ominous disease processes and warrant further workup.

Preeclampsia is more severe on the spectrum of hypertensive disorders in pregnancy (HDP). Preeclampsia is characterized by a blood pressure measurement 140/90 mm Hg or higher in a patient without a hypertensive history and proteinuria of 0.3 g or more in 24 hours. Preeclampsia can have a variety of other severe features (described in Fig. 29.4), such as kidney injury, thrombocytopenia (decreased platelets), liver injury, vision changes, headaches, and pulmonary edema.

Eclampsia is preeclampsia plus seizures. You should have the same approach of assessing blood pressure and urine protein levels, but the history of seizures will come from patient or emergency medical service reports or presentation in the ED. It is important to note that a patient with a history of seizure disorder is different than a patient who began having seizures during pregnancy.

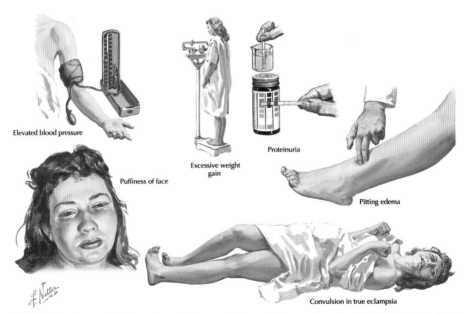

Elevated blood pressure

Puffiness of face

Excessive weight gain

Proteinuria

Pitting edema

Convulsion in true eclampsia

Fig. 29.4 Preeclampsia/eclampsia patient presentations in the emergency department. (From Smith RP. Preeclampsia and eclampsia. In: Smith RP, ed. *Netter's Obstetrics and Gynecology*. 3rd ed. Elsevier; 2018:494–497.)

The job of the EDT will be to collect information to aid in establishing the diagnosis. This entails taking the initial blood pressure at triage and then repeating the blood pressure (if abnormal) 15 minutes following the initial elevated blood pressure. If it is consistently high, a urine sample should be taken to assess for protein levels. IV access for patients with HDP is important in order to provide acute management with IV benzodiazepines, magnesium, and antihypertensive medications, as well as to perform the necessary lab work to fully establish the patient's diagnosis. Basic laboratory evaluation in patients with hypertensive disorders in pregnancy includes complete blood cell count that includes a white cell count, hemoglobin, hematocrit, and platelets, electrolytes, kidney and liver function studies, random urine protein and creatinine testing, and an electrocardiogram.

If a patient is found to have preeclampsia or eclampsia, they will be started on boluses of magnesium and antihypertensive medicines. Continued monitoring of blood pressure is essential to measure treatment efficacy, and values 140/90 mm Hg or higher should be reported quickly. Patients with preeclampsia or eclampsia are often treated with large doses of magnesium, which can result in toxicity including respiratory depression and heart block, which, if present, should be rapidly brought to the attention of the treating team.

Trauma in Pregnancy

Trauma patients come into the ED and receive the "standard ABC" (Airway, Breathing, Circulation) (ABC) initial assessment. If there are any obvious skin or clothing contaminants, the patient should be cleaned and then assessed for any other injuries.

Specifically for pregnant patients, a β-HCG blood test to confirm pregnancy is an important step to take in any trauma. While making sure the mother is stable, the team will want to use ultrasound imaging to assess the status of the baby. Ultrasound with Doppler can be used at the bedside to assess fetal heart function and determine if there are any gross abnormalities or changes from previous imaging. In situations in which trauma-related imaging is important to assess the injuries of the mother, ensure the fetus is protected with lead gowns before x-ray imaging or computed tomography scans of the head, neck, or chest.

Patient in Active Labor

Patients in late stages of pregnancy (late second or third trimester) may present to the ED in active labor. On triage assessment, they may complain of severe intermittent abdominal pain or pelvic pressure, clear vaginal discharge ("my water broke"), or a single episode of bloody vaginal discharge ("bloody show"). If a patient who reports or appears to be in the late stages of pregnancy presents to triage with these symptoms, it is important to call for assistance to help move the patient to a room for immediate pelvic examination to make sure that the baby's head is not visible at the vaginal opening (crowning). In institutions with in-house OBGYN services, patients in active labor without a crowning fetus or other emergent medical comorbidities can be immediately transferred to the L&D for further evaluation and management.

For laboring patients that are crowning in the ED, many institutions have a "code labor" that will mobilize personnel and material to treat the laboring patient. Patients who are going to deliver in the ED can suffer from several complications, including vaginal or cervical lacerations, postpartum bleeding, or shoulder dystocia, which is a form of arrested labor in which the baby's shoulder is caught on the pelvic brim.

Because of the potential for decompensation, bleeding, and hypotension, IV access at the head of the bed should be a priority while delivery occurs at the foot of the bed. Monitoring during delivery should be secured both for mother and fetus. Fetal heart monitoring helps clinicians to recognize fetal distress during delivery. If resources are mobilized with a code labor, L&D nurses may be available at bedside to assist with fetal monitoring, and EDTs should be available to help position the patient for optimal monitoring and delivery. After birth, the baby will be moved to the mother's chest and assessed for muscle tone, skin color, and cry. Another essential aspect of monitoring will be to place the newborn into the warmer apparatus after their initial evaluation and skin-to-skin time with the mother. EDTs should ensure the machine is in the room with the warmer active before delivery so that fetal monitoring can be quickly established. After delivery of the newborn, collection of cord blood for initial blood gases and a sample of the cord for pathology takes place, followed by delivery of the placenta. After delivery, both mother and baby should be transferred to the L&D and neonatal intensive care unit for evaluation by the OBGYN and pediatrics, respectively.

Gynecologic Complaints in the Nonpregnant Patient

VAGINAL BLEEDING, NOT PREGNANT

Vaginal bleeding in the nonpregnant woman can cause hemodynamic instability, chronic anemia without hypotension, or can be an early sign of cervical or uterine cancer. The speed and extent of the workup will vary according to the clinical context. All postmenopausal bleeding is considered abnormal and will require a thorough gynecologic evaluation. This is often done as an outpatient.

Premenopausal uterine bleeding can have several causes, including irregular menstrual cycles that are caused by irregular ovulation, structural abnormalities of the uterus such as fibroids (benign smooth muscle tumors of the uterine wall), endometrial polyps, or cervical abnormalities that bleed. The general workup for these issues is to perform an exam, check the patient's hematocrit, and order a pelvic ultrasound.

Chronically bleeding patients can have significant symptoms of anemia, including skin or conjunctival pallor, fatigue, generalized weakness, or chest pain or shortness of breath with exertion. At times they may require blood transfusions, and iron supplementation is often prescribed.

PELVIC PAIN SYNDROMES

There are two major types of issues that present with gynecologic pain: ovarian pathology and infection. The ovary is an active organ that extrudes an ovum approximately every month, which is picked up by the opening of the fallopian tube. The area from which the egg came now becomes the corpus luteum, a series of cells that produce the progesterone that would be required if a pregnancy resulted during this cycle. On occasion, the corpus luteum becomes a cystic structure that can "rupture" into the abdominal cavity. When this happens, the woman feels sudden onset of unilateral pelvic pain. This may happen during intercourse, which can lead to great anxiety for the patient. The pain does not often last long, and it may be gone by the time the patient arrives in the ED. A pelvic ultrasound often shows free fluid in the pelvis but no cystic structures in the ovary.

Another significant non–pregnancy-related ovarian problem is ovarian torsion. This condition often presents with severe unilateral pelvic pain resulting from a twisting of the ovary that cuts off the arterial circulation to and venous return from the ovary. The underlying cause of the torsion may be related to some type of cystic structure(s) on the ovary. The diagnosis is made a bit more difficult because the ovary can spontaneously torse and detorse leading to intermittent, severe pain. Color-flow Doppler sonography is needed to confirm the diagnosis, and surgery may be required if the ovary remains torsed and ischemic.

Pelvic infections are most common in young women who are sexually active with multiple partners and do not use any barrier methods of contraception. The cervix becomes infected with gonorrhea or chlamydia during intercourse, and if untreated, the infection can ascend from the cervix to infect the linings of both the uterus and fallopian tubes. When this occurs, the patient is said to have salpingitis or pelvic inflammatory disease. The patient will often complain of lower abdominal pain with a vaginal discharge and may have a fever. The diagnosis can be made clinically or by pelvic sonogram. Depending on the clinical severity and history of prior episodes, the patient may require IV antibiotics and admission. Tuboovarian abscesses, which may be seen on sonogram, may require surgical drainage.

Vaginal and Labial Problems

Patients may complain of vaginal discharge or pain in the rectogenital region. Both of these complaints most frequently require a pelvic exam and visualization of the external genitalia, vaginal walls, and uterine cervix. Depending on the findings, the physician may take swabs from the vaginal walls (looking for yeast or *Trichomonas*) and cervix (looking for gonorrhea or chlamydia). The labia can be the site for two types of abscesses:

1. A labial abscess, which originates from the base of the hair follicles similar to the way abscesses can form in other parts of the body
2. An infected Bartholin gland duct cyst; the Bartholin duct, the secretions of which help lubricate the vagina, becomes obstructed and abscess formation follows.

Both of these conditions require drainage that can be done in the ED.

Conclusion

Depending on their symptoms, when women of childbearing age present to the ED, it is important to gather an appropriate triage history with pertinent information, such as LMP; perform bedside pregnancy testing; and monitor vital signs closely. Vital sign abnormalities in pregnant patients should be reported quickly, especially elevated blood pressures (>140/90 mm Hg) and signs of shock, such as hypotension or tachycardia. Promptly secure IV access in bleeding patients, and make sure that they are quickly transported to ultrasound. Maintain patient privacy, and always consider advocating for private rooms for patients who will likely need a pelvic exam.

References for Additional Reading

About Pregnancy [WWW Document], n.d. https://www.nichd.nih.gov/. URL https://www.nichd.nih.gov/health/topics/pregnancy/conditioninfo (accessed August 6, 2022).

Cunningham FG, Leveno KJ, Dashe JS, Hoffman BL, Spong CY, Casey BM. *Ectopic Pregnancy. Williams Obstetrics.* New York, NY: McGraw Hill; 2022.

Definition of Term Pregnancy [WWW Document], n.d. URL https://www.acog.org/en/clinical/clinical-guidance/committee-opinion/articles/2013/11/definition-of-term-pregnancy (accessed August 6, 2022).

Fetal development: Month-By-Month Stages of Pregnancy [WWW Document], n.d. Clevel. Clin. URL https://my.clevelandclinic.org/health/articles/7247-fetal-development-stages-of-growth (accessed August 6, 2022).

NVSS - Birth Data [WWW Document], 2022. URL https://www.cdc.gov/nchs/nvss/births.htm (accessed August 6, 2022).

Rogers VL, Roberts SW. Preeclampsia-Eclampsia. In: Papadakis MA, McPhee SJ, Rabow MW, McQuaid KR, eds. *Current Medical Diagnosis & Treatment.* New York, NY: McGraw-Hill Education; 2022.

Sanghavi M, Rutherford JD. Cardiovascular physiology of pregnancy. *Circulation.* 2014;130(12):1003–1008.

Amputation: removal of a limb by trauma, medical illness, or surgery
Angiogenesis: development of new blood vessels

Barotrauma: injury due to changes (up or down) in surrounding air or water pressure
Blanchable: loss of vascular pink coloration of tissue that occurs when capillaries of the skin are compressed (as opposed to no color change, which is termed *nonblanchable*)

Caustic: able to burn or corrode organic tissue by chemical action
Cerumen: earwax
Claudication: cramping muscle pain that occurs during exertion that is associated with inadequate peripheral arterial blood flow as metabolic demands increase
Conductive hearing: movement of sound through the external and middle ears
Contracture: fixed tightening of muscle, tendons, ligaments, or skin that prevents normal range of motion
Cricothyroidotomy: an incision in the neck to establish an emergency airway

Debridement: the mechanical removal of dead or damaged tissue or foreign objects from a wound
Dehiscence: separation of previously approximated wound edges
Dermis: thick layer of living tissue below the epidermis containing blood capillaries, nerve endings, sweat glands, hair follicles, and other structures
Desiccation: drying out of tissue
Devascularization: loss of the blood supply to a bodily part due to destruction or obstruction of blood vessels
Dysphagia: difficulty swallowing

Edema: swelling caused by excess fluid trapped in body's tissues
Endoscopy: a procedure which uses a long, flexible tube with a camera on it (an *endoscope*) inserted into a body opening to visualize and evaluate distal structures
Epidermis: outer-most layer of the skin; overlies the dermis
Epistaxis: bleeding from the nose
Erythematous: redness of the skin or mucous membranes caused by increased blood flow in superficial capillaries
Eschar: a dry, dark scab or falling away of dead skin
Escharotomy: surgical incision through the eschar to release the constriction, thereby restoring distal circulation and allowing for adequate ventilation
Exudate: a mass of cells and fluid that has seeped out of blood vessels or an organ, especially in inflammation

Fluctuance: yielding to pressure on palpation, suggesting a fluid collection

Gangrene: tissue necrosis that results from loss of blood flow secondary to infection, illness, or injury
Granulation tissue: highly vascularized new tissue growth

Induration: increased tissue firmness resulting from inflammatory responses
Ischemia: inadequate blood supply to an organ or part of the body

Laryngoscopy: examination procedure to view the back of the throat using lights, mirrors, and/or a small camera attached to a flexible, fiberoptic tube
Lymphangitis: inflammation of the peripheral lymphatic channels, typically secondary to an infectious cause, that presents as linear erythema spreading proximally from the site of infection

Maceration: degradation of tissue from prolonged excessive moisture
Mastoidectomy: surgical removal of the mastoid
Myringotomy: an incision of the tympanic membrane to drain fluid and relieve pressure

Necrosis: the death of most or all of the cells in an organ or tissue due to disease, injury, or failure of the blood supply

Otalgia: ear pain

Reepithelization: the process of creating a new barrier between wound and environment through epithelial cell migration

Sensorineural hearing: transmission of sound from the inner ear to the brain via nerve pathways
Snellen chart: eye chart used to measure visual acuity

Tinnitus: ringing sound in the ear
Trismus: difficulty opening the mouth

Urticaria: red, itchy hives

INDEX

Page number followed by "*f*" indicates figures, and "*t*" indicates tables.